AF442675

AIRWAY REMODELING

LUNG BIOLOGY IN HEALTH AND DISEASE

Executive Editor

Claude Lenfant
Director, National Heart, Lung and Blood Institute
National Institutes of Health
Bethesda, Maryland

86. Severe Asthma: Pathogenesis and Clinical Management, *edited by S. J. Szefler and D. Y. M. Leung*
87. *Mycobacterium avium*–Complex Infection: Progress in Research and Treatment, *edited by J. A. Korvick and C. A. Benson*
88. Alpha 1–Antitrypsin Deficiency: Biology • Pathogenesis • Clinical Manifestations • Therapy, *edited by R. G. Crystal*
89. Adhesion Molecules and the Lung, *edited by P. A. Ward and J. C. Fantone*
90. Respiratory Sensation, *edited by L. Adams and A. Guz*
91. Pulmonary Rehabilitation, *edited by A. P. Fishman*
92. Acute Respiratory Failure in Chronic Obstructive Pulmonary Disease, *edited by J.-P. Derenne, W. A. Whitelaw, and T. Similowski*
93. Environmental Impact on the Airways: From Injury to Repair, *edited by J. Chrétien and D. Dusser*
94. Inhalation Aerosols: Physical and Biological Basis for Therapy, *edited by A. J. Hickey*
95. Tissue Oxygen Deprivation: From Molecular to Integrated Function, *edited by G. G. Haddad and G. Lister*
96. The Genetics of Asthma, *edited by S. B. Liggett and D. A. Meyers*
97. Inhaled Glucocorticoids in Asthma: Mechanisms and Clinical Actions, *edited by R. P. Schleimer, W. W. Busse, and P. M. O'Byrne*
98. Nitric Oxide and the Lung, *edited by W. M. Zapol and K. D. Bloch*
99. Primary Pulmonary Hypertension, *edited by L. J. Rubin and S. Rich*
100. Lung Growth and Development, *edited by J. A. McDonald*
101. Parasitic Lung Diseases, *edited by A. A. F. Mahmoud*
102. Lung Macrophages and Dendritic Cells in Health and Disease, *edited by M. F. Lipscomb and S. W. Russell*
103. Pulmonary and Cardiac Imaging, *edited by C. Chiles and C. E. Putman*
104. Gene Therapy for Diseases of the Lung, *edited by K. L. Brigham*
105. Oxygen, Gene Expression, and Cellular Function, *edited by L. Biadasz Clerch and D. J. Massaro*
106. Beta$_2$-Agonists in Asthma Treatment, *edited by R. Pauwels and P. M. O'Byrne*
107. Inhalation Delivery of Therapeutic Peptides and Proteins, *edited by A. L. Adjei and P. K. Gupta*
108. Asthma in the Elderly, *edited by R. A. Barbee and J. W. Bloom*
109. Treatment of the Hospitalized Cystic Fibrosis Patient, *edited by D. M. Orenstein and R. C. Stern*
110. Asthma and Immunological Diseases in Pregnancy and Early Infancy, *edited by M. Schatz, R. S. Zeiger, and H. N. Claman*
111. Dyspnea, *edited by D. A. Mahler*
112. Proinflammatory and Antiinflammatory Peptides, *edited by S. I. Said*
113. Self-Management of Asthma, *edited by H. Kotses and A. Harver*
114. Eicosanoids, Aspirin, and Asthma, *edited by A. Szczeklik, R. J. Gryglewski, and J. R. Vane*
115. Fatal Asthma, *edited by A. L. Sheffer*
116. Pulmonary Edema, *edited by M. A. Matthay and D. H. Ingbar*
117. Inflammatory Mechanisms in Asthma, *edited by S. T. Holgate and W. W. Busse*
118. Physiological Basis of Ventilatory Support, *edited by J. J. Marini and A. S. Slutsky*

148. Pulmonary and Peripheral Gas Exchange in Health and Disease, *edited by J. Roca, R. Rodriguez-Roisen, and P. D. Wagner*
149. Lung Surfactants: Basic Science and Clinical Applications, *R. H. Notter*
150. Nosocomial Pneumonia, *edited by W. R. Jarvis*
151. Fetal Origins of Cardiovascular and Lung Disease, *edited by David J. P. Barker*
152. Long-Term Mechanical Ventilation, *edited by N. S. Hill*
153. Environmental Asthma, *edited by R. K. Bush*
154. Asthma and Respiratory Infections, *edited by D. P. Skoner*
155. Airway Remodeling, *edited by P. H. Howarth, J. W. Wilson, J. Bousquet, S. Rak, and R. A. Pauwels*

ADDITIONAL VOLUMES IN PREPARATION

Respiratory-Circulatory Interactions in Health and Disease, *edited by S. M. Scharf, M. R. Pinsky, and S. Magder*

The Lung at High Altitudes, *edited by T. F. Hornbein and R. B. Schoene*

Genetic Models in Cardiorespiratory Biology, *edited by G. G. Haddad and T. Xu*

Ventilator Management Strategies for Clinical Care, *edited N. S. Hill and M. Levy*

Drug Delivery to the Lung, *edited by H. Bisgaard, C. O'Callaghan, and G. C. Smaldone*

Severe Asthma: Pathogenesis and Clinical Management, *edited by S. J. Szefler and D. Y. M. Leung*

The opinions expressed in these volumes do not necessarily represent the views of the National Institutes of Health.

AIRWAY REMODELING

Edited by

Peter H. Howarth
Southampton General Hospital
Southampton, England

John W. Wilson
Monash University and
The Alfred Hospital
Prahran, Australia

Jean Bousquet
Montpellier University and
Service des Maladies Respiratoires–INSERM U454
Montpellier, France

Sabina Rak
Göteborg University and
Sahlgrenska University Hospital
Göteborg, Sweden

Romain A. Pauwels
Ghent University and
Ghent University Hospital
Ghent, Belgium

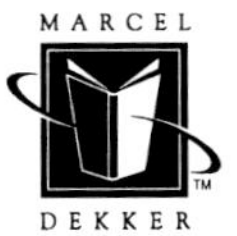

MARCEL DEKKER, INC.   NEW YORK · BASEL

ISBN: 0-8247-0448-7

This book is printed on acid-free paper.

Headquarters
Marcel Dekker, Inc.
270 Madison Avenue, New York, NY 10016
tel: 212-696-9000; fax: 212-685-4540

Eastern Hemisphere Distribution
Marcel Dekker AG
Hutgasse 4, Postfach 812, CH-4001 Basel, Switzerland
tel. 41-61-261-8482; fax: 41-61-261-8896

World Wide Web
http://www.dekker.com

The publisher offers discounts on this book when ordered in bulk quantities. For more information, write to Special Sales/Professional Marketing at the headquarters address above.

Current printing (last digit):
10 9 8 7 6 5 4 3 2 1

PRINTED IN THE UNITED STATES OF AMERICA

INTRODUCTION

Remodeling is defined as a change in size, structure, or composition of . . . you name it! If you are remodeling a building or house, this is very nice and most would expect to see an improvement. However, if you are speaking of remodeling a tissue, then it is cause for concern. In biology, remodeling represents an adaptive response of tissues to injury or disease.

The term may have been coined as far back as 1966 by Lynne Reid with regard to lung development (1) and later, again, in 1978 as a result of observation of the structural changes that occur in the pulmonary vessels during pulmonary hypertension (2). Over the years, significant progress has been made in understanding the remodeling process that develops in the vascular tree—for example, in the coronary artery affected by atherosclerosis or in the pulmonary vessels subjected to an increase in blood pressure. It also occurs in the myocardium itself during heart failure.

In the airways, our understanding of the remodeling process has been and remains much more limited. Airway obstruction, which is the distinctive feature of asthma, has long been considered reversible. However, the observation that lung function is permanently altered in asthma has led to the conclusion that the causal factors are airway injury and repair, all as a consequence of airway inflammation. Everyone recognizes that the mechanisms responsible for the structural alterations, their physiological and biological consequences, the role of these changes in the natural history of asthma, and the amenability of these changes to therapeutic intervention are all issues at the forefront of asthma research. Progress is being made and remodeling of the airway is unquestionably at the cutting edge of basic and clinical investigation.

When the opportunity occurred to include a volume on this topic in the Lung Biology in Health and Disease series, it was clear that a void would be filled. Furthermore, it was certain that a remarkable gestalt would be created, given the involvement of experts such as Peter H. Howarth, John W. Wilson, Jean Bousquet, and Romain A. Pauwels, who each have authored or contributed extensively to the most noted work in airway modeling. And, indeed, the product is much greater than the sum of its component parts! As a result, I am privileged to present to the reader a unique and novel volume that covers remodeling from the basic mechanisms to its physiological consequences and to therapeutic control. The authorship is international; thus it brings to this volume the breadth of what is known today, irrespective of where the work was done. Clinicians and, more important, patients can only benefit from this book by understanding the alterations that occur in asthma. This will undoubtedly lead to a better therapy.

I am grateful to all the editors and contributors for the opportunity to present this volume to the series' readership.

Claude Lenfant, M.D.
Bethesda, Maryland

References

1. Reid LM. The embryology of the lung in: de Reuck AVS, Porter R, eds. Ciba Foundation Symposium on Development of the Lung. J. & A. Churchill, London, 1966:109–124.
2. Reid LM. The Pulmonary Circulation: Remodeling in Growth and Disease. The 1978 J. Burns Amberson Lecture. Am Rev Resp Dis 1979; 119:531–546.

PREFACE

Major advances have been made in the last decade in the implementation of guidelines for asthma, emphasizing the importance of treating the underlying airway inflammatory process. This has led to the greater use of regular prophylactic therapy—in particular, inhaled corticosteroids—and improved asthma control with a reduction in exacerbations; less need for emergency care, hospital admissions, and systemic steroid administration; and improved lung function and quality of life. It has been apparent from a range of studies, however, that even with inhaled corticosteroid therapy there is room for further improvement in asthma care. Add-on studies with additional bronchodilator medication on a regular basis, such as with long-acting β-agonists, leukotriene receptor antagonists, and theophyllines, have all demonstrated that combination therapy provides better lung function, further reduces symptoms, and decreases the risk of disease exacerbation.

It is also apparent, however, that there is more to asthma than simple airway inflammation and bronchoconstriction. Well-defined structural airway changes occur within the airway wall in asthma. These structural alterations, which include glandular increases within the airways, enhanced collagen deposition within the lamina propria, and an increase in the airway vasculature along with airway smooth muscle hypertrophy and hyperplasia, have been encompassed under the term *airway remodeling*. These remodeling processes are evident throughout the airways, involving the large as well as the small distal airways, and have been implicated in the chronicity and persistence of disease. The structural changes, which lead to airway wall thickening, have been shown mathematically to contribute to the development and maintenance of bronchial hyperresponsiveness and theoretically can account for the exaggerated decline in lung function and loss of reversibility that is evident in asthma of long duration. The awareness of these changes is not new. Indeed, morphological abnormalities were well described early in the last century. It is, however, the realization of the implications of these changes that has focused attention in this area.

The prevention or resolution of these structural airway changes thus represents a third important target in asthma management, in addition to inflammation and bronchosconstriction. This book brings together expertise in basic science, physiology, morphology, pharmacology, and clinical medicine to discuss the nature of the remodeling process within the airways in asthma, the mechanisms involved, and the impact of remodeling on airway function and on clinical disease expression. The impact of the currently available pharmacological therapies for asthma on the remodeling process is discussed and these considerations are extended to consider potential future targets that may be relevant to the regulation of the remodeling process within the airways.

Chronic and persistent asthma is a both debilitating and life-threatening and in addition represents a spectrum of the asthma disease that carries a considerable burden of the health care costs. The implications of the remodeling process are not, however, limited to such patients as, if the progression from mild disease is to be prevented, an understanding of the risk factors and mechanisms that lead to the remodeled airway has to be applied to the milder disease to allow early intervention to stop disease progression. This book is thus relevant to all with an interest in asthma and we hope that it stimulates and interests a broad readership.

It would not have been possible to publish this book without the help of many to whom we would like to express our thanks and gratitude. The meeting on which this book is based arose following discussion with Dr. Malcolm Johnson, Director of Respiratory Science at GlaxoWellcome, owing to the increasing awareness of chronic structural changes and their relevance to persistence of the disease. This project would not have been possible without his support and that of Mr. Alan Wright and Ms. Rosemary Docherty. The meeting on which this book is based took part in Göteburg, Sweden, and we are grateful to those who graciously hosted the event. Finally, we would like to thank the editor of this series, Dr. Claude Lenfant.

Peter H. Howarth
John W. Wilson
Jean Bousquet
Sabina Rak
Romain A. Pauwels

CONTRIBUTORS

Tony R. Bai, M.D., F.R.A.C.P., F.R.C.P.C.   Professor, Respiratory Division, Department of Medicine, University of British Columbia, and St. Paul's Hospital, Vancouver, British Columbia, Canada

Giovanni Bonsignore, M.D.   Professor of Pneumology, Institute of Lung Pathophysiology, Italian National Research Council (CNR), Palermo, Italy

Jean Bousquet, M.D., Ph.D.   Professor, Department of Respiratory Medicine, Montpellier University, and Head, Department of Allergy and Clinical Immunology, Service des Maladies Respiratoires–INSERM U454, Hôpital Arnaud de Villeneuve, Montpellier, France

Neil G. Carroll, Ph.D.   Department of Pulmonary Physiology, Sir Charles Gairdner Hospital, Nedlands, Western Australia, Australia

Pascal Chanez, M.D., Ph.D.   Service des Maladies Respiratoires–INSERM U454, Hôpital Arnaud de Villeneuve, Montpellier, France

Rosalia Gagliardo   Institute of Lung Pathophysiology, Italian National Research Council (CNR), Palermo, Italy

Philippe Godard, Ph.D.   Professor, Montpellier University, and Service des Maladies Respiratoires–INSERM U454, Hôpital Arnaud de Villeneuve, Montpellier, France

Tari Haahtela, M.D., Ph.D.   Assistant Professor, Helsinki University, and Division of Allergology, Skin and Allergy Hospital, Helsinki University Central Hospital, Helsinki, Finland

Peter H. Howarth, B.Sc.(Hons), M.B.B.S., D.M., F.R.C.P.   Reader in Medicine, Division of Respiratory Cell and Molecular Biology, Department of Medical Specialties, Southampton General Hospital, Southampton, England

Dany Jaffuel, M.D., Ph.D.   Service des Maladies Respiratoires–INSERM U454, Hôpital Arnaud de Villeneuve, Montpellier, France

Alan Lloyd James, M.D., F.R.A.C.P.   Department of Pulmonary Physiology, Sir Charles Gairdner Hospital, Nedlands, Western Australia, Australia

Björn Jonson, M.D., Ph.D., F.C.C.P.   Professor, Department of Clinical Physiology, University of Lund, Lund, Sweden

Johan C. Kips, M.D., Ph.D.   Professor, Department of Respiratory Diseases, Ghent University, and Ghent University Hospital, Ghent, Belgium

Darryl A. Knight, Ph.D.   Senior Research Officer and Adjunct Lecturer, Asthma and Allergy Research Institute and Department of Medicine, University of Western Australia, Perth, Western Australia, Australia

Aili L. Lazaar, M.D.   Assistant Professor, Pulmonary, Allergy and Critical Care Division, Department of Medicine, University of Pennsylvania Medical Center, Philadelphia, Pennsylvania

Xun Li, M.D.   Department of Respiratory Medicine, The Alfred Campus, Monash University, Prahran, Australia

Gisele Mautino, Ph.D.   Cell Biologist, Service des Maladies Respiratoires–INSERM U454, Hôpital Arnaud de Villeneuve, Montpellier, France

Fabrice Jean Paganin, M.D., Ph.D.   Service de Réanimation, CHD (Intensive Care Unit) Felix Guyon, St. Denis Réunion, France

Els Palmans, M.Sc.   Department of Respiratory Diseases, Ghent University Hospital, Ghent, Belgium

Reynold A. Panettieri, Jr., M.D.   Associate Professor, Pulmonary, Allergy, and Critical Care Division, Department of Medicine, University of Pennsylvania Medical Center, Philadelphia, Pennsylvania

Romain A. Pauwels, M.D., Ph.D.   Professor and Head, Department of Respiratory Diseases, Ghent University, and Ghent University Hospital, Ghent, Belgium

William R. Roche, M.D., Ph.D.   Professor, Department of Medicine, University of Southampton, and Southampton General Hospital, Southampton, England

Gagliardo Rosalia, Ph.D.   Cell Biologist, Institute of Lung Pathophysiology, Italian National Research Council (CNR), Palermo, Italy

Janis K. Shute, Ph.D.   Department of Medical Specialties, Southampton General Hospital, Southampton, England

Liboria Siena, Ph.D.   Cell Biologist, Institute of Lung Pathophysiology, Italian National Research Council (CNR), Palermo, Italy

Alastair G. Stewart, Ph.D.   Associate Professor and Reader in Pharmacology, Department of Pharmacology, University of Melbourne, Parkville, Victoria, Australia

Nele Vanacker, B.Pharm.   Department of Respiratory Diseases, Ghent University Hospital, Ghent, Belgium

Per Venge, M.D., Ph.D.   Professor, Division of Clinical Chemistry, Department of Medical Science, University of Uppsala, Uppsala, Sweden

Antonio Maurizio Vignola, M.D., Ph.D.   Professor of Pneumology, Institute of Lung Pathophysiology, Italian National Research Council (CNR), Palermo, Italy

John W. Wilson, B.Sc.(Hons), M.B.B.S., Ph.D., F.R.A.C.P., F.C.C.P. Associate Professor, Department of Respiratory Medicine, The Alfred Campus, Monash University, Prahran, Australia

CONTENTS

1

What Does Airway Remodeling Mean?

Its Relevance to Asthma

JEAN BOUSQUET

Montpellier University and
Service des Maladies Respiratoires–
  INSERM U454
Hôpital Arnaud de Villeneuve
Montpellier, France

ANTONIO MAURIZIO VIGNOLA

Institute of Lung Pathophysiology
Italian National Research Council (CNR)
Palermo, Italy

For decades, asthma has been considered a condition of reversible airflow obstruction, and in the majority of patients, complete reversiblity of long-standing abnormal spirometric measurements, such as FEV_1, may be observed after treatment. However, many asthmatics, both children and adults, have evidence of residual airway obstruction, which may even be detected in asymptomatic patients. This clinically demonstrable irreversible component of the airways obstruction was observed on pathological findings at the turn of the century (1) and already proposed in the definition of asthma in 1962 (2). However, these features were almost completely ignored for a long time and the concept of airway remodeling in asthma was only proposed in 1992 (3).

Remodeling is defined in the *Concise Oxford Dictionary* as "model again or differently, reconstruct." This is a critical aspect of wound repair in all organs representing a dynamic process that associates matrix production and degradation in reaction to an inflammatory insult (4) leading to a normal reconstruction process (model again) or a pathological one (model differently). Asthma is a chronic inflammatory disease of the airways, the evolution of which follows the natural course of chronic inflammation. This is always followed by healing, which begins very early and results in either tissue repair, a tightly regulated salutary biological response, or fibrosis, an unregulated pathological process.

Structural changes in the airway walls are essential features of asthma (5) and include extracellular matrix remodeling, epithelial desquamation, goblet cell hyperplasia, prominent smooth muscle, vascular remodeling, collagen deposition below the basement membrane, and elastolysis (6).

It is critical to understand the regulation of airway remodeling in asthma but its initiation and progression are not yet understood. Apoptosis functions to efficiently eliminate normal cells no longer required in remodeling tissues (7). The balance of cell recruitment and apoptosis during the healing response, and aberrations of this process, appear to be important factors in lesion progression. Matrix metalloproteinases (MMPs) are a class of structurally related enzymes that function in the degradation of extracellular matrix proteins and are likely to be involved in the remodeling of asthma (8,9).

Is remodeling of the airways a proven clinical concept? It is clear that changes in the extracellular matrix have the capacity to influence airway function in asthma. However, it is not known how each of the many changes that occur in the airway wall contribute to altered airway function in asthma. In asthma, remodeling is almost always present in biopsies, e.g., collagen deposition on basement membrane (10), but is not always clinically demonstrated. Destruction and subsequent remodeling of the normal bronchial architecture are manifested by an accelerated decline in FEV_1. This irreversible component of the airway obstruction is more prominent in severe patients and persists even after aggressive anti-inflammatory treatment. What is clear, however, is that asthmatics, children or adults, are heterogeneous with regard to complete reversiblity of airflow limitation. Radiographic studies using CT scans confirm the presence of airways remodeling in asthma (11). There are other clinical consequences of remodeling (12). The increase in smooth muscle mass can lead to a severe bronchial obstruction during an asthma attack. Mucous glands are sometimes enlarged and may induce excessive mucous production. The ongoing inflammation and subepithelial fibrosis are linked with the persistence of exacerbations and nonspecific bronchial hyperresponsiveness (13). Degradation and/or reorganization of elastin and cartilage may result in decreased airway wall stiffness and increased airway narrowing for a given amount of force generated by the smooth muscle (14).

Airway remodeling in asthma: no doubt, no more (15). This process appears to be of great importance for understanding the long-term follow-up of the patients (16), but there are major gaps in our knowledge. Inflammation is usually a self-limiting process and it is possible that some cells like the eosinophils may be both deleterious and protective as they can release metalloproteases that may limit the remodeling of the airways (17) and some anti-inflammatory agents. Physiological correlations with pathology represent a major missing link that should be filled. The heterogeneity of structural changes in patients also should be better understood, and although some patients present extensive airway remodeling a few months after the apparent occurrence of asthma, others do not appear to have any clinically relevant remodeling after a course of several decades of the disease. More long-term studies are needed to appreciate the prevention and treatment of remodeling (18). Future research should therefore provide better methods for limiting airway remodeling in asthma.

References

1. Ellis A. The pathological anatomy of bronchial asthma. Am J Med Sci 1908; 136:407–429.
2. American Thoracic Society. Definitions and classifications of chronic bronchitis, asthma and emphysema. Am Rev Respir Dis 1962; 85:762–768.
3. Bousquet J, Chanez P, Lacoste JY, et al. Asthma: a disease remodeling the airways. Allergy 1992; 47:3–11.
4. Cotran R, Kumar V, Robin S. Inflammation and repair. In: Cotran R, Kumar V, Robin S, eds. Robbins Pathologic Basis of Disease. Philadephia: WB Saunders, 1989:39–87.
5. Jeffery P. Bronchial biopsies and airway inflammation. Eur Respir J 1996; 9: 1583–1587.
6. Redington AE, Howarth PH. Airway wall remodelling in asthma. Thorax 1997; 52:310–312.
7. Haslett C, Savill JS, Whyte MK, Stern M, Dransfield I, Meagher LC. Granulocyte apoptosis and the control of inflammation. Philos Trans R Soc Lond B Biol Sci 1994; 345:327–333.
8. Mautino G, Oliver N, Chanez P, Bousquet J, Capony F. Increased release of matrix metalloproteinase-9 in bronchoalveolar lavage fluid and by alveolar macrophages of asthmatics. Am J Respir Cell Mol Biol 1997; 17:583–591.
9. Vignola A, Riccobono L, Mirabella A, et al. Sputum TIMP-1 to MMP-9 ratio correlates with airflow obstruction in asthma and COPD. Am J Respir Crit Care Med 1998; 158:1945–1950.

10. Roche WR, Beasley R, Williams JH, Holgate ST. Subepithelial fibrosis in the bronchi of asthmatics. Lancet 1989; 1:520–524.

11. Paganin F, Mariottini C, Brousse C, et al. Non-allergic asthma induces a high prevalence of CT-scan permanent abnormalities. Am J Respir Crit Care Med 1995; 153:110–116.

12. Pare PD, Bai TR, Roberts CR. The structural and functional consequences of chronic allergic inflammation of the airways. Ciba Found Symp 1997; 206:71–86.

13. Vignola M, Kips J, Bousquet J. Tissue remodeling as a feature of persistent asthma. J Allergy Clin Immunol 2000; 105:1041–1053.

14. Bousquet J, Jeffery PK, Busse WW, Johnson M, Vignola M. Asthma: from bronchoconstriction to airways inflammation and remodeling. Am J Respir Crit Care Med 2000; 161:1720–1745.

15. Bousquet J, Vignola AM, Chanez P, Campbell AM, Bonsignore G, Michel FB. Airways remodelling in asthma: no doubt, no more? Int Arch Allergy Immunol 1995; 107:211–214.

16. Haahtela T. Airway remodelling takes place in asthma—what are the clinical implications? Clin Exp Allergy 1997; 27:351–353.

17. Ohno I, Ohtani H, Nitta Y, et al. Eosinophils as a source of matrix metalloproteinase-9 in asthmatic airway inflammation. Am J Respir Cell Mol Biol 1997; 16:212–219.

18. Olivieri D, Chetta A, Del-Donno M, et al. Effect of short-term treatment with low-dose inhaled fluticasone propionate on airway inflammation and remodeling in mild asthma: a placebo-controlled study. Am J Respir Crit Care Med 1997; 155:1864–1871.

2

How Can We Assess Airway Remodeling Using Imaging?

DANY JAFFUEL

Service des Maladies Respiratoires–
 INSERM U454
Hôpital Arnaud de Villeneuve
Montpellier, France

FABRICE JEAN PAGANIN

CHD Felix Guyon
St. Denis Réunion, France

JEAN BOUSQUET

Montpellier University and
Service des Maladies Respiratoires–
 INSERM U454
Hôpital Arnaud de Villeneuve
Montpellier, France

I. Introduction

Asthma is a clinical syndrome characterized by its reversibility of airway obstruction, but several studies suggest that chronic asthma may be associated with the development of irreversible airway obstruction (1,2). In 1962, the American Thoracic Society noted that some asthmatics, particularly those who have had asthma for many years and/or present a severe form of the disease, may have persistent airflow obstruction (3). The pathophysiological mechanism of asthma classically includes bronchospasm, hypersecretion, and chronic inflammation. More recently, attention has been focused on "airway remodeling." Healing begins in the early stage in any inflammatory process and results in repair, inducing a regeneration that leaves no residual trace of the previous injury and/or the replacement of injured tissue by connective tissue. In asthma, the most common changes accounting for a remodeling of the airways (2) include subepithelial fibrosis (4), activation of myofibroblasts

"

(5), hypertrophy or hyperplasia of smooth muscle and mucous glands (6–8), and elastic fiber disruption (9).

At a macroscopic step, computerized tomography (CT scan) has been used in the diagnosis of airway diseases because of the high degree of anatomical detail provided and because CT scan is considered more sensitive than other imaging techniques. In asthma, high-resolution CT scan (HRCT scan) has been used to measure the internal size of the airways at baseline, during challenge, or after bronchodilatation. Moreover, it has been consistently observed that some asthmatic patients present abnormalities related to fixed airway remodeling such as emphysema, bronchiectasis, and bronchial wall thickening.

II. Imaging Techniques and Airway Remodeling

A. CT Scan and HRCT Scan

Owing to the high degree of anatomical detail provided and a greater sensibility, most of the studies published used the technique of HRCT scanning of the lungs. There are many protocols of high resolution. The most commonly used is the protocol developed by Mayo and colleagues (10), adapted or not with some variation in several studies. The characteristics of the original protocol are as follows: the matrix size is 512×512 at a pixel of 0.5 mm, a gantry ($20°$) is used to improve the visualization of subsegmental bronchi, and the scanning time is about 3 sec. The 1-mm scans are obtained at 15-mm increments from the upper to the lower part of the lungs. Scans are performed without contrast during full deep inspiration, and images are recorded at a window width of 1.600 HU and a window level of -600 HU and then reconstructed using a sharp bone algorithm.

B. Other Imaging Techniques

The first and most widely used imaging technique for assessing asthma is the chest roentgenogram. Chest roentgenograms continue to be obtained on asthmatic patients during exacerbation. Abnormalities observed are hyperinflation, bronchial wall thickening, pneumonia, and complications such as atelectasis and pneumothorax. However, chest roentgenograms have two characteristics that limit their sensitivity and specificity for detecting and diagnosing early lung disease. First, they have relatively low attenuation density resolution (i.e., small differences in attenuation between normal and abnormal lungs are difficult to observe). Second, many structures are superimposed on the two-dimensional projected chest radiographic image, making it difficult to decide what the abnormality represents anatomically. In chronic asthma, comparative studies with HRCT have shown that the use of chest roentgenograms provided little information on the bronchi except in cases of major lesions such as seen in allergic bronchial aspergillosis. Therefore, although chest roentgenograms have relatively low cost and wide availability, they have little utility for the evaluation of airway remodeling as compare to HRCT scan.

Additional noninvasive radiological methods have been developed that can be applied to assess asthma on a research basis. These newer methods include magnetic resonance imaging (MRI), positron emission tomography (PET), gamma-camera imaging using two-dimensional (2-D) and three-dimensional imaging, and single photon emission computed tomography (SPECT) imaging (11). MRI of the lung is severely limited by low proton density, cardiac and respiratory motion, and susceptibility effects induced by multiple air/tissue interfaces. The portions of the tree demonstrated on routine spin-echo images include only the trachea, major bronchi, intermediate bronchus on the right side, and lobar bronchi. Imaging of the intrapulmonary airways responsible for obstructive disease such as asthma is not yet feasible. These inconveniences must, therefore, be overcome before this technology can perhaps attain significant use for the appreciation of airway remodeling. As with MRI, the large air-to-tissue ratio of the lungs limits the use of PET technology for the appreciation of airway remodeling. PET scanning is currently limited to measure pulmonary β-adrenoreceptor density and regional pulmonary extravascular density or blood volume. Gamma-camera imaging of the lungs has been used as a research tool to assess regional aerosol deposition in the lungs and mucociliary clearance in asthmatics. Tomographic imaging using SPECT is better suited to distinguish between deposition in the small and large airways than conventional 2-D images. However, 2-D and SPECT gamma-camera imaging have no utility for the evaluation of airway remodeling.

III. Importance of HRCT Scan in the Diagnosis of Emphysema

Pulmonary emphysema is a pathological diagnosis defined as ''a condition of the lung characterised by abnormal permanent enlargement of the airspaces distal to terminal bronchioles accompanied by destruction of their walls.'' While several studies tried to assess the presence and severity of emphysema by clinical examination, pulmonary function test, and chest roentgenogram, it appears to be difficult to distinguish patients with moderate emphysema from those with mild or no emphysema by these methods. Moreover, lung function tests are not specific for emphysema and alteration of transfer of the lung for carbon monoxide (TLCO) may be due to cardiogenic edema or interstitial disease. Despite the fact that very mild emphysema goes undetected and the severity of the disease underestimated, HRCT scan is the most sensitive radiographic method to assess emphysema and has been shown to be more sensitive than pulmonary function tests or TLCO (12). Moreover, some studies have demonstrated that a good correlation between the HRCT and pathological findings of emphysema (13,14).

Using HRCT scan, the presence and extent of emphysema can be determined by visual assessment of areas of abnormally low attenuation or by objective quantification based on the attenuation values. HRCT scans at 1-cm intervals have been used to detect whether the relative area of lung occupied by attenuation values lower than a given threshold would be a measure of emphysema (15). The strongest correlation was found for -950 HU and this study also revealed that the TLCO associated with HRCT-scan quantification is sufficient to predict microscopic measurements. A subsequent study from the same group suggests that HRCT scan is also influenced by total lung capacity and, to a lesser degree, by age (16). However, normal CT attenuation values for the lung have not yet been established. Millimetric slices are more accurate than centrimetric ones in the diagnosis of emphysema but not all studies found a major difference between the two techniques. This is probably because CT scan explores only a small part of the whole parenchyma and pulmonary involvement in emphysema is indeed irregular and not homogeneous (17). Recently, a new technique of CT scan such as the sliding thin slab, minimum intensity projection (STS-MIP) has been used to improve the accuracy of CT scans (18). Moreover, CT scans performed in full expiration can reveal emphysema ignored by conventional HR technique in full inspiration (15,19,20). However, care must be taken as the images observed in full expiration that are not visible at full inspiration may reflect air trapping rather than true emphysema. These results were subsequently confirmed in asthmatics (21).

IV. Importance of HRCT Scan in the Diagnosis of Bronchiectasis

Bronchiectasis is a pathological diagnosis defined as ''a condition characterised by abnormal and permanent dilatation of pulmonary airways.'' The clinical findings in patients with bronchiectasis (chronic cough, sputum production, airway obstruction on lung function test) are characteristics, though not specific. Because the definition of bronchiectasis is a morphological one, imaging has a key role in its identification. Chest roentgenogram is very helpful because it is rarely without positive findings such as atelectasis, honeycomb-like structure, and increased pulmonary markings. However, the diagnosis of bronchiectasis is confirmed by HRCT scan performed with millimetric slices, which shows dilated bronchi (cystic, cylindrical, varicose), mucoid impaction, areas of pneumonitis, and atelectasis. When investigators have compared CT scan and bronchography, they have shown that CT scans are specific in greater than 90% and sensible in greater than 95% of cases when the high-resolution CT-scan technique is used (22). Bronchography is valuable in confirming the location of the bronchiectasis only if surgery is contemplated for a localized bronchiectasis and to exclude the presence of significant disease elsewhere. In the other cases, bronchography is considered a tool of the past.

V. Demonstration of Irreversible Abnormalities Using HRCT Scan in Asthma

Several studies (Table 1) have shown that irreversible abnormalities are observed in the lungs of asthmatic patients on a CT scan such as emphysema, bronchiectasis, bronchial wall thickening, and sequelar linear shadows. However, some aspects remain to be clearly established and less controversial. Reversible abnormalities usually include mucoid impactions, acinar pattern, and lobar collapse (23).

A. Emphysema

CT Scan Findings

Using HRCT scan and visual assessment, emphysema-like images were found in 9–53% of asthmatic patients (23–28). When HRCT scans were performed before and after medical treatment (corticosteroid or β_2-agonist), the emphysema-like images were found to be fixed abnormalities (23,28). In the largest study published (126 patients), emphysema was found in 39.3% of asthmatic patients, correlated with the severity of the disease and the nonatopic status (24). However, a study of 62 patients (27) found emphysema only in current or ex-smokers and no correlation of emphysema with the duration or the severity of asthma. The difference between these two studies might be attributed to differences in the population studied and particularly the difference in crite-

Table 1 Summary of CT-Scan Studies in Asthma

Author, year	Clinical characteristics of patients	CT-scan technique	Results of study
Kinsella et al., 1988 (41)	10 asthmatic patients (mean FEV_1: 56.4%), nonsmokers 10 patients (mean FEV_1: 53.4%), smokers	Conventional CT scan Sections cut of 10-mm collimation at 10-mm increments Vital assessment	Emphysema score significantly more important in smoking patients than in nonsmoking asthmatic patients. DLCO/VA significantly more important in nonsmoking asthmatic patients than in smoking patients. Correlation between DLCO/VA and emphysema score not shown.
Neeld et al., 1990 (37)	8 patients with ABPA; 8 asthmatic patients (with skin test positive to *Aspergillus*); mean FEV_1 not shown; tobacco status not shown	High resolution Sections cut of 1.5-mm collimation at 10- or 20-mm increments Visual assessment	Bronchiectasis in 41% of patients with ABPA significantly different from 15% in asthmatic patients without ABPA. Bronchial thickening in 30% of patients with ABPA not significantly different from 23% in asthmatic patients without ABPA.
Kondoh et al., 1990 (42)	17 asthmatic patients (mean FEV_1: 68%), nonsmokers 18 asthmatic patients (mean FEV_1: 67%), smokers	Conventional CT scans Sections cut of 10-mm collimation at 15-mm increments Visual assessment	Emphysema score significantly more important in smoking asthmatic patients than in nonsmoking asthmatic patients. Emphysema score correlated with DLCO/VA (not correlated with FEV_1 and total lung capacity).

| Paganin et al., 1992 (23) | 61 asthmatic patients (mean FEV_1: 70.12% ± 23) (10 asthmatics have CT scan during exacerbation and after treatment); 10 adult control subjects (mean FEV_1: ND), nonsmokers | High resolution
Sections cut of 1-mm collimation at 15-mm increments
Visual assessment | Abnormal CT-scan finding in asthmatics:
Bronchial wall thickening in 16%
Bronchiectasis in 65%
Emphysema in 18%
After treatment:
Mucoid impaction, acinar patterns, lobar collapses disappeared.
Bronchiectasis, emphysema remain unchanged. |
| Lynch et al., 1993 (25) | 48 asthmatic patients (mean FEV_1: 63%), 21 current or ex-smokers 22 adult control subjects; FEV_1: not shown; 4 current smokers | High-resolution and conventional CT scans
Sections cut of 1.5-mm or 2-mm and 20-mm collimation at 20-mm increments
Visual assessment | Abnormal CT-scan finding in asthmatics:
Bronchial wall thickening in 92%
Bronchial dilatation in 31% not correlated with airflow obstruction, not significantly more frequent in asthmatic patients than in control subjects.
Emphysema in 19%, correlated with FEV_1, DLCO/VA, functional residual capacity and tobacco status; more frequent in asthmatic patients than in control subjects. |

Table 1 Continued

Author, year	Clinical characteristics of patients	CT-scan technique	Results of study
Newman et al., 1994 (21)	18 asthmatic patients (mean FEV_1: 61.1%) 22 adult control subjects (mean FEV_1: 93.3%) All nonsmokers	High-resolution and conventional CT scans Sections cut of 1.5 and 10-mm collimation at the level of the transverse aorta and just above the diaphragm Quantitative CT at both end expiration and end inspiration (% of pixel below -900 HU = pixel index)	The best discriminator between asthmatic and normal subject is the 1.5-mm HRCT expiratory inferior scan. Pixel index on expiration correlated with: Residual volume FEV_1 Functional residual capacity.
Angus et al., 1994 (26)	17 patients with ABPA (mean FEV_1: 49.4%), 11 current or ex-smokers 11 asthmatic patients (with skin test positive to *Aspergillus*) (mean FEV_1: 75.5%) 4 current or ex-smokers	High resolution Sections cut of 3-mm collimation at 9-mm increments Visual assessment	Bronchiectasis in 82% of patients with ABPA significantly different from 18% in asthmatic patients without ABPA. Emphysema in 53% of patients with ABPA significantly different from 9% in asthmatic patients without ABPA.
Paganin et al., 1996 (24)	70 asthmatic patients with atopy; 56 asthmatic patients nonatopics; nonsmokers; AAS score: 1–5; FEV_1: 35–120%	High resolution Sections cut of 1-mm collimation at 15-mm increments Visual assessment	AAS score correlated with: Emphysema Sequella linear shadow Varicose bronchiectasis Cylindrical bronchiectasis

| Grenier et al., 1996 (38) | 50 asthmatic patients; 12 current or ex-smokers; AAS score: 1–5; FEV_1: 25–115%
 10 adult control subjects (mean FEV_1: not shown), nonsmokers | High resolution
 Sections cut of 1.5-mm collimation at 10-mm increments
 Visual assessment | Abnormal CT-scan finding in asthmatics:
 Bronchial wall thickening in 82%
 Bronchiectasis in 28.5%
 Decreased lung attenuation in 30%
 Bronchial wall thickening, decreased lung attenuation, small centrilobular opacities, extent of bronchiectasis more frequently observed in patients with greater AAS score.
 Clinically acceptable observer variability.
 Intra- and interobserver agreements measured by kappa statistics ranging from 0.6 to 0.79 and from 0.4 to 0.64 respectively. |
| Mochizuki et al., 1997 (27) | 62 asthmatic patients; 34 current or ex-smokers (mean FEV_1: not shown) | High resolution
 Sections cut of 1-mm collimation at 15-mm increments
 Visual assessment | Emphysema score > 0 in 23% of the patients.
 No emphysema in nonsmoking asthmatic patients.
 Emphysema score correlated with: DLCO/VA, FEV_1, and age but not with the duration or the severity of the disease.
 Clinically acceptable observer variability.
 Intra- and interobserver agreements measured by kappa statistics are 0.99 and 0.93, respectively. |

Table 1 Continued

Author, year	Clinical characteristics of patients	CT-scan technique	Results of study
Biernacki et al., 1997 (28)	17 asthmatic patients (mean FEV_1 65%, 33–105%), nonsmokers 17 COPD patients (mean FEV_1 32%, 15–68%), nonsmokers 7 adult control subjects (mean FEV_1 103%, 90–110%), nonsmokers	Conventional CT scans Sections cut of 10-mm collimation at 30-mm increments CT lung density	Asthmatics and COPD patients have lower CT lung density than control subjects. No correlation of lung density with FEV_1, DLCO/VA. No modification of lung density after β_2-agonist nebulization.
Park et al., 1997 (39)	39 asthmatic patients (mean FEV_1 not shown, 27–128%), nonsmokers 22 adult control subjects (mean FEV_1 not shown, 82–102%), nonsmokers	High resolution Sections cut of 1-mm collimation at the level of the aortic arch, the tracheal carina, 1 cm below the carina, the inferior pulmonary veins, 2 cm above the diaphragm at both end expiration and end inspiration Visual assessment	Abnormal CT-scan finding in asthmatics: Bronchial wall thickening in 44% correlated with airflow obstruction; more frequent in asthmatic patients than in control subjects. Bronchial dilatation in 31% not correlated with airflow obstruction, but more frequent in asthmatic patients than in control subjects. Mosaic lung attenuation in 18% correlated with airflow obstruction. Air trapping in 50% not correlated with airflow obstruction and the predicted residual volume, but more frequent on expiratory CT scan in asthmatic patients than in control subjects.

Awadh et al., 1998 (29)	15 asthmatic patients with near fatal asthma (mean FEV_1 68%); 13 asthmatic patients with moderate asthma (mean FEV_1 73%); 12 asthmatic patients with mild asthma (mean FEV_1 102%); 14 adult control subjects (mean FEV_1 103%); all nonsmokers	High resolution Sections cut of 1-mm collimation at the level of the aortic arch, the tracheal carina, 1 cm below the carina, the inferior pulmonary veins, 2 cm above the diaphragm at both end expiration and end inspiration Visual assessment	Patients with more severe asthma have more airway wall thickening than those with mild asthma.
Carr et al., 1998 (40)	24 asthmatic patients (mean FEV_1 56.5, AAS 4), nonsmokers	High resolution Sections cut of 3-mm collimation at 10-mm increments on full inspiration and at 30 mm on full expiration Visual assessment	Abnormal CT-scan finding in asthmatics: Bronchial wall thickening in 63% Bronchial dilatation in 66% Air trapping on inspiratory scan in 25% and on expiratory scan in 83% Interobserver agreements for bronchial dilatation, bronchial thickening, air trapping on inspiration and on expiration measured by kappa statistics are 0.73, 0.78, 0.99, 0.79, respectively.

ria for airway obstruction. Their criterion for reversibility of airway obstruction was an increase exceeding 20% in FEV_1, whereas ours was 12%. Patients with severe asthma occasionally experience a decrease in reversibility. Moreover, patients who were unable to maintain full inspiration necessary to produce HRCT scan are sometimes excluded from the studies. Thus, some studies might have been biased against patients with severe asthma.

Other CT-scan techniques have been used to evaluate emphysema in asthmatic patients. CT scans performed in full expiration can reveal emphysema ignored by conventional HR technique in full inspiration, but the images observed in full expiration that are not seen in full inspiration may reflect air trapping rather than true emphysema in asthmatic patients (29,30). Measuring lung density, Biernacki et al. (28) found that both asthmatics and COPD patients had a lower lung density than normal healthy subjects. Moreover, COPD patients had a lower lung density than asthmatics, but there was an overlap between the two groups and asthmatics were analyzed together although FEV_1 values ranged from 33% to 105%. Low CT lung density may also result from air trapping and TLCO may be used to differentiate air trapping and emphysema (30).

Significance of CT Scan Findings

The significance of these CT-scan abnormalities remains to be fully elucidated (31). In the pathological examination of asthmatic lungs, true emphysema, a destructive process focusing on the acinus, was observed in some cases (32,33) but is not a common feature (6) and is never extensive. Moreover, in most of the patients studied, smoking habits were not assessed so that it is not fully clear whether the emphysema was really due to asthma. In the study by Sobonya (32), one of seven nonsmoking asthmatics showed histological features of mild emphysema. Parenchymal destruction has been observed in a fatal case of a nonsmoking asthmatic with toluene-di-isocyanate sensitivity (34), but the mechanisms of this occupational form of asthma may differ from those of other forms of the disease.

Bronchial gland duct ectasia has been described in fatal bronchial asthma (6,35) and was associated with emphysema. The histological features of patients in whom death was considered to be due to asthma were studied (36). Bronchial gland duct ectasia was diagnosed if there was more than one abnormally dilated epithelial lined protrusion from a bronchus, extending through the smooth muscle layer. Interstitial emphysema was present in 10/53 clinical cases of fatal asthma, all of whom had bronchial gland duct ectasia

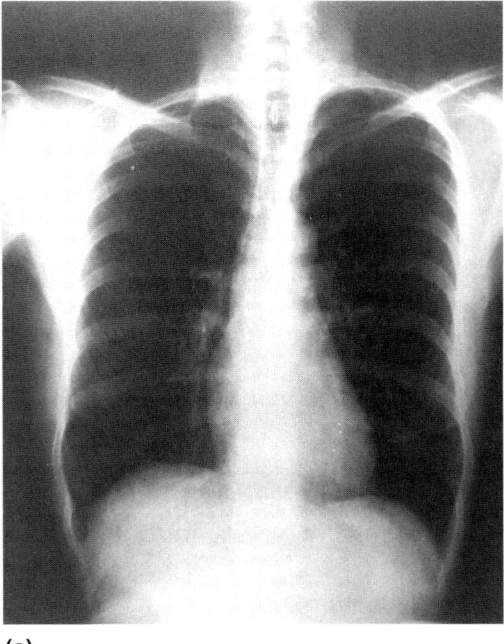

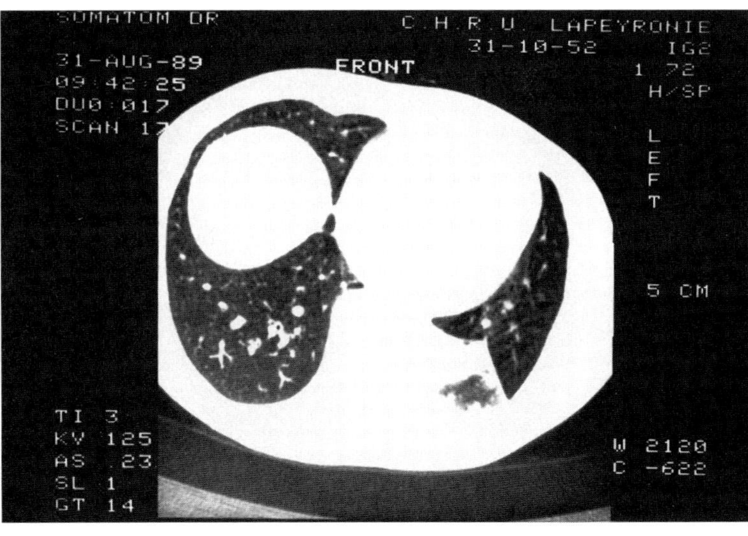

Figure 1 (a) Chest X-ray of an asthmatic patient presenting an acute exacerbation showing hyperinflation. (b) HRCT scan of the same asthmatic patient, the same day as the chest X-ray, showing an alveolar syndrome of the left lower lobe and filled cylindrical bronchiectases of the right lower lobe (W 2120, C-622).

(a)

SOMATOM DR
C.H.R.U. LAPEYRONIE
11-11-47
IG2
17-JUL-89
1 73
17:30:27
H/SP
DU0:019
SCAN 20
LEFT
5 CM
TI 3
KV 125
W 2100
AS .23
C -600
SL 1
GT 15
TP 250
Aiguelongue
VT/JL

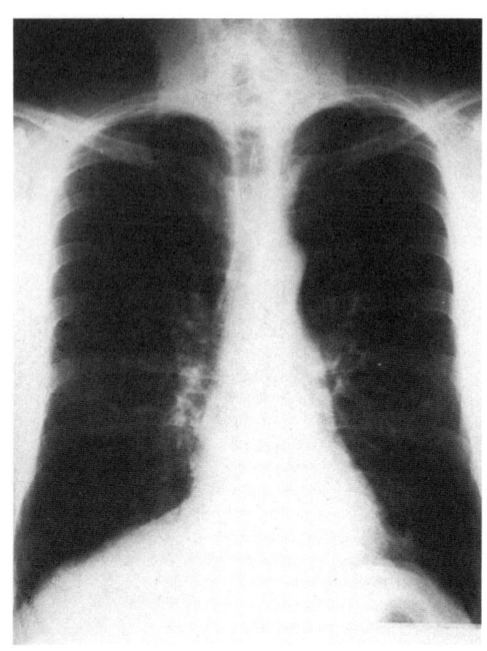

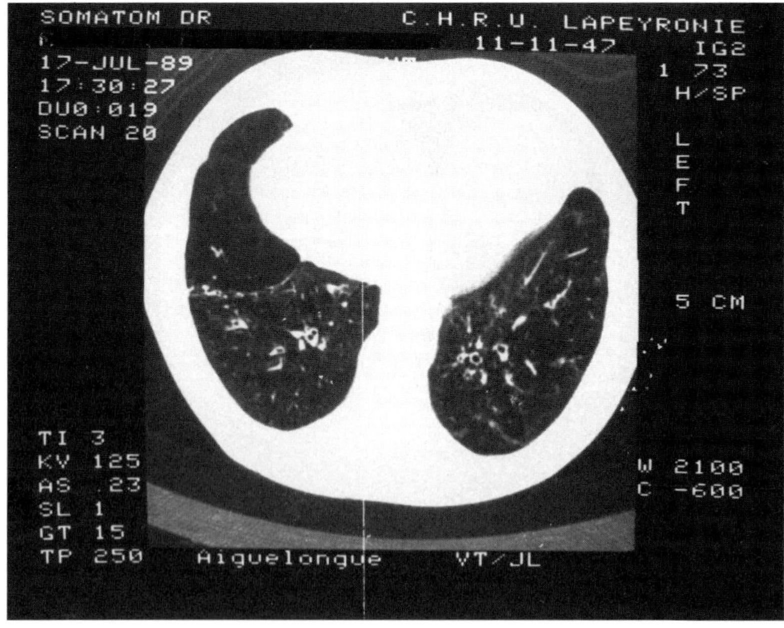

(b)

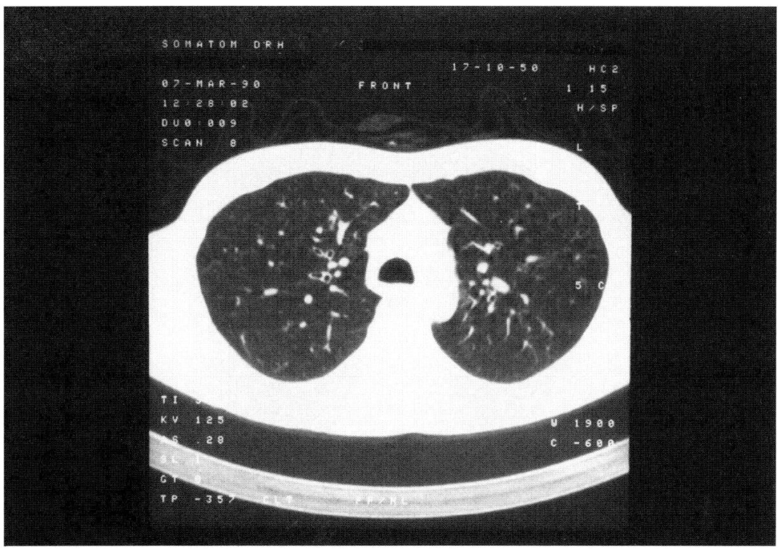

Figure 3 HRCT scan of the mild asthmatic patient showing a cylindrical bronchiectasis of both upper lobes (W 1900, C −600).

and a histological diagnosis of asthma. Interstitial emphysema was not observed in control subjects. The authors concluded that bronchial gland duct ectasia is a common histological feature of severe asthma, and that interstitial emphysema may be a consequence of rupture of these dilated gland ducts. However, the relationships between these histological features and CT-scan emphysema-like images are unknown.

B. Bronchiectasis

CT Scan Findings

Using HRCT scan and millimetric slices, bronchiectasis were found in 15–82% of asthmatic patients (23–26,37–39) (Figs. 1–3). When HRCT scans

---

Figure 2 (a) Chest X-ray of a severe asthmatic patient showing no major abnormality. (b) HRCT scan of the same asthmatic patient, the same day as the chest X-ray, showing cylindrical and varicose bronchiectases in both lower lobes and complete destruction of the middle lobe (W 2100, C −600).

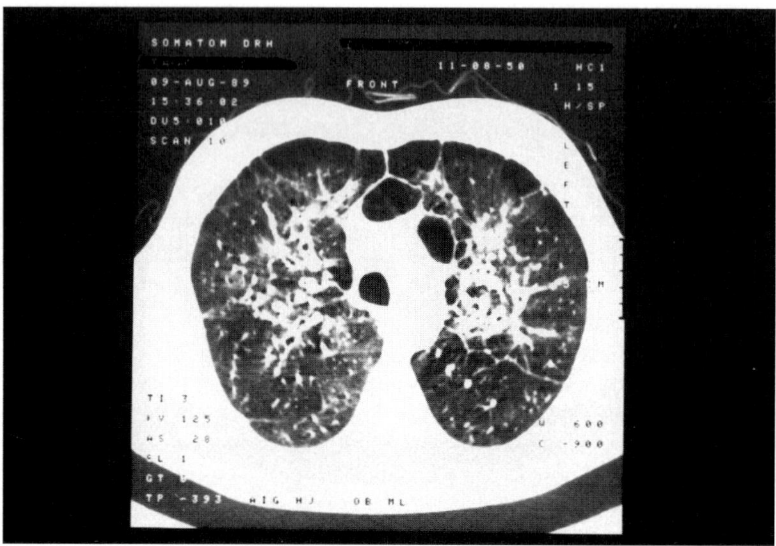

Figure 4   HRCT scan of a patient with stage 5 allergic bronchopulmonary aspergillosis showing bullous and paraseptal emphysema of the upper lobes and bronchi filled with secretions (W 1600, C −900).

were performed before and after medical treatment (corticosteroid and β_2-agonist), bronchiectases were found to be fixed abnormalities (23). We found cylindrical and varicose bronchiectasis correlated with the severity of asthma and the nonatopic status (24) whereas others did not (25,38,39). The discrepancies between the results of these studies may be explained by differences in populations or in CT-scan criteria for diagnosis of bronchiectasis. Indeed, the best CT-scan criterion for diagnosis of bronchiectasis is probably the assessment of the diameter of the bronchus on several successive slices with very small interspace intervals (5 mm) and not the commonly used comparison of the diameter of the bronchus with that of the homologous pulmonary artery. In fact, there are several possible reasons why the bronchus may be larger than its adjacent pulmonary artery without indicating true bronchiectasis: division of the artery but not that of the homologous bronchus, variation of the pulmonary artery with changes in blood volume or hypoxia. Moreover, some studies concerned asthmatic patients with allergic bronchopulmonary aspergillosis (ABPA) (26,37), a disease characterized by the presence of extensive bronchiectasis (Fig. 4).

Significance of CT-Scan Findings

The significance of bronchiectasis in asthma remains nuclear. These lesions were observed in nonsmoking patients who had apparently never suffered from the pulmonary diseases in childhood that might account for their presence. To explain bronchiectasis in non-ABPA patients, Neeld et al. (37) hypothesized that some asthmatic subjects might have subclinical ABPA, but this is unlikely to be the case. Moreover, in our studies, skin tests to *Aspergillus fumigatus* have been carried out in all patients and were always negative. Moreover, in these patients, total serum IgE levels were often normal ruling out the diagnosis of ABPA.

Bronchectasis found using CT scans in asthma are rarely associated with cough and sputum. They are not as extensive as in ABPA or true bronchiectasis. Cylindrical bronchiectasis occurs frequently and was found in patients with variable severity. Varicous and cystic bronchectases are rare and observed only in the most severe patients (23,24). These may be sequelae of mucoid impactions and bronchial hypersecretion. It is possible that bronchial dilatation may be due to progressive bronchial destruction and therefore remodeling of the airways.

C. Bronchial Wall Thickening

Using HRCT scan and millimetric slices, bronchial wall thickening was found in 16–92% of asthmatic patients (23–25,37,39,40). The discrepancy for the prevalence of bronchial wall thickening in asthma can probably be explained by the subjectivity of the finding. Moreover, HRCT-scan assessment of the bronchial wall may be impaired by the use of inappropriate window setting. Bronchial wall thickening in asthma may reflect bronchial and peribronchial inflammation. Moreover, it has been reported that in pathological specimens of asthmatic lungs, the increases in smooth muscle, mucous gland, and cartilage contributed to the increased total wall thickness of the bronchi (8). We and others found bronchial wall thickening correlated with the severity of asthma (23–25). The failure of response to oral steroids (23) supports the concept that bronchial wall thickening is a fixed structural change in the lung and a marker of airway remodeling.

VI. HRCT-Scan Abnormalities and Asthma Severity

A total score of permanent CT-scan abnormalities was calculated by simple summation (24). This score increased significantly with the severity of asthma

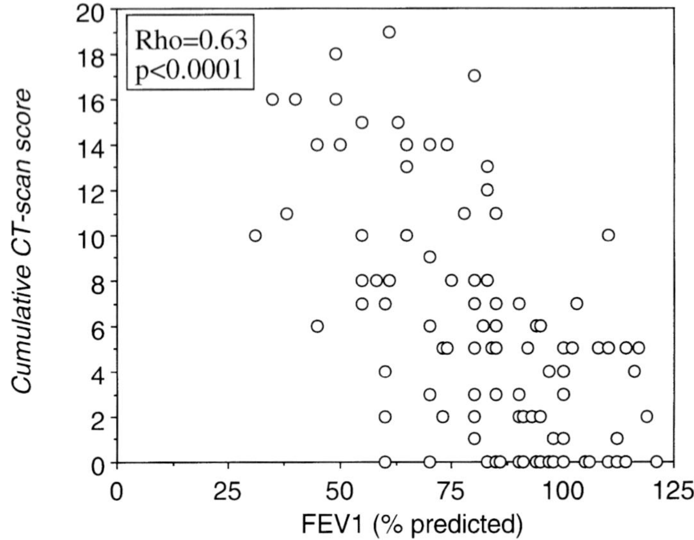

Figure 5 Correlation between a cumulative CT-scan score and FEV_1 in 136 asthmatics of variable severity and etiology. (From Ref. 24.)

in both allergic and nonallergic asthmatic patients and was significantly correlated with FEV_1 (Fig. 5). Patients with brittle asthma had a low cumulated CT-scan score. Moreover, for a similar clinical severity and duration of the disease, patients with nonallergic asthma presented more abnormalities on their CT scan than those with allergic asthma although the duration of the disease was apparently similar.

VII. Conclusion

The approach to better understand and evaluate the complexity of asthma and in particular that of airway remodeling required new tools. Macroscopic appreciation by HRCT scan may bring new and valuable information. Anatomical pulmonary changes, including bronchial wall thickening, emphysema, and bronchiectasis, have been demonstrated by HRCT scan. These abnormalities seem to be more extensive in severe forms of asthma and in nonallergic rather than in allergic patients. However, the place of HRCT scan in the assessment of a patient in the clinical routine remains to be clearly established. HRCT scan may be an advantage in patients with severe asthma in order to evaluate permanent and irreversible airway abnormalities.

References

1. Brown PJ, Greville HW, Finucane KE. Asthma and irreversible airflow obstruction. Thorax 1984; 39:131–136.
2. Bousquet J, Chanez P, Lacoste JY, et al. Asthma: a disease remodeling the airways. Allergy 1992; 47:3–11.
3. American Thoracic Society. Definitions and classifications of chronic bronchitis, asthma and emphysema. Am Rev Respir Dis 1962; 85:762–768.
4. Roche WR, Beasley R, Williams JH, Holgate ST. Subepithelial fibrosis in the bronchi of asthmatics. Lancet 1989; 1:520–524.
5. Brewster CE, Howarth PH, Djukanovic R, Wilson J, Holgate ST, Roche WR. Myofibroblasts and subepithelial fibrosis in bronchial asthma. Am J Respir Cell Mol Biol 1990; 3:507–511.
6. Dunnill M, Massarella G, Anderson J. Comparison of the quantitative anatomy of the bronchi in normal subjects, in status asthmaticus, in chronic bronchitis, and in emphysema. Thorax 1969; 24:176–179.
7. Bai TR. Abnormalities in airway smooth muscle in fatal asthma. Am Rev Respir Dis 1990; 141:552–557.
8. Carrol N, Elliot J, Morton A, James A. The structure of large and small airways in nonfatal and fatal asthma. Am Rev Respir Dis 1993; 147:405–410.
9. Bousquet J, Lacoste JY, Chanez P, Vic P, Godard P, Michel FB. Bronchial elastic fibers in normal subjects and asthmatic patients. Am J Respir Crit Care Med 1996; 153:1648–1654.
10. Mayo JR, Webb WR, Gould R, et al. High-resolution CT of the lungs: an optimal approach. Radiology 1987; 163:507–510.
11. Woolcock AJ. Effect of drugs on small airways. Am J Respir Crit Care Med 1998; 157:S203–S207.
12. Klein JS, Gamsu G, Webb WR, Golden JA, Muller NL. High-resolution CT diagnosis of emphysema in symptomatic patients with normal chest radiographs and isolated low diffusing capacity. Radiology 1992; 182:817–821.
13. Foster W, Jr., Pratt PC, Roggli VL, Godwin JD, Halvorsen R, Jr, Putman CE. Centrilobular emphysema: CT-pathologic correlation. Radiology 1986; 159:27–32.
14. Bergin CJ, Muller NL, Miller RR. CT in the qualitative assessment of emphysema. J Thorac Imaging 1986; 1:94–103.
15. Gevenois PA, De-Vuyst P, de-Maertelaer V, et al. Comparison of computed density and microscopic morphometry in pulmonary emphysema. Am J Respir Crit Care Med 1996; 154:187–192.

16.   Gevenois PA, Scillia P, de-Maertelaer V, Michils A, De-Vuyst P, Yernault JC. The effects of age, sex, lung size, and hyperinflation on CT lung densitometry. Am J Roentgenol 1996; 167:1169–1173.

17.   Kuwano K, Matsuba K, Ikeda T, et al. The diagnosis of mild emphysema. Correlation of computed tomography and pathology scores. Am Rev Respir Dis 1990; 141:169–178.

18.   Remy-Jardin M, Remy J, Gosselin B, Copin MC, Wurtz A, Duhamel A. Sliding thin slab, minimum intensity projection technique in the diagnosis of emphysema: histopathologic-CT correlation. Radiology 1996; 200:665–671.

19.   Miniati M, Filippi E, Falaschi F, et al. Radiologic evaluation of emphysema in patients with chronic obstructive pulmonary disease. Chest radiography versus high resolution computed tomography. Am J Respir Crit Care Med 1995; 151: 1359–1367.

20.   Eda S, Kubo K, Fujimoto K, Matsuzawa Y, Sekiguchi M, Sakai F. The relations between expiratory chest CT using helical CT and pulmonary function tests in emphysema. Am J Respir Crit Care Med 1997; 155:1290–1294.

21.   Newman KB, Lynch DA, Newman LS, Ellegood D, Newell J, Jr. Quantitative computed tomography detects air trapping due to asthma. Chest 1994; 106:105– 109.

22.   Grenier P, Maurice F, Musset D, Menu Y, Nahum H. Bronchiectasis: assessment by thin-section CT. Radiology 1986; 161:95–99.

23.   Paganin F, Trussard V, Seneterre E, et al. Chest radiography and high resolution computed tomography of the lungs in asthma. Am Rev Respir Dis 1992; 146: 1084–1087.

24.   Paganin F, Mariottini C, Brousse C, et al. Non-allergic asthma induces a high prevalence of CT-scan permanent abnormalities. Am J Respir Crit Care Med 1996; 153:110–114.

25.   Lynch DA, Newell JD, Tschomper BA, Cink TM, Newman LS, Bethel R. Uncomplicated asthma in adults: comparison of CT appearance of the lungs in asthmatic and healthy subjects. Radiology 1993; 188:829–833.

26.   Angus RM, Davies ML, Cowan MD, McSharry C, Thomson NC. Computed tomographic scanning of the lung in patients with allergic bronchopulmonary aspergillosis and in asthmatic patients with a positive skin test to *Aspergillus fumigatus*. Thorax 1994; 49:586–589.

27.   Mochizuki T, Nakajima H, Kokubu F, Kushihashi T, Adachi M. Evaluation of emphysema in patients with reversible airway obstruction using high-resolution CT. Chest 1997; 112:1522–1526.

28.   Biernacki W, Redpath AT, Best JJ, MacNee W. Measurement of CT lung density in patients with chronic asthma. Eur Respir J 1997; 10:2455–2459.

29.   Awadh N, Muller N, Park C, Abboud R, Fitzegrald J. Airway wall thickness in patients with near fatal asthma and control groups: assessment with high resolution computed tomographic scanning. Thorax 1998; 53:248–263.

30.   Gould GA, Redpath AT, Ryan M, et al. Lung CT density correlates with mea-

surements of airflow limitation and the diffusing capacity. Eur Respir J 1991; 4:141–146.

31. Paganin F, Jaffuel D, Bousquet J. Significance of emphysema observed on computed tomography scan in asthma. Eur Respir J 1997; 10:2446–2448.

32. Sobonya RE. Quantitative structural alterations in long-standing allergic asthma. Am Rev Respir Dis 1984; 130:289–292.

33. Messer J, Peters G, Bennett W. Causes of deaths and pathological findings in 304 cases of bronchial asthma. Br J Dis Chest 1960; 38:616–624.

34. Fabbri LM, Danieli D, Crescioli S, et al. Fatal asthma in a subject sensitized to toluene diisocyanate. Am Rev Respir Dis 1988; 137:1494–1498.

35. Huber H, Koessler K. The pathology of bronchial asthma. Arch Intern Med 1922; 30:689–696.

36. Cluroe A, Holloway L, Thomson K, Purdie G, Beasley R. Bronchial gland duct ectasia in fatal bronchial asthma: association with interstitial emphysema. J Clin Pathol 1989; 42:1026–1031.

37. Neeld DA, Goodman LR, Gurney JW, Greenberger PA, Fink JN. Computerized tomography in the evaluation of allergic bronchopulmonary aspergillosis. Am Rev Respir Dis 1990; 142:1200–1205.

38. Grenier P, Mourey-Gerosa I, Benali K, et al. Abnormalities of the airways and lung parenchyma in asthmatics: CT observations in 50 patients and inter- and intraobserver variability. Eur Radiol 1996; 6:199–206.

39. Park CS, Muller NL, Worthy SA, Kim JS, Awadh N, Fitzgerald M. Airway obstruction in asthmatic and healthy individuals: inspiratory and expiratory thin section CT findings. Radiology 1997; 203:361–367.

40. Carr D, Hibon S, Rubens M, Chung K. Peripheral airways obstruction on high-resolution computed tomography in chronic severe asthma. Respir Med 1998; 92:448–453.

41. Kinsella M, Muller NL, Staples C, Vedal S, Chan-Yeung M. Hyperinflation in asthma and emphysema. Assessment by pulmonary function testing and computed tomography. Chest 1988; 94:286–289.

42. Kondoh Y, Taniguchi H, Yokoyama S, Taki F, Takagi K, Satake T. Emphysematous change in chronic asthma in relation to cigarette smoking. Assessment by computed tomography. Chest 1990; 97:845–849.

3

The Use of Morphometry to Assess Airway Wall Remodeling in Asthma

NEIL G. CARROLL and ALAN LLOYD JAMES

Sir Charles Gairdner Hospital
Nedlands, Western Australia, Australia

I. Introduction

The use of morphometric techniques to study the airways allows us to quantify descriptive pathology by a variety of measurement techniques that assist our understanding of airway function in terms of structural organization. In the lung it provides us with a reasonable interpretation of airway structure in vivo, and the observations made at a single time point or over time can provide important information on the natural history of asthma.

The term ''remodeling'' has been used to describe the structural alterations that have been observed in the airways of patients with asthma. It is commonly assumed that remodeling of the airways is a dynamic event and occurs as a response to both intermittent inflammatory stimuli and the persistent presence and activation of a range of infiltrating inflammatory cells. It is also possible that proinflammatory actions of tissue-resident (i.e., structural) cells within the airway wall may be important in the remodeling process. Remodeling implies that tissue homeostasis is not preserved following injury or insult. Inflammation in the airway may cause or be in response to tissue injury. Normal tissue homeostasis would result in normal airway architecture being preserved after the repair phase following tissue injury. It may well be that airway wall remodeling may occur not as a result of tissue damage but in response to various inflammatory mediators acting on a range of tissue subtypes.

It is important to differentiate between acute and chronic changes in airway structure. Acute changes such as mucus secretion, cellular infiltration, accumulation of edema fluid, and changes in vessel caliber are usually reversible either spontaneously or in response to treatment. Chronic changes in airway structure may develop or resolve more slowly and may become irreversible. Chronic changes might involve an increase in the size and/or number of tissue elements, alterations due to resolution from acute injury, long-term changes in the function of airway-resident cells, and formation of new structures within the tissue milieu. The potential targets for remodeling in the airway wall are the airway epithelium, the basement membrane, smooth muscle, mucus glands, cartilage, blood vessels, nerves, and the extracellular matrix (Fig. 1). A variety of morphometric techniques, each with its own intrinsic

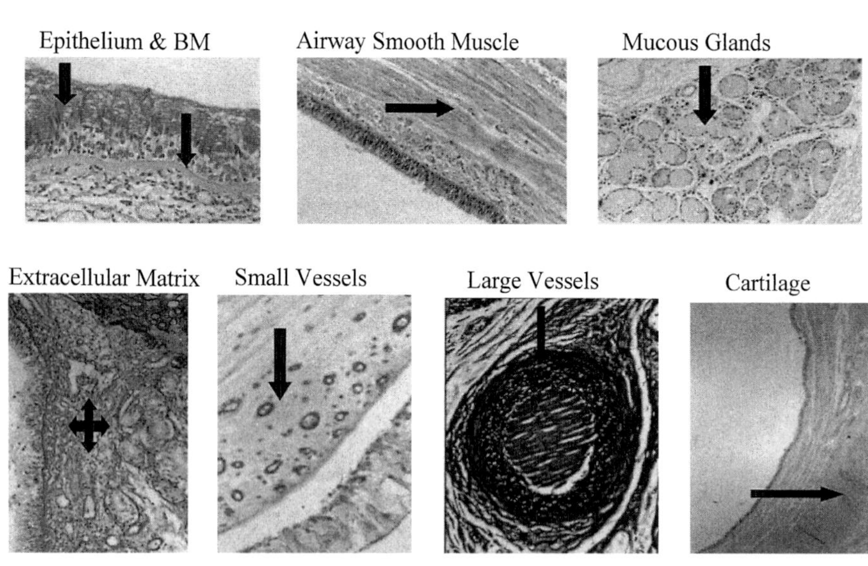

Figure 1 Potential sites for airway wall remodeling in patients with asthma. These structures are able to be quantified using morphometric techniques.

advantages and disadvantages, have been used to assess airway structure in patients with asthma. Morphometry quantifies airway structures that enable the modeling of the effects of airway structure on airway function (1–3). This allows comparison of airway structure between groups of patients with and without asthma or before and after treatment. This chapter will summarize previous studies that have quantified airway structure of patients with asthma, attempt to compare the results of these different studies with one another, and discuss the advantages and limitations of the methodologies used to assess airway structure.

II. Epithelium

Owing to the variable preservation of airway epithelium in both bronchial biopsy specimens and autopsy specimens, only one study (4) quantifying epithelial thickness has been published. Compared with control cases, the area of epithelium in cases of asthma was increased in all airway sizes: small membranous bronchioles, 126% (of control); small cartilaginous airways, 156%; and large cartilaginous airways, 57%. A number of quantitative studies have been made of airway epithelial integrity and damage in asthmatic and nonasthmatic cases. Bronchial biopsy studies have shown increased epithelial damage in asthma (5), although this has not been observed in all studies (6,7). Using a semiquantitative method in cases obtained at autopsy, no differences were found in epithelial damage or desquamation between nonasthmatic cases and cases of fatal and nonfatal asthma (8). Omari et al. (9) showed a correlation between epithelial damage and in vitro responsiveness in human bronchial segments, suggesting that the epithelium acts as a barrier to limit the access of stimulants to smooth muscle when they are applied to the airway lumen. Epithelial damage measured by bronchial biopsy has been related to in vivo airway responsiveness in some studies (6), but not others (5). Soderberg et al. (10) obtained bronchial biopsies to characterize the structure of the airway epithelium in healthy nonasthmatic volunteers using light and electron microscopy. This study showed that mechanical damage of bronchial biopsies caused by the forceps should be considered before alterations in structural integrity of the epithelium are attributed to asthma or other pulmonary disease.

III. Smooth Muscle

Ten studies (4,8,11–18) have quantitatively compared the area of airway smooth muscle (ASM) in asthmatic with that in nonasthmatic cases, mostly in fatal cases, although some studies have included nonfatal cases (4,8,15,16). In the study of Ebina et al. (17) membranous and cartilaginous airways were examined in control cases and cases of fatal asthma. They observed that in some of their cases of asthma the area of smooth muscle was increased in both large and small airways and that in others the increase in area of smooth muscle was confined to central airways. In their study, multiple serial sections of airways were cut and measured to reconstruct a three-dimensional image of the ASM cells and then a three-dimensional sampling area of known volume (a "dissector") (19) (see Fig. 2) was used to determine the volume fraction of muscle in cases of fatal asthma. By counting the area and number of smooth muscle cells within the spatial probe they showed that ASM is both hypertrophic and hyperplastic in these cases. As the authors allude to in these comprehensive studies, these techniques are very tedious and very time consuming, thereby reducing the likelihood of examining a large number of cases and airways.

The study by Thomson et al. (18) found no differences between cases of fatal asthma and control cases. They measured ASM using a longitudinal orientation for the tissue sections that displayed the smooth muscle in a transverse orientation (Fig. 3a) in contrast to the longitudinal orientation of muscle fibers observed in transverse airway sections (Fig. 3b). They used a point-counting procedure, which differentiated between connective tissue elements, extracellular matrix, and muscle fibers and normalized the data by total cross-sectional tissue area. When the proportion of smooth muscle was counted in this manner, they found no difference between the amount of ASM in patients with asthma compared with nonasthmatic control cases. This study was limited to 5 cases in each group, which may reduce the power of the observations. In 1973, Heard and Hossain (12) employed a point-counting technique across multiple serial sections over a 2-mm length of airway and they too differentiated between muscle fibers and nonmuscle areas in transverse sections of airways. They showed clear differences in ASM thickness between asthmatics and nonasthmatics. They also counted ASM nuclei and showed that the numbers of nuclei were greatly increased in patients with asthma compared with nonasthmatics. The study by Carroll et al. (8) sampled large and small airways from patients with fatal (severe) and nonfatal (mild) asthma and measured the total area of muscle in transverse sections of airway by tracing the area of muscle onto a digitizing tablet (Fig. 3c) and standardized the area of muscle by dividing by the basement membrane perimeter to correct for airway size. This technique showed that compared with control cases, ASM was increased in cases of fatal asthma in large and small airways in cases of fatal asthma and only in small airway in cases of nonfatal asthma. This study also

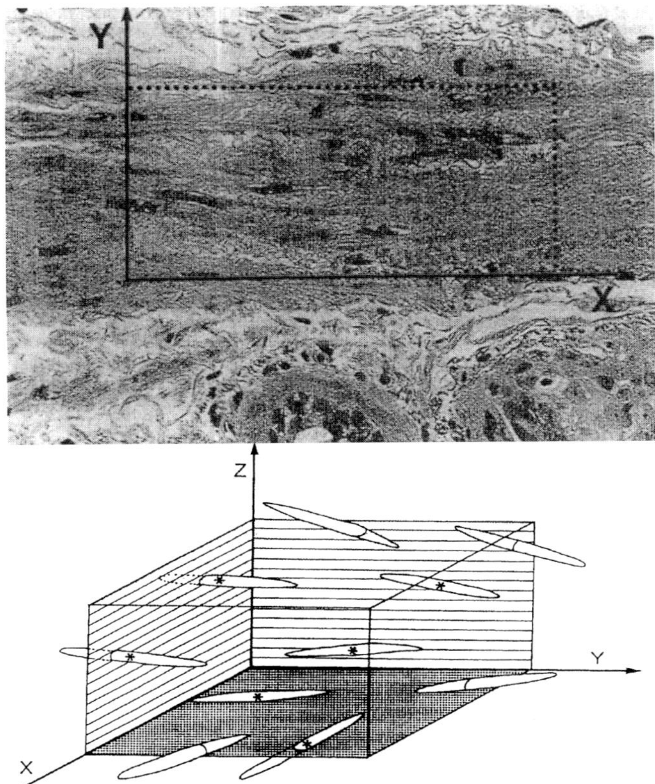

Figure 2 Transverse section of a large airway (upper panel) from which smooth muscle cells are traced in serial sections to reproduce a three-dimensional image (lower panel). A three-dimensional spatial probe (a ''dissector'') of known volume is applied to the image to estimate the volume fraction of smooth muscle in the airway. (From Ref. 17.)

showed that midsized central airways had the most marked increase in muscle area.

IV. Mucous Glands

Five studies (8,11,14,15,20) of mucous gland area in asthma have been undertaken. In cases of fatal asthma the average increase in mucous gland area

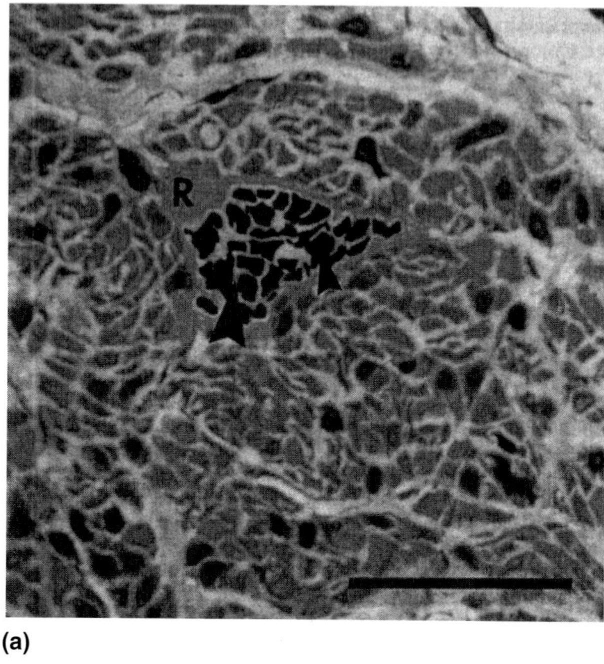

(a)

Figure 3   (a) Smooth muscle orientation from axially sectioned large airways. The muscle fibers are cut in a transverse plane. (From Ref. 18 [overleaf].) (b) Smooth muscle orientation from a large airway cut in transverse section. The muscle fibers are cut in a longitudinal plane. (From Ref. 18.) (c) Smooth muscle cells in a longitudinal plane. The thick black continuous line around the muscle fibers demonstrates how smooth muscle area is measured using planimetry. (From Ref. 18.)

compared with controls was 151% (range 61–285%) and in nonfatal cases was 25% (22–27%). Extraparenchymal cartilaginous airways were predominantly examined, although in some studies any airway containing cartilage or glands was included. This could result in bias if mucous glands are present in a greater number of distal (smaller) airways in patients with asthma than in control cases. This would result in an underestimation of the average area of mucous glands in central airways for cases of asthma. It is unknown if the distribution of mucous glands down the bronchial tree changes in asthma. The use of point counting and the ''Reid index'' (14) to quantify mucous gland volume

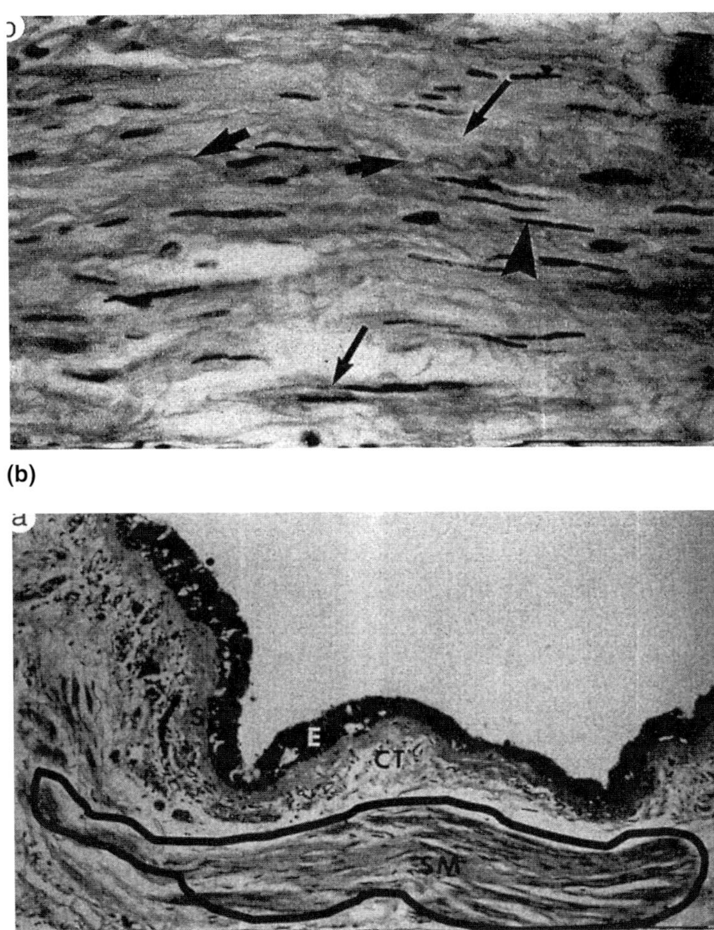

(b)

(c)

essentially express the mucous gland area as a proportion of the airway wall area. Using these techniques to assess mucous gland structure does not allow for changes in the volume of the airway wall, which might also be increased in asthma. Therefore, it may be more reliable to express the volume of the glands relative to the basement membrane (BM) perimeter as this is similar in patients with and without asthma (8).

V. Cartilage

The area of cartilage in the airway wall of patients with asthma has been measured in only a few studies (8,11,14) and there are few data regarding the distribution of cartilage down the bronchial tree in asthma. The data from these few studies show a wide variation with only the study of Carroll et al. (8) showing an increase in the area of cartilage in asthma. The study by Carroll et al. (8) measured the area of cartilage directly using a digitizing tablet and expressed the area per millimeter of the BM perimeter rather than adopt a point-counting technique. This method is independent of changes in airway wall thickness.

VI. Sub-basement Membrane Connective Tissue and Extracellular Matrix

Early studies noted that thickening of the basement membrane (BM) was a characteristic feature of asthma (11,13,21), although not confined to this disease. It was later confirmed that, in fact, the BM, or lamina reticularis, is not thicker in cases of asthma but that there is substantial deposition of collagen types III and V and fibronectin beneath the BM giving rise to the thickened appearance on light microscopy (22). A number of studies have measured the thickness of the connective tissue below the BM in cases of nonfatal, generally mild asthma (6,11,22–25). These show an increased thickness of 60–90% compared with control cases. The increased thickness of the BM in cases of fatal asthma has been invariably commented on, but infrequently measured. In the study of Huber and Koessler (13) the thickness of the BM in cases of fatal asthma was similar to that seen in cases of nonfatal asthma. Wilson and Li (25) showed that reliable measurements of the reticular BM can be made using light microscopy (Fig. 4) and give similar results to those obtained using electron microscopy. Accurate measurement of BM thickness requires the tissue sections to be oriented in a transverse plane. In addition to tissue orientation, which might variably affect the thickness of the measured collagen layer below the BM, so too might the angle of measurement (Fig. 5). The study by Sullivan et al. (26) showed that the error caused by small change in measurement angle transecting the BM is likely to be trivial and that approximately 70–100 measurements of BM thickness will give a precision of 10% for the measurement. Laitinen et al. (27) have demonstrated that the extracellular matrix glycoprotein tenascin is also expressed in the BM of patients with asthma

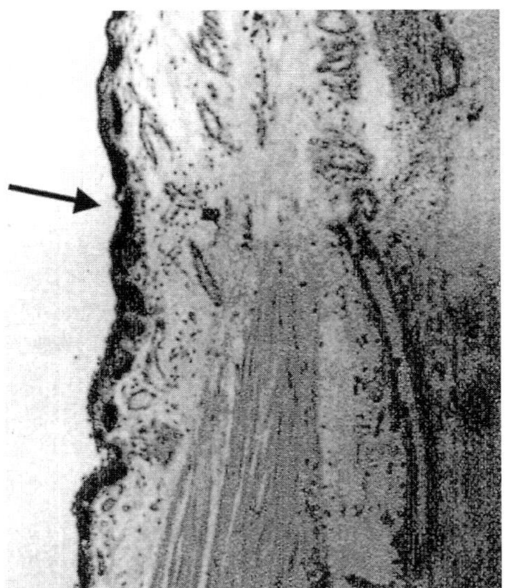

Figure 4 Irregular pattern of staining for collagen below the basement membrane (arrow). Reliable measurements of ''basement membrane'' thickness can be made using a light microscope in this way.

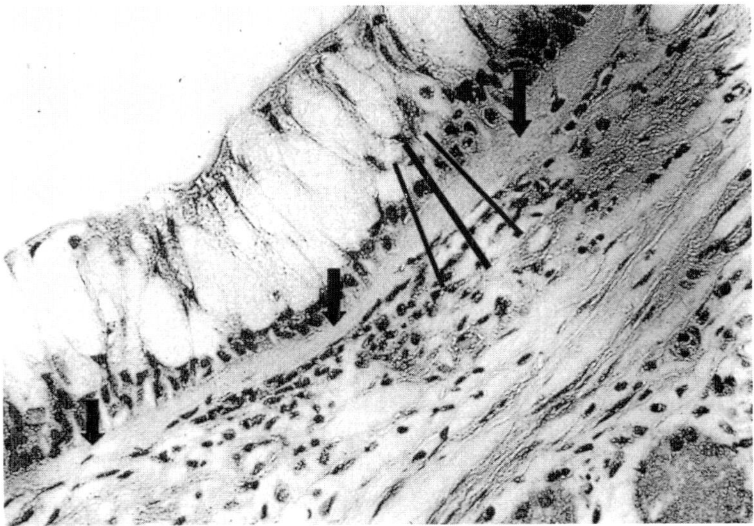

Figure 5 Thickened ''basement membrane'' (thick arrows) from a case of fatal asthma. The three single lines show the perpendicular angle of measurement used to assess basement membrane thickness.

to a greater extent than in nonasthmatics suggesting a remodeling process rather than injury to the BM itself. In addition to increased collagen deposition below the BM, Wilson and Li (25) also demonstrated that the airway submucosa contains significantly more type III collagen and type V collagen than in nonasthmatics. This may have important functional implications in patients with asthma (28).

VII. Blood Vessels

Five quantitative studies of blood vessels within the airway walls of asthmatic and nonasthmatic subjects have been published (16,29–32). Using bronchial biopsy, Beasley et al. (29) found similar numbers of submucosal blood vessels in asthmatic (mean 142, range 108–171 vessels/mm^2) and nonasthmatic (123, 106–135) subjects. Saetta et al. (31) examined the muscular arteries adjacent to membranous bronchioles in cases of fatal asthma. They found them to have similar thickness to those in control cases, despite infiltration of inflammatory cells, predominantly into the wall adjacent to the airway wall. Kuwano et al. (16) measured the number and areas of blood vessels in the adventitia and submucosa of membranous bronchioles in cases of asthma (fatal and nonfatal) and compared them with control cases. They found that although the number of vessels per area of tissue in each group was similar, the area (as a percent of the tissue area, mean $\pm$ SD) was increased in asthma, both in the adventitia (12 $\pm$ 8% vs. 8 $\pm$ 4%) and in the submucosa (3 $\pm$ 1% vs. 1 $\pm$ 1%). These findings suggest that congestion of blood vessels is present in cases of asthma. These data are supported by findings of Carroll et al. (30) in which the number of blood vessels was not different between patients with asthma and controls but the patients with asthma had significantly more large blood vessels and less small blood vessels, suggesting distension of existing vessels. A more recent study by Li and Wilson (32) examined bronchial biopsy specimens from 12 subjects with mild asthma and showed that both the number of blood vessels per square millimeter and the percent of biopsy area occupied by vessels was significantly greater in the patients with asthma compared with healthy control subjects. At least some of the variability between the results of these different studies may be due to different methodologies employed in each study. The study of Beasley et al. (29) used airway sections stained with haematoxylin and eosin. The study by Kuwano et al. (16) stained the sections with both Masson's trichrome and Factor VIII, which gave significantly different results for vessel numbers and area. Carroll et al (30) stained tissue sections with Factor VIII, which resulted in very similar results for blood vessel numbers to the study of Kuwano et al. (16). The study by Li and Wilson (32) used type IV collagen to identify the blood vessels. Beasley et al. (29) and Li and Wilson (32) measured blood vessel dimensions in bronchial biopsy specimens while Carroll et al. (30) and Kuwano et al. (16) used whole transverse sections of airways obtained at autopsy. These methodological differences require consideration when interpreting and comparing the results from these different studies.

VIII. Inner Wall Area

Three studies (4,8,16) have measured the inner wall area (i.e., the area between the BM and the outer border of the airway smooth muscle) in asthma. Two of these studies included cases of nonfatal asthma (8,16), and the study of Kuwano et al. (16) included only membranous airways. Compared with control cases, in cases of fatal asthma the mean (range) increase in inner wall area was 64% (range 55–95%) in small membranous airways, 146% (133–162%) in large membranous airways, 280% (258–302%) in small cartilaginous airways, and 80% (41–119%) in large cartilaginous airways. Compared with control cases, in cases of nonfatal asthma, the mean increase in inner wall area was 48% (33–64%) in small membranous airways, 38% (24–52%) in large membranous airways, 120% in small cartilaginous airways, and 20% in large cartilaginous airways. The epithelium was not included in the measurement of inner wall area in the study of Kuwano et al. (16) because of its variable loss from the BM. In the other two studies, if more than 25% of the BM was covered by epithelium, internal perimeter was estimated by extrapolating the epithelial surface between intact areas of epithelium. This was shown to be highly reproducible. The exclusion or inclusion of the thickness of the epithelium will result in variations in wall thickness that will be relatively greater in the peripheral airways, where the epithelium makes up a larger proportion of the airway wall. However, the qualitative differences between asthmatic and nonasthmatic cases are likely to be the same.

IX. Outer Wall Area

Only two studies (8,16) have compared the outer wall area from the outer border of the airway smooth muscle to the adventitial surface in asthmatic and nonasthmatic cases. Only the study of Carroll et al. (8) included large airways. Compared with control cases, in cases of fatal asthma the increase in outer wall area was 85% and 91%, respectively, in small membranous airways, 93% and 156% in large membranous airways, 105% in small cartilaginous airways, and 41% in large cartilaginous airways. Compared with control cases, in cases of nonfatal asthma, the mean increase in outer wall area was −11% and 51%, respectively, in small membranous airways, 21% and 60% in large membranous airways, 38% in small cartilaginous airways, and 7% in large cartilaginous airways.

X. Total Wall Area

Four studies (8,13,16,31) have examined the entire wall area in asthmatic and nonasthmatic subjects, although only two included large airways (8,13). Compared with control cases, in cases of fatal asthma the mean increase in total wall area was 72% (range 45–100%) in small membranous airways, 108% (46–231%) in large membranous airways, 80% and 157%, respectively, in small cartilaginous airways, and 44% and 57% in large cartilaginous airways. Compared with control cases, in cases of nonfatal asthma, the mean increase in total wall area was 95% (−7–102%) in small membranous airways, 17% (2–32%) in large membranous airways, 68% in small cartilaginous airways, and 2% in large cartilaginous airways.

XI. Methodological Issues

Airway structure and dimensions vary depending on what level within the bronchial tree they are measured at (Fig. 6). For example, the inner airway wall, the airway epithelium, and the smooth muscle layer occupy a significantly greater proportion of the total cross-sectional area of the entire airway in peripheral airways compared to central airways. Mucous glands and cartilage are not present in the peripheral airways (<4 mm BM perimeter). The arrangement of smooth muscle is a circumferential, almost continuous layer in peripheral airways while it is discontinuous and may only be present between cartilage plates in large central airways. Therefore, the extent to which bronchial biopsy of the proximal bronchial tree is representative of the smaller and more numerous distal airways may be limited. Bronchial biopsy specimens from different levels of the central bronchial tree of patients with asthma yield similar results in terms of inflammatory cell profile and numbers (33). The density of eosinophils and lymphomononuclear cells and the numbers and blood vessels square millimeter of airway wall are different for small membranous airways compared with large cartilaginous airways (34,35). However, the relationship between cell and vessel densities between cases of asthma and control cases remains unchanged (30,34). A recent study by Haley et

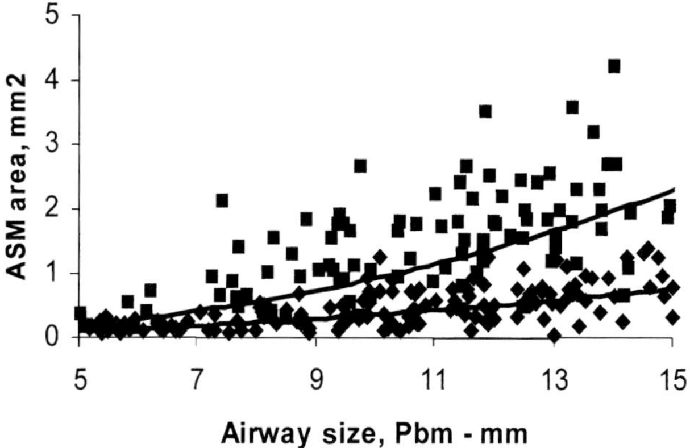

Figure 6 Effect of increasing airway size (measured as the basement membrane perimeter) on the x-axis on smooth muscle area (y-axis) measured in transverse sections of airways from cases of fatal asthma (squares) and control cases (diamonds). Note the considerable variation in smooth muscle area in different-sized airways within the bronchial tree.

al. (36) observed regional variations in inflammatory cell distribution when comparing large versus small airways of patients with asthma. This study also showed differences in cell distributions between the inner and outer airway wall. On the other hand, increases in airway wall thickness and smooth muscle area have been shown to be confined to membranous airways in cases of nonfatal asthma compared with control cases (8). Therefore, when comparing different airways from different individuals it is important to compare airways of similar sizes if the airway dimensions are going to be comparable. Airway size is usually measured as a diameter or by the measured perimeter of the BM. Measuring the diameter of the airway is confounded by smooth muscle tone and lung volume and may underestimate airway size if the lung is not fully inflated or the smooth muscle not fully relaxed. In whole airway sections, it is preferable to use the basement perimeter as a marker of airway size as this measurement has been shown to be independent of muscle tone and lung volume (37).

The number of subjects and observations required for comparisons between case groups needs to be carefully considered to enable a representative and powerful sample to be obtained. This will depend on what aspect of airway structure is being measured as well as the amount of intrasubject and intersubject variability (26,38–40).

Currently, bronchial biopsy, surgical resection, and tissue obtained at autopsy are used to assess airway wall remodeling in patients with asthma. New techniques for assessing airway structure in vivo include high-resolution computed tomography (HRCT) (41) and optical coherence tomography (OCT) (42), which may well prove to be useful tools for assessing airway remodeling in patients with asthma in the future. These techniques have the advantage of being repeatable and can assess variations in airway structure throughout the lung. The disadvantages appear to be the limited range of airway sizes that measurements can be made on, especially for OCT. The current limitations of HRCT appear to be that one can only examine total airway wall thickness and cannot differentiate changes within the airway wall from those around it.

The type of fixation medium used during tissue processing will determine how the tissue might be subsequently stained and what sort of artifact might occur as a result of such fixation techniques (43). The use of frozen sections enhances antigen preservation but often at the expense of morphological integrity. The use of paraffin to embed tissue makes it difficult to obtain thin sections and may result in some degree of three-dimensional artifact occurring owing to the thickness of the sections. The use of harder compounds such as methacrylate and epoxy resins to embed tissue sections will allow for thinner sections to be cut, which helps overcome the problems associated with thicker airway sectioning. A variety of routine histochemical stains can be employed to identify different airway structures but provide little information about important structural proteins that may be involved in airway remodeling. Immunohistochemistry allows the use of a vast array of monoclonal and polyclonal antibodies to detect specific cellular components of the remodeling process but variations in tissue fixation and tissue processing can variably alter antigen preservation and may reduce the sensitivity and/or specificity of detection. Immunofluorescent techniques are often used but can make it more difficult to be precise about surrounding airway structure and the specific sites involved within the airway wall. In situ hybridization allows the examination of molecular events, localized to the airway, which may well regulate the whole remodeling process. The time and cost efficiency of these procedures varies greatly as well.

Routine light microscopy provides a two-dimensional image of medium resolution and magnification. The use of confocal microscopy enables three-dimensional reconstruction of whole airways providing good spatial resolution. Electron microscopic analysis provides images at very high magnification and resolution allowing extrafine details of airway structure and cellular morphology to be examined. Common methods of measuring airway structure include direct measurement of the area of interest using appropriate image analysis software. If the sampling technique provides a truly representative sample of the airway structures of interest, point counting or use of the mean linear intercept may be useful. Point counting adopts a procedure where the number of points falling on the area of interest is divided by the total number of points occupying the total area and can provide an accurate estimate of the volume fraction of the tissue component of interest. The mean linear intercept employs a similar principle in which the number of times a grid of lines of known length intercept the area of interest gives a volume fraction. These methods are employed in a two-dimensional aspect and assume an isotropic uniform random (IUR) distribution of the tissue of interest within the area sampled.

Airway dimensions are also influenced by factors such as age, gender, treatment, disease, and smoking status and these factors need to be either matched or allowed for when analyzing morphometric data. Morphometric measurements are often expressed as a component fraction or volume in terms of densities, percentages, or proportions. If measurements are made over time or after a period of treatment, it is important to consider whether it is the numerator or the denominator that is changing. It is feasible that acute structural changes due to acute inflammatory events might resolve rapidly either spontaneously or in response to treatment and variably affect both the component of interest and/or the area over which it is sampled. Different methods of expressing proportions or densities can give markedly different results. Consider the following example. An airway with a basement membrane perimeter of 1 mm has an inner wall area of 0.025 mm^2. An airway with a basement membrane perimeter of 16 mm has an inner wall area of 8 mm^2. If one inflammatory cell was counted in the 1-mm airway the number of cells per mm^2 would be 40 cells/mm^2. If 320 cells were counted in the 16-mm airway, the number of cells per mm^2 would be 40 cells/mm^2. On the other hand, if the same cell counts were expressed per mm^1 of the BM perimeter, the 1-mm airway would have a cell count of 1 cell/mm^1 while the airway with a Pbm of 16 mm would have a cell count of 20 cells/mm^1. Thus the same cell counts in the same airways can result in different answers depending on how the results are normalized and expressed. This example illustrates the relative differences in airway dimensions at different sites in the bronchial tree and again should be considered when interpreting results and comparing different studies.

Finally, when comparing airway structure between different groups or individuals to examine airway wall remodeling, one cannot exclude host airway structure as a potential confounding factor. It is likely that initial airway structure in any individual has the same degree of variation as the human body somatotype itself. It may be that people with a certain type of airway structure are susceptible to developing hyperresponsive airways and subsequently asthma. The normal range of airway structure in individuals with no history of respiratory disease in addition to the structure of airways in patients with asthma still requires further examination.

References

1. Freedman RJ. The functional geometry of the bronchi. The relationship between changes in external diameter and calibre, and a consideration of the passive role played by the mucosa in bronchoconstriction. Bull Eur Physiolpathol Respir 1972; 8:45–52.
2. Moreno RH, Hogg JC, Pare PD. Mechanics of airway narrowing. Am Rev Respir Dis 1986; 133:1171–1180.
3. Wiggs BR, Bosken C, Pare PD, James AL, Hogg JC. A model of airway narrowing in asthma and in chronic obstructive pulmonary disease. Am Rev Respir Dis 1992; 145:1251–1258.
4. James AL, Pare PD, Hogg JC. The mechanics of airway narrowing in asthma. Am Rev Respir Dis 1989; 139:242–246.
5. Laitinen LA, Heino M, Laitenen A, Kava T, Haahtela T. Damage of the airway epithelium and bronchial reactivity in patients with asthma. Am Rev Respir Dis 1985; 131:599–606.
6. Jeffery PK, Wardlaw AJ, Nelson FC, Collins JV, Kay AB. Bronchial biopsies in asthma: an ultrastructural, quantitative study and correlation with hyperreactivity. Am Rev Respir Dis 1989; 140:1745–1753.
7. Lozewicz S, Wells C, Gomez E, et al. Morphological integrity of the bronchial epithelium in mild asthma. Thorax 1990; 45:12–15.
8. Carroll NG, Elliot J, Morton AR, James AL. The structure of large and small airways in nonfatal and fatal asthma. Am Rev Respir Dis 1993; 147:405–410.
9. Omari TI, Sparrow MP, Mitchell HW. Responsiveness of human isolated bronchial segments and its relationship to epithelial loss. Br J Clin Pharmacol 1993; 35:357–365.
10. Soderberg M, Hellstrom S, Sandstrom T, Lundgren R, Bergh A. Structural characterization of bronchial mucosal biopsies from healthy volunteers: a light and electron microscopical study. Eur Respir J 1990; 3:261–266.
11. Dunnill MS, Massarella GR, Anderson JA. A comparison of the quantitative anatomy of the bronchi in normal subjects, in status asthmaticus, in chronic bronchitis, and in emphysema. Thorax 1969; 24:176–179.
12. Heard BE, Hossain S. Hyperplasia of bronchial muscle in asthma. J Pathol 1973; 110:319–331.
13. Huber HL, Koessler KK. The pathology of bronchial asthma. Arch Intern Med 1922; 30:689.
14. Takizawa T, Thurlbeck WM. Muscle and mucous gland size in the major bronchi

of patients with chronic bronchitis, asthma, and asthmatic bronchitis. Am Rev Respir Dis 1971; 104:331–336.

15. Sobonya RE. Quantitative structural alterations in long-standing allergic asthma. Am Rev Respir Dis 1984; 130:289–292.

16. Kuwano K, Bosken CH, Pare PD, Bai TR, Wiggs BR, Hogg JC. Small airways dimensions in asthma and in chronic obstructive pulmonary disease. Am Rev Respir Dis 1993; 148:1220–1225.

17. Ebina M, Takahashi T, Chiba T, Motomiya M. Cellular hypertrophy and hyperplasia of airway smooth muscles underlying bronchial asthma. Am Rev Respir Dis 1993; 148:720–726.

18. Thomson RJ, Bramley AM, Schellenburg RR. Airway muscle stereology: Implications for increased shortening in asthma. Am J Respir Crit Care Med 1996; 154:749–757.

19. Sterio DC. The unbiased estimation of number and size of arbitary particles using the disector. J Microsc 1984; 134:127–136.

20. Aikawa T, Shimura S, Sasaki H, Ebina M, Takishima T. Marked goblet cell hyperplasia with mucus accumulation in the airways of patients who died of severe acute asthma attack. Chest 1992; 101:916–921.

21. Houston JC, De Navasquez S, Trounce JR. A clinical and pathological study of fatal cases of status asthmaticus. Histopathology 1953; 2:407–421.

22. Roche WR, Williams JH, Beasley R, Holgate ST. Subepithelial fibrosis in the bronchi of asthmatics. Lancet 1989; 1:520–524.

23. Brewster CEP, Howarth PH, Djukanovich R, Wilson J, Holgate ST, Roche WR. Myofibroblasts and subepithelial fibrosis in bronchial asthma. Am J Respir Cell Mol Biol 1990; 3:507–511.

24. Jeffery PK, Godfrey RW, Adelroth E, Nelson F, Rogers A, Johansson SA. Effects of treatment on airway inflammation and thickening of basement membrane reticular collagen in asthma. A quantitative light and electron microscopic study. Am Rev Respir Dis 1992; 145:890–899.

25. Wilson JW, Li X. The measurement of reticular basement membrane and submucosal collagen in the asthmatic airway. Clin Exp Allergy 1997; 27:363–371.

26. Sullivan P, Stephens D, Ansari T, Costello J, Jeffery P. Variation in the measurements of basement membrane thickness and inflammatory cell number in bronchial biopsies. Eur Respir J 1998; 12:811–815.

27. Laitinen A, Altraja A, Kampe M, Linden M, Virtanen I, Laitinen L. Tenascin is increased in airway basement membrane of asthmatics and decreased by an inhaled steroid. Am J Respir Crit Care Med 1997; 156:951–958.

28. Wilson JW, Li X, Pain CF. The lack of distensibility of asthmatic airways. Am Rev Respir Dis 1993; 148:806–809.

29. Beasley R, Roche W, Roberts JA, Holgate ST. Cellular events in the bronchi in mild asthma and after bronchial provocation. Am Rev Respir Dis 1989; 139: 806–817.

30. Carroll NG, Cooke C, James AL. Bronchial blood vessel dimensions in asthma. Am J Respir Crit Care Med 1997; 155:689–695.

31. Saetta M, Di Stefano AD, Rosina C, Thiene G, Fabbri LM. Quantitative structural analysis of peripheral airways and arteries in sudden fatal asthma. Am Rev Respir Dis 1991; 143:138–143.

32. Li X, Wilson JW. Increased vascularity of the bronchial mucosa in mild asthma. Am J Respir Crit Care Med 1997; 156:229–233.

33. Azzawi M, Bradley B, Jefffery PK, et al. Identification of activated T lymphocytes and eosinophils in bronchial biopsies in stable atopic asthma. Am Rev Respir Dis 1990; 142:1407–1413.

34. Carroll NG, Cooke C, James AL. The distribution of eosinophils and lymphocytes in the large and small airways of asthmatics. Eur Respir J 1997; 10:292–300.

35. Synek M, Beasley R, Frew AJ, et al. Cellular infiltration of the airways in asthma of varying severity. Am J Respir Crit Care Med 1996; 154:224–230.

36. Haley KJ, Sunday ME, Wiggs BR, et al. Inflammatory cell distribution within and along asthmatic airways. Am J Respir Crit Care Med 1998; 158:565–572.

37. James AL, Hogg JC, Dunn LA, Pare PD. The use of the internal perimeter to compare airway size and to calculate smooth muscle shortening. Am Rev Respir Dis 1988; 138:136–139.

38. Carroll NG, Lehman E, Barret J, Morton AR, Cooke C, James AL. Variability of airway structure and inflammation in normal subjects and in cases of nonfatal and fatal asthma. Pathol Res Pract 1996; 192/3:238–248.

39. Richmond I, Booth H, Ward C, Walters EH. Intrasubject variability in airway inflammation in biopsies in mild to moderate stable asthma. Am J Respir Crit Care Med 1996; 153:899–903.

40. Sont JK, Willems LNA, Evertse CE, Hooijer R, Sterk PJ, van Krieken JHJM. Repeatability of measures of inflammatory cell number in bronchial biopsies in atopic asthma. Eur Respir J 1997; 10:2602–2608.

41. Seneterre E, Paganin F, Bruel JM, Michel FB, Bousquet J. Measurement of the internal size of bronchi using high resolution computed tomography. Eur Respir J 1994; 7:596–600.

42. Pitris C, Brezinski ME, Bouma BE, Tearney GJ, Southern JF, Fujimoto JG. High resolution imaging of the upper respiratory tract with optical coherence tomography. Am J Respir Crit Care Med 1998; 157:1640–1644.

43. Lum H, Mitzner W. Effects of 10% formalin fixation on fixed lung volume and lung tissue shrinkage. Am Rev Respir Dis 1985; 132:1078–1083.

4

Physiological Consequences of Lung Remodeling in Asthma

BJÖRN JONSON

University of Lund
Lund, Sweden

I. Introduction

Airway remodeling in asthma was originally observed in fatal cases (1) but has been confirmed in other materials (2,3). An abnormal decline in FEV_1 with age has been found particularly important in nonallergic asthma (4). Clinical observations have indicated that not only airways but also lung parenchyma is remodeled in long-lasting asthma. Paganin et al. (5) showed with high-resolution computed tomography that permanent abnormalities occur with respect to both bronchi and parenchyma. They confirmed that the pathology is more pronounced in nonallergic asthma. Signs of fibrosis and peribronchial thickening were frequently observed. Emphysema was another common finding.

Bronchial obstruction, which is not reversible after a prolonged period of efficient treatment with corticoseroids and other drugs, may be a consequence of several factors, e.g., bronchial wall thickening (6) and reduced airway distensibility (7). Reduced pulmonary elastic recoil due to emphysematous parenchymal remodeling is another reason for fixed bronchial obstruction. An uncoupling between the parenchyma and the airways, which would abolish the dilating forces of the parenchyma, is another possible cause (8).

In efforts to prevent permanent ventilatory incapacity in asthma it is important to know whether the problems are caused by airway or lung parenchyma remodeling or uncoupling between the two. It appears that few data are available that can shred light on the problem. This reflects that ordinary methods for studies of ventilation do not allow distinction between mechanisms behind bronchial narrowing.

II. Relationship Between Lung Elastic Recoil and Bronchial Dimensions

The dimension of a bronchus depends on its intrinsic properties, which are of morphological and functional nature. The inherent contractile forces within the bronchus represent functional aspects. These forces depend on the surface tension of the liquid lining, elastic tension within the bronchial wall, and the tone of the smooth bronchial muscles. Small bronchi, unsupported by cartilage, would close under the influences of intrinsic forces if left alone. The only force that balances the intrinsic closing forces is caused by the elastic recoil of the alveolar attachments to the bronchi, (Fig. 1, left panel). The right

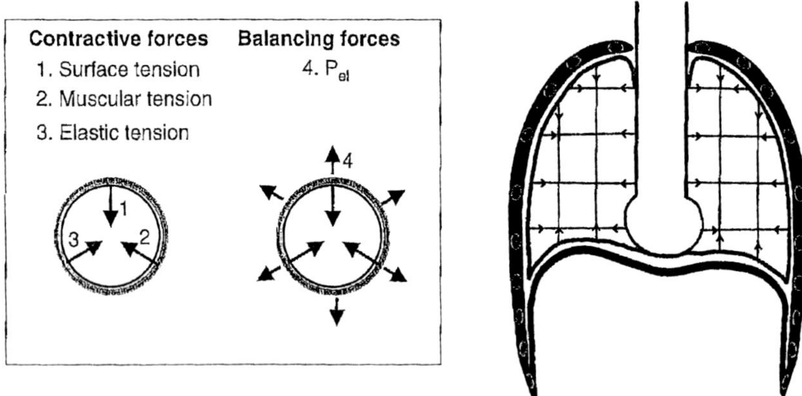

Figure 1   The forces tending to contract and close an airway, and the only balancing force, which is the elastic recoil pressure of the surrounding lung parenchyma, P_{el} (left panel). The force dilating the airways is the same one that lowers pleural pressure, i.e., P_{el} (right panel).

panel of Figure 1 illustrates that the elastic recoil force of the lung that leads to a negative pleural pressure also dilates the bronchi. Under static conditions the elastic recoil pressure of the lung, P_{el}, can be measured as a difference between the airway pressure and the pleural (or esophageal) pressure.

Obviously, airway resistance depends on P_{el}. Resistance also depends upon flow rate because a higher flow rate increases turbulence in the airway. During expiration the resistive pressure drop along the airway and the Bernoulli effect together cause a reduction in intraluminal pressure of intrathoracic airways relative to the external pressure. This phenomenon will tend to narrow the airway in a flow dependent way. When flow becomes high enough the airway will be subjected to dynamic compression. Accordingly, to draw conclusions about intrinsic airway properties from values of lung resistance, R_L, we must standardize for P_{el} and for flow rate.

III. The Flow Regulator Method

Figure 2 illustrates that the transpulmonary pressure was measured during a long expiration during which flow rate was restricted to 1 L/sec and also caused intermittent flow interruptions (9). P_{el} was measured during each interruption. During each square flow pulse the resistive pressure, superimposed upon P_{el}, was measured and pulmonary resistance, R_L, was calculated. A diagram was obtained in which R_L, measured at 1 L/sec, was plotted against P_{el}. Lung volume was measured with body plethysmography. Thus, a diagram over P_{el} against lung volume was also obtained.

R_L was determined at a standardized flow rate and was related to P_{el}. As P_{el} represents the force that dilates the intrathoracic airways, the R_L/P_{el} diagram is a specific indicator of intrinsic airway obstruction. The P_{el}/V diagram, on the other hand, is an indicator of parenchyma pathology reflecting fibrosis and emphysema.

IV. A Study of Bronchial and Parenchymal Physiology in Chronic Asthma

As only few data in the literature allow differentiation between functional consequences of airway and parenchyma remodeling, a reanalysis of an old study was performed (10). Simultaneous information about the static pulmonary elastic recoil pressure and the lung resistance in relation to P_{el} at standardized flow rate was obtained with the flow regulator method.

It must be emphasized that the study does not meet modern standards,

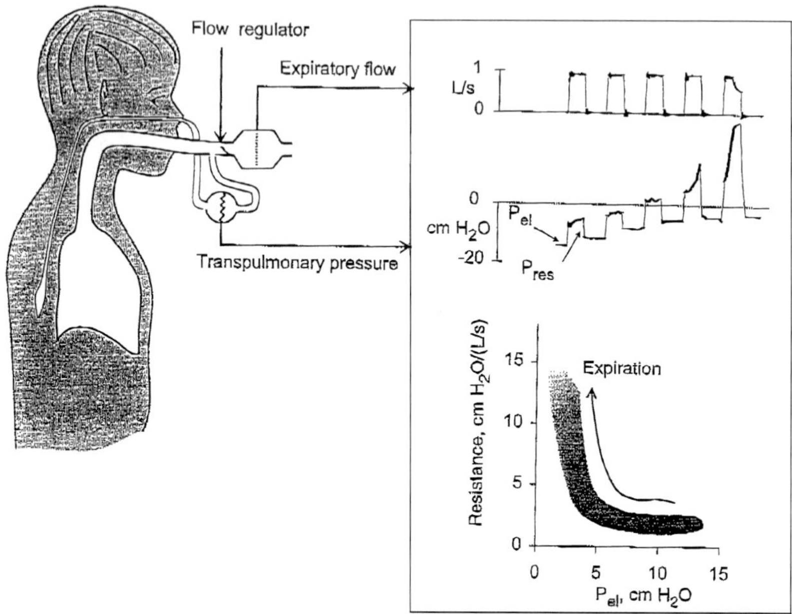

Figure 2   The flow regulator method is based upon a deep expiration. The flow regulator controls the expiratory flow to 1 L/sec and intermittently closes the airway. During flow interruptions the elastic recoil pressure, P_{el}, is read from the measured transpulmonary pressure. The pressure increment during the periods of flow is the resistive pressure, P_{res}. Resistance is plotted against P_{el}. Shadowed area corresponds to the normal range.

for example, with respect to nomenclature and diagnostic criteria. Anyway, the study provides some unique information, which at least illustrates that further studies are needed.

V.   Material

Sixteen men, age 40–54 years, were treated in an outpatient asthma ward. The duration of clinical symptoms was 3–49 years, median 13 years. The diagnosis asthma was retrospectively established from four criteria: All patients had clinical symptoms of asthma. In eight or nine patients allergic asthma was indicated by provocation tests; seven of them were undergoing hyposensitization. Spirometry and pulmonary resistance, R_L, were normal after epinephrine had been given subcutaneously in 10 subjects and improved quite significantly in three others. Eleven patients were treated with peroral steroids. The patients were treated by the same physician and were vigorously attended for the époque. The patients were studied when they were in a stable clinical condition as free of symptoms as their disease made possible. In 13 patients the study was repeated 2 years after the initial study.

Twelve healthy men matched for age, height, and weight served as controls.

VI. Results

The R_L/P_{el} diagrams indicated none to very important intrinsic bronchial obstruction (Fig. 3). In some subjects R_L in relation to P_{el} remained very high

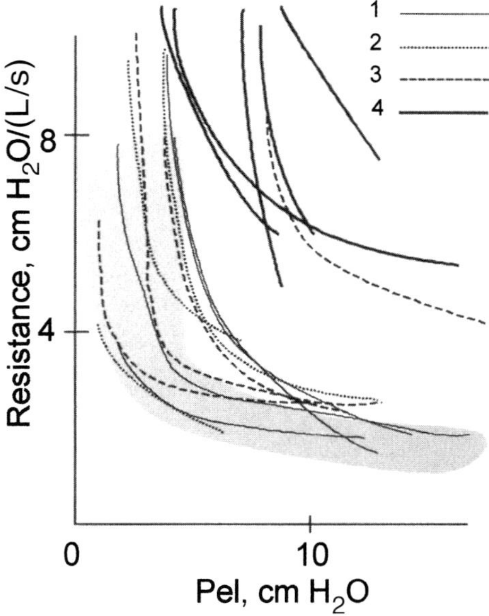

Figure 3 Pulmonary resistance plotted against P_{el} in the asthmatic subjects divided into four groups. Below, D indicates duration in years. (1) Moderate nocturnal asthma and asthma related to infections, D = 4–11. (2) Moderate asthma of nonspecific nature, D = 4–7. (3) Allergic asthma D = 12–29. (4) Allergic asthma with perennial symptoms, D = 26–49 years. Shadowed area corresponds to the normal range.

after subcutaneous injection of 0.5 mg of epinephrine, particularly in patients with a long history of asthma.

The P_{el}/V diagrams showed a loss of elastic recoil in relation to volume in most subjects (Fig. 4). Two subjects had rather high recoil pressures. Most P_{el}/V curves showed a slope that was normal, which translates into normal lung compliance. However, some subjects with particularly long duration of the asthmatic disease had lower than normal compliance. After epinephrine injection the static pressure volume curve often changed its slope and position, as shown in Figure 5. The upper panel shows an example of how the volume at which the P_{el} equaled 4 cm H_2O, $V_{Pel=4}$, decreased after epinephrine. The lower panel shows that the residual volume, RV, decreased in proportion to the change in $V_{Pel=4}$. RV was about 2 L lower than $V_{Pel=4}$.

Forced expired volume in 1 sec, FEV_1 in liters, reflected both intrinsic bronchial obstruction expressed as R_L at a P_{el} of 7.5 cm H_2O and the bronchial dilating force expressed as P_{el} at a volume equal to (TLC-3) L.

$$FEV_1 = 3.3 - 0.29\ R_{Pel=7.5} + 0.2\ Pel_{TLC-3}$$
$$RSD = 0.43$$
$$\text{(1)}$$

Likewise FEV_1 in percent of vital capacity, FEV%, was significantly correlated to both $R_{Pel=7.5}$ and P_{el} measured at 50% of the vital capacity, VC.

$$FEV\% = 67.6 - 3.5\ R_{Pel=7.5} + 2.2\ Pel_{50\%\ of\ VC}$$
$$RSD = 8.5\%$$
$$\text{(2)}$$

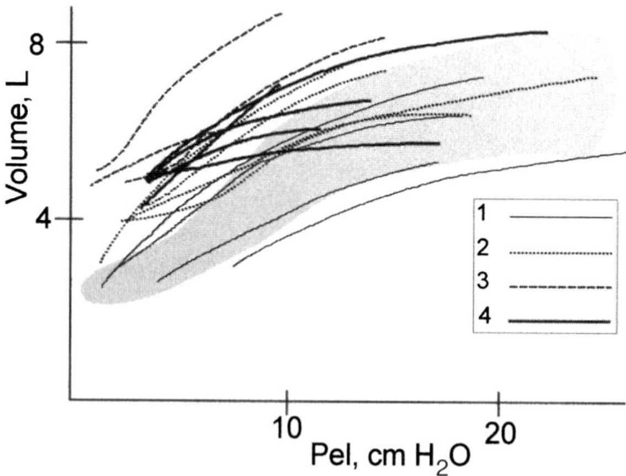

Figure 4 Static elastic pressure volume diagrams in the asthmatic subjects. Groups as in Figure 3. Shadowed area corresponds to the normal range.

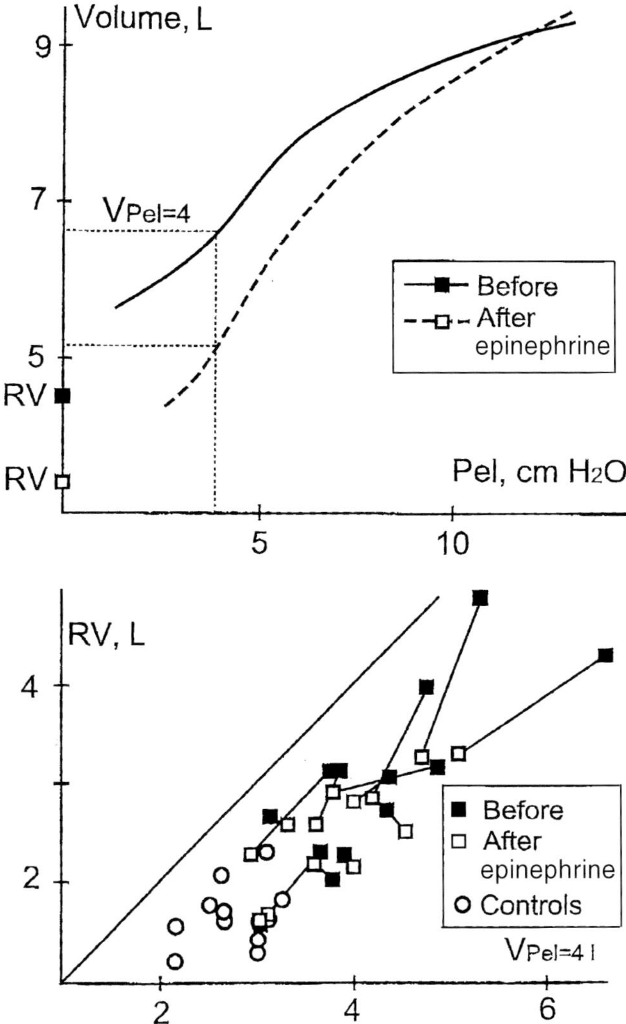

Figure 5 The P_{el}/V curve in one of the subjects shifted toward lower volumes after bronchodilatation with epinephrine. A corresponding decrease was observed in residual volume, RV (upper panel). RV was in the control subjects as well as in the asthmatics about 2 L lower than the volume at which P_{el} was 4 cm H_2O, $V_{Pel=4}$ (lower panel). In asthmatics after bronchodilatation RV and $V_{Pel=4}$ decreased to a similar extent.

Pel$_{TLC-3}$ and Pel$_{50\% \text{ of VC}}$ were used in the analysis as these values were considered representative for P$_{el}$ during the segment of the flow/volume curve of particular importance for FEV$_1$ and FEV%, respectively. RSD is the residual standard deviation.

When the study was repeated 2 years later, essentially similar results were obtained.

VII. Discussion

A. Airways and Lung Parenchyma

The subjects of the study had long-standing asthma and were, when necessary, treated with peroral steroids. Smoking habits were not adequately reported but were of low prevalence. The main findings, particularly after epinephrine injection and similar on two occasions with 2 years' interval, reasonably represent remodeling of airways and parenchyma in asthma. Intrinsic bronchial properties and parenchymal recoil, represented by R$_L$ and P$_{el}$, respectively, had about equally large influence of ventilatory capacity estimated as FEV$_1$ and FEV%. In the material comprising patients with moderate to severe disease it is notable that the residual standard deviations of FEV$_1$ and FEV% after correlation to resistive and elastic properties were not larger than the standard deviation of normal values in a group of healthy subjects. The shift after epinephrine in the static P$_{el}$/V curve (Fig. 4) and the related change in residual volume (Fig. 4) indicate a complex nature of lung mechanics in asthma. The static P$_{el}$/V curve is probably largely influenced by small airway closure, which implies that it does not offer a straightforward description of elastic properties of the lung parenchyma.

Remodeling of lung parenchyma leads to loss of elastic recoils as in emphysema or to an increase of recoil or reduced compliance as in fibrosis. Similar findings have more recently been reported by Dutu et al. (11). The data serve as physiological correlates to observations made, e.g., with computer tomography (5).

The results illustrated by Eq. (1) and (2) strongly indicate that the functional coupling between airways and parenchyma is preserved in chronic asthma. From physical aspects it is difficult to conceive that the parenchymal recoil, which acts either directly through alveolar attachments or indirectly by lowering the intrathoracic pressure, should not influence a bronchus.

Available data merit that emphasis is paid to the airways and to the parenchyma when functional consequences of lung remodeling are studied in asthma.

B. Small and Large Airways: Airway Hyperresponsiveness

Most standard lung function tests like FEV_1 and resistance measurement reflect large rather than small airways. However, an increasing number of studies show that small airways are involved in the inflammatory process as much as large airways (12,13). Many different physiological tests have over the years been suggested to differentiate between small and large airway involvement, often without adequate theoretical or laboratory support. Tests indicating closure of airways appear from that aspect to be the most applicable. In a prospective study of laboratory animal workers Sjöstedt et al. (14) showed that the volume of trapped gas, a measure of closed lung zones during ordinary tidal breathing, increased after 7 years of follow-up. The responsiveness with respect to methacholine was high already at the start of the study and remained so, while the responsiveness with respect to FEV_1 increased in sensitized workers. The results supported the hypothesis that allergic asthma might start in small airways. Wagner et al. (15) measured directly peripheral airway resistance and responsiveness to histamine in normal smokers and in symptom-free asthmatics. The asthmatic subjects had higher initial resistance and higher peripheral airway responsiveness than the controls. The referred studies and another recent study by Burns et al. (16) finally prove that airways, notably small airways, are hyperresponsive in early stages of asthma.

A question that is much more complex is to which extent hyperresponsiveness is a factor in long-standing asthma and its relationship to remodeling. An increased elastic recoil pressure tends to attenuate bronchoconstriction induced with methacholine (17), while a reduced elastic recoil pressure leads to an increased airway responsiveness (18). In asthma, parenchyma remodeling may lead to both fibrosis, with high elastic recoil pressure, and emphysema, with a reduced recoil pressure. The two phenomena may exist to a varying degree in different lung regions in the individual patient. Our knowledge is too limited even to speculate about the role of hyperresponsiveness in small and large airways in chronic asthma.

As has been emphasized in recent years, airway remodeling in asthma is a reality (19,20). So is parenchyma remodeling. The present review shows that the functional consequences are far from adequately studied.

Acknowledgments

The Swedish Medical Research Council (02872), the Swedish Heart Lung Foundation, and the Medical Faculty of Lund supported the study.

References

1. Huber HL, Koessler KK. The pathology of bronchial asthma. Arch Intern Med 1922; 30:689–760.
2. Kuwano K, Bosken CH, Paré PD, Bai TR, Wiggs BR, Hogg JC. Small airways dimensions in asthma and in chronic obstructive pulmonasry disease. Am Rev Respir Dis 1993; 148:1220–1225.
3. Carroll N, Elliot J, Morton A, James A. The structure of large and small airways in nonfatal and fatal asthma. Am Rev Respir Dis 1993; 147:405–410.
4. Ulrik CS, Backer V, Dirksen A. A 10 year follow up of 180 adults with bronchial asthma: factors important for the decline in lung function. Thorax 1992; 47:14–18.
5. Paganin F, Séneterre E, Chanez P, Daurés JP, Bruel JM, Michel FB, Bousquet J. Computed tomography of the lungs in asthma; influence of disease severity and etiology. Am J Respir Crit Care Med 1996; 153:110–114.
6. Roche WR, Beasley R, Williams JH, Holgate ST. Subepithelial fibrosis in the bronchi of asthmatics. Lancet 1989; 1:520–524.
7. Wilson JW, Li X, Pain MC. The lack of distensibility of asthmatic airways. Am Rev Respir Dis 1993; 148:806–809.
8. Moreno RH, Hogg JC, Paré PD. Mechanics of airway narrowing. Am Rev Respir Dis 1986; 133:1171–1180.
9. Jonson B. A method for determination of pulmonary elastic recoil and resistance at a regulated flow rate. Scand J Clin Lab Invest 1969; 24:115–125.
10. Jonson B. Pulmonary mechanics in patients with pulmonary disease, studied with the flow regulator method. Scand J Clin Lab Invest 1970; 25:375–390.
11. Dutu S, Jienescu Z, Basca N. Pulmonary mechanics in patients with asthma bronchiale in symptom-free interval. Pneumoftiziologia 1995; 44:49–52.
12. Caroll N, Cooke C, James A. The distribution of eosinophils and lymphocytes in the large and small airways of asthmatics, Eur Respir J 1997; 10:292–300.
13. Haley KJ, Sunday ME, Wiggs BR, Kozakewich HP, Reilly JJ, Mentzer SJ, Sugarbaker DJ, Doerschuk CM, Drazen JM. Inflammatory cell distribution within and along asthmatic airways. Am J Respir Crit Care Med 1998; 158:565–572.
14. Sjöstedt L, Willers S, Orbaek P, Wollmer P. A seven-year follow-up study of lung function and methacholine responsiveness in sensitized and non-sensitized workers handling laboratory animals. J Occup Environ Med 1998; 40:118–124.
15. Wagner EM, Bleecker ER, Permutt S, Liu MC. Direct assessment of small airways reactivity in human subjects. Am J Respir Crit Care Med 1998; 157:447–452.
16. Burns GP, Gibson GJ. Airway hyperresponsiveness in asthma. Not just a problem of smooth muscle relaxation with inspiration. Am J Respir Crit Care Med 1998; 158:203–206.
17. Ding DJ, Martin JG, Macklem PT. Effects of lung volume on maximal methacholine-induced bronchoconstriction in normal humans. J Appl Physiol 1987; 62:1324–1330.

18. Bellofiore S, Eidelman DH, Macklem PT, Martin JG. Effects of elastase-induced emphysema on airway responsiveness to methacholine in rats. J Appl Physiol 1989; 66:606–612.
19. Haahtela T. Airway remodelling takes place in asthma—what are the clinical implications? Clin Exp Allergy 1997; 27:351–353.
20. Paré PD, Bai TR, Roberts CR. The Structural and Functional Consequences of Chronic Allergic Inflammation of the Airways. The Rising Trends in Asthma. Ciba Foundation Symposium 206. Chichester: Wiley, 1997:71–89.

5

Consequences of Airway Remodeling to the Patient

TARI HAAHTELA

Helsinki University and
Helsinki University Central Hospital
Helsinki, Finland

I. Introduction

There is a wide range of clinical stages in the asthmatic population, e.g., a patient with 50 years' symptom history and a patient who has wheezed for a week. The two patients need different treatment strategies, but anti-inflammatory medication is essential for both. Some patients seem to have severe and chronic asthma from the very beginning (many of them having nonallergic asthma manifested in association with a respiratory infection). But many patients have a mild disease for decades and no signs of progressive airway changes.

In the same patient, the disease severity may fluctuate considerably, and the course of the asthma is difficult to predict. Even persistent asthma may have more favorable natural course than expected. After a 25-year follow-up, 12% of 285 adult asthmatics were symptom-free and showed normal lung function (1). About two-thirds of mildly asthmatic children will outgrow the disease, while the third with more severe asthma will have persistent symptoms in adult life (2).

Pharmacological treatments depend on the severity of symptoms and functional abnormality. A patient who has recovered from newly acquired asthma, is free of symptoms, and has normal bronchial responsiveness does not necessarily need any medication. But a patient with severe everyday symptoms and marked fluctuation of peak expiratory flow rates may need a wide range of drugs to prevent life-threatening exacerbations.

Very little data exists on the impact of various treatments on the "natural" course of childhood or adult-onset asthma. Also the data available on the long-term benefits of different interventions are few.

II. From Individuals to Populations

Three patients illustrate the different course of asthma and eosinophilic airway inflammation.

Patient 1 is 29 years of age. He has had nonallergic asthma from early childhood, has never smoked, has always had poor compliance to drug treatment, and used alternative therapies like homeopathy. Figure 1 shows progres-

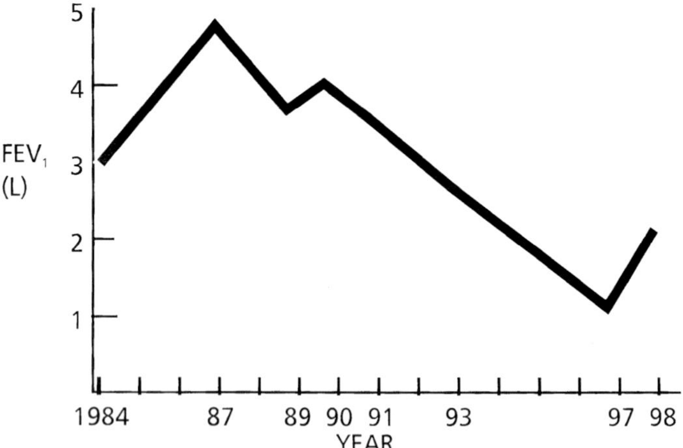

Figure 1   Patient example: 29-year-old man, with lifelong asthma, nonsmoker, poor compliance, alternative treatments. Progressive decline of FEV_1 during 10 years.

sive decline of FEV$_1$ over time. The lung function was well preserved up to the age of 20, but then recoveries after exacerbations were slow and an irreversible obstructive component appeared. The response to short-acting β$_2$-agonist diminished, and the morning/evening amplitude of the PEF curve flattened. In 1996 the best PEF values reached barely half of those observed in 1984 (Fig. 2).

The patient has major structural changes in the airways, which have become persistent and resulted in marked physiological consequences. He is unable to work and the disease seriously limits the daily activities. The exacerbations are life-threatening.

Patient 2 is 23 years of age. From age 9 months to 2 years she had several episodes of so-called obstructive bronchitis. She said, ''My mother asked the doctors if I had asthma, but they did not think so.'' Up to the age of 10 she suffered from cough and episodes of wheezing and was irregularly

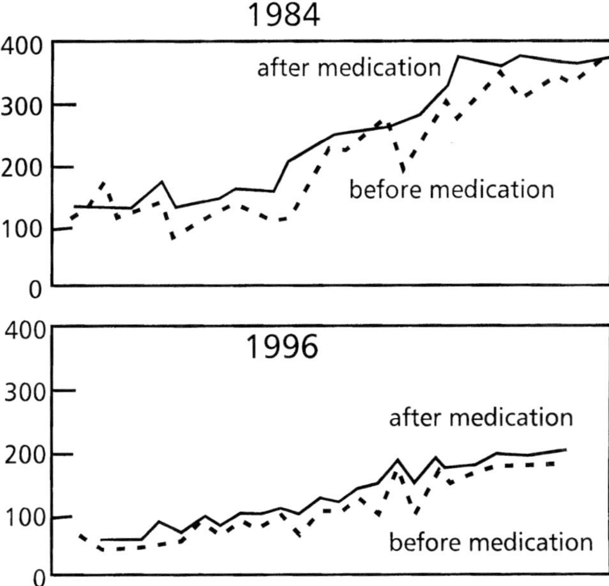

Figure 2 Same patient as in Figure 1. Peak expiratory flow values for 2 weeks during severe exacerbation of asthma in 1984 and in 1996. The lower curves are recordings before, and the upper curves after, inhaling short-acting β$_2$-agonist.

treated with inhaled β_2-agonists and theophylline. At the age of 11 the diagnosis of allergic asthma was eventually made, and a small dose of inhaled beclomethasone (50 µg twice daily) was introduced. Six months later there was a note in her files: ''Cannot use beclomethasone because of continuous cough and problems with breathing.'' This probably happened because her airways were so inflamed that a small dose of steroid with freon propellants caused irritation first; the parents stopped the treatment. At the age of 22 she was doing well, had a permanent job, and lived a normal life but said that she always wheezes when exercising, especially during cold weather. Her lung function was: FVC 4.04 L (93% of predicted), FEV_1 2.85 L (74% of predicted), FEV% 79, and $PD_{15}FEV_1$ 0.08 (severely increased bronchial responsiveness). A high dose of inhaled steroid, budesonide 1600 µg/day was started. Over a year she improved clinically, and her exercise tolerance was better. $PD_{15}FEV_1$ also improved to 0.17, but still showed moderately increased responsiveness.

For years the patient did not receive adequate treatment and her lung function was permanently affected: no pharmacological therapy can reverse the marked hyperresponsiveness back to normal. Nevertheless, lung volumes are near reference values and the clinical outcome seems good. The patient had experienced a lot of unnecessary suffering during the years because of delayed diagnosis, and she will probably always need some medication to control the condition.

Patient 3 is 52 years of age. At the age of 40 he started to have prolonged coughs after respiratory infections. Asthma was suspected, but never diagnosed because lung function was normal. He was nonatopic. A slightly increased number of eosinophils in blood and sputum was, however, found. No regular medication was prescribed. Perennial rhinitis appeared as well. He exercised actively and kept fit, but the symptoms continued, and sputum production along with cough increased. He used the word ''slimy'' to describe his state for years. After 12 years his lung function was still in the normal range, but a severe eosinophilic inflammation was observed (Fig. 3). The patient was free of symptoms after 2 weeks' treatment with inhaled steroids.

The patient has a syndrome that does not even have an agreed diagnostic label or definition. We have called the syndrome ''asthma-like inflammation'' implying the close relationship of the airway pathology to asthma (3). The example also shows that even severe eosinophilic inflammation for years does not always result in significant changes in airway physiology.

Patient 1 illustrates that severe and poorly controlled asthma may pro-

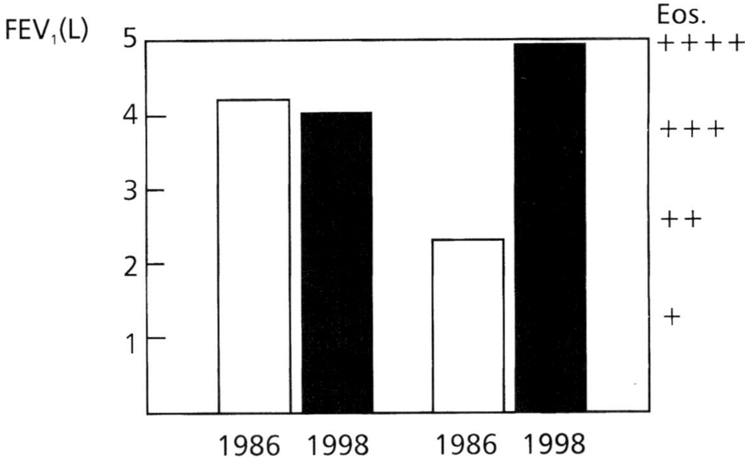

Figure 3 Patient example: 52-year-old man, nonsmoker, nonatopic, symptoms for 12 years, PD_{15} > 1.60 mg. FEV_1 has remained constant and in the normal range from 1986 to 1998 in spite of chronic cough and sputum production. The number of eosinophils was increased in sputum in 1986, and even more so in 1998.

gress to an increasingly irreversible state. This has, indeed, been confirmed epidemiologically in elderly patients during a longitudinal study of a general population sample (4). A gradual decline of FEV_1 over time seems to take place in an asthmatic population compared with normal subjects (5). Kelly et al. (6) showed in a case-control study that FEV% declined more in 7-year-old asthmatic children compared with normal subjects when they were reexamined at the age of 10, 14, 21, and 28 years of age. The outcome of lung function correlated to the frequency of wheezing implying that symptomatic episodes—probably associated with increase in inflammatory cell influx into the airways—may cause permanent damage, which is reflected in lung function. Paganin et al. (7) reported a number of lung abnormalities in nonsmoking asthmatics by using computed tomography. These changes included bronchial thickening, linear shadows, bronchiectasis, and emphysema, which were more pronounced in severe than in mild disease and in nonallergic than allergic patients.

The possible clinical consequences of airway remodeling are outlined in Table 1.

Table 1 Clinical Consequences of Airway Remodeling

Structural change	Clinical outcome
1. Goblet cell and mucous gland increase	Mucus secretion, cough
2. Persistence of inflammatory cells	Escalation of symptoms
3. Fibrogenic growth factor release, collagen deposition, neovascularization	Increased bronchial responsiveness
4. Mucosal thickening, smooth muscle increase	Persistent airflow limitation, severe bronchospasm during exacerbations
5. Lysis of elastic fibers, damage of airway and lung tissue	Reduced elasticity—dynamic collapse

III. Delayed Diagnosis

Bronchial obstruction and increased bronchial responsiveness are outcomes of the inflammatory process, and it may be argued that at the time asthma is diagnosed, detection of eosinophilic inflammation is always late.

In September 1997 the clinicians of the outpatient department of allergology in Helsinki explored retrospectively the delay from the start of symptoms indicating asthma to the actual diagnosis made by physician. The estimate was based on patient files and personal interview. The average delay in children aged 6 months–16 years was 1 year 7 months (range 0–6 years, $n = 34$). In adults aged 16–70 years the average delay was 5 years 4 months (range 0–30, $n = 36$). In patients treated in the same department in 1992–1993 ($n = 333$, mean age 34 years), the delay from symptoms to diagnosis estimated from the patient files was found to be 3.6 years on average (range 0–30).

Irwin et al. (8) studied thoroughly 102 patients who had had cough for more than 53 months. Of these patients 31% had, in fact, asthma, and the average length of the disease at the time of the diagnosis was 4 years. Puolijoki and Lahdensuo (9) studied 147 patients who had had prolonged cough for more than 2 months. During a 1-year follow-up 31% were shown to have asthma. They also studied another 182 patients with unexplained cough for more than 2 months; patients with asthma were carefully ruled out (10). After a follow-up of 4.4 years 16% turned out to be asthmatics. History of atopy, allergic rhinitis, or asthmatic family members increased the risk from three- to fourfold. The increased number of eosinophils in blood, sputum, or nasal secretion also increased the risk three- to fourfold.

In Sweden Larsson et al. (11) made a population-based survey in a small community and could detect 666 asthmatics of whom two-thirds had clinically mild disease, which nevertheless had a significant impact on the patients' everyday life. Of these ''mild'' patients 71% had consulted a doctor, but in only 19% had the correct diagnosis of asthma been made. Asthma was also seriously underdiagnosed among Danish adolescents (12).

Siponen (13) made a psychosocial study of asthmatics and concluded: 1) the patients hesitate to search for help, 2) do not easily go to a doctor, 3) pretend to have common cold, 4) pretend to have allergy, not asthma, 5) deny the possibility of asthma, 6) try to preserve the identity of a healthy person, and 7) fear the label of a chronic disease. Asthma has a reputation of a severe, lifelong disease among the general public.

IV. Anti-inflammatory Treatment Is Late

The delay in making the diagnosis of asthma results in ineffective treatment for long periods. This is especially true in general practice, where large numbers of coughing and wheezing patients are treated inadequately. Most patients with prolonged cough and mucus production, but with normal or close to normal lung function, receive repeated courses of antibiotics, expectorants, antitussives, antihistamines, bronchodilators, but not adequate anti-inflammatory medication. This kind of treatment not affecting eosinophilic inflammation can continue for years.

Anti-inflammatory medication with inhaled steroids or cromones or even with theophylline and leukotriene antagonists is not usually considered before the patient shows definite signs of asthma observed with lung function measurements. This is understandable because of the lack of readily available diagnostic methods of eosinophilic inflammation; bronchofiberoscopy is not such a method. However, the intensive research on the mucosal inflammatory process may offer new methods. Analysis of induced sputum samples is one of the keys to improved diagnostics of eosinophilic airway inflammation. Sputum induced by hypertonic saline has been shown to be similar to lower respiratory secretions expectorated spontaneously (14), and to give comparable results to bronchoscopic methods (15).

The long-term effect of pharmacological, and especially steroid, intervention may be quite different in patients with a new disease (16) compared to patients with a more prolonged history (17,18). Whether steroids are only suppressing the disease or also modifying the outcome may depend on timing of the intervention. The observation that inhaled steroids do not seem to have any permanent effect on the degree of increased bronchial responsiveness may be due to patients having an asthma history for years before intervention with effective anti-inflammatory therapy (19,20). For the same reason inhaled steroids have not consistently influenced the thickness of the reticular basement layer, or the other elements of airway remodeling (17,21,22). "Scar" formation of the airways is probably a result of airway remodeling via chronic release of various inflammatory mediators and cytokines, and once established may not be readily reversible with any kind of pharmacological intervention.

Increased bronchial responsiveness is probably a consequence of long-lasting or recurrent airways inflammation in liable individuals. Results from cross-sectional studies have shown a moderate correlation between the two (23–25). Boulet et al. (23) showed by high-resolution computed tomography that in subjects with a fixed component of airflow obstruction, the thicker the airway wall, the lower was the PC_{20} for methacholine. Treatment aimed at increasing bronchial responsiveness reduced the number of activated eosinophils in bronchial lamina propria and subepithelial collagen thickness (26). Hoshino et al. (27) were able to show that 800 µg of beclomethasone for 6 months to chronic asthmatics reduced the thickness of the lamina reticularis when placebo did not. However, early treatment of eosinophilic inflammation is probably more efficient in preventing development of increased bronchial responsiveness caused by changes in airway structure.

V. Long-Term Effect of Treatment May Depend on Timing of Intervention

One possibility in exploring the long-term influence of treatment is to study what happens when treatment is stopped. Few studies address these issues in adults or in children (Table 2).

Short-term studies on the withdrawal of inhaled steroid therapy after treatment for 4 weeks or less suggest that bronchial responsiveness increases within weeks of inhaled steroid reduction or withdrawal (28,29). However, patients in these studies have had persistent asthma with a long symptom history. It has been shown that periods of treatment considerably longer than 4 weeks do not fully reverse the inflammatory changes in the airways, even in patients with relatively mild asthma (30,31).

Table 2 Stopping the Treatment with Inhaled Steroids: Long-Term Studies in the 1990s

Study	Duration of intervention and effect on lung function after withdrawal

Juniper et al., 1991 (19)
  Adults
	1 yr treatment, 3 mo follow-up
	  Effect: 3 mo in most

van Essen-Zandvliet et al., 1994 (20)
  Children
	28–36 mo treatment, 6 mo follow-up
	  Effect: gradual worsening back to baseline

Haahtela et al., 1994 (36)
  Adults
	2 yr treatment, 1 yr follow-up
	  Effect: 50% of improvement maintained,
	  in one-third no deterioration

van Schayck et al., 1995 (32)
  Adults
	4 yr treatment, 1 yr follow-up
	  Effect: 1 yr for some

Osterman et al., 1997 (33)
  Adults
	1 yr treatment, 6 mo follow-up
	  Effect: 50% of improvement maintained

Simons, 1997 (34)
  Children
	1 yr treatment, 2 week follow-up
	  Effect: lost in two weeks

Juniper et al. (19) showed that the improvements in bronchial responsiveness induced by treatment with budesonide for 1 year were maintained for at least 3 months after cessation of or reduction in treatment with an inhaled steroid. As mentioned earlier, the patients did not have early asthma, but rather a chronic disease with at least moderate severity.

Van Schayck et al. (32) withdrew inhaled bechlomethasone from a group of patients after 4 years of treatment. Before that, they were treated with bronchodilators for the first 2 years, and with beclomethasone for the third and fourth year. Some patients with poor lung function showed an accelerated rate of decline after withdrawal of the inhaled steroid, but those with good lung function showed no increase in the rate of decline of lung function. The investigators concluded that patients in the latter group could stop inhaled steroid after treatment for 2 years. Again, the patients had persistent asthma with a long history.

Osterman et al. (33) followed their patients after the treatment year for another 6 months without steroids. The budesonide-treated patients maintained about 50% of their achieved improvement in bronchial responsiveness during the follow-up period, but only the patients with milder disease remained in the study, which somewhat invalidated the observations. Overall, the effects of low-dose budesonide treatment for a year were mainly temporary. Again, most of the patients did not have a "new" disease.

van Essen-Zandvliet et al. (20) included children with chronic obstruction and severe asthma. After treatment with inhaled budesonide (600 µg daily) for 28–36 months only about 60% of children had reached normal FEV_1. When the steroid therapy was tapered off in some of the children over 6 months, a gradual worsening of the disease occurred. All the patients used regular salbutamol while decreasing the dose of budesonide.

Simons (34) treated children with mild or moderate persistent asthma with beclomethasone 400 µg daily for 1 year. The beneficial effect on increased bronchial responsiveness disappeared 2 weeks after cessation of treatment.

The studies of Haahtela et al. (35,36) differed from all the above-mentioned studies by accepting only patients who had had asthmatic symptoms less than a year and no previous anti-inflammatory treatment. Two treatment strategies were compared: initial treatment with inhaled steroid or with β_2-agonist alone. The patients inhaled either budesonide 1200 µg or terbutaline 750 µg daily as the first and only regular medication. Two years' treatment with inhaled budesonide resulted in almost complete clinical recovery and normalization of lung function, and it was superior compared with β_2-agonist treatment. Bronchial biopsies were taken from a subgroup of patients, and after 3 months the budesonide-treated subjects had a significantly greater fall in the numbers of inflammatory cells than the terbutaline-treated patients (16).

The study was continued for a third year to investigate the effects of dose reduction or discontinuation of steroid treatment. A delayed introduction of inhaled steroid was also examined. The lung function was well maintained for the third year in patients in whom the daily budesonide dose was reduced from 1200 µg (by Nebuhaler) to 400 µg (by Turbuhaler) (step-down strategy). Most of those patients who switched from budesonide to placebo showed a slight decline in lung function, which for PC_{15} became significant toward the end of the third year, but six patients did not deteriorate at all (36). The patients who were first treated with a β_2-agonist, terbutaline, for 2 years, and only subsequently treated with budesonide, did not reach the same level of lung function within the third year as those who were treated with budesonide from the beginning of the study. Some functional reversibility was lost by delaying the start of steroid treatment (Fig. 4).

Selroos and co-workers (37) examined retrospectively the influence of the duration of pretreatment symptoms on the response to inhaled steroid treatment in steroid-naive adult patients with asthma. The duration of symptoms

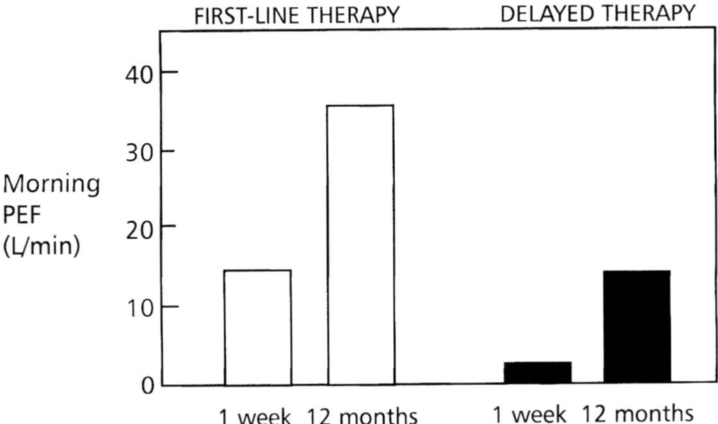

Figure 4 Improvements in morning PEF values in patients with budesonide as first-line therapy within 1 year of start of asthma symptoms and in patients treated only more than 2 years after start of symptoms (delayed therapy). (Modified from Ref. 36.)

ranged from less than 6 months to more than 10 years. The response to budesonide was best in patients with the shortest history of symptoms before intervention.

Agertoft and Pedersen (38) measured lung function and growth in 278 children with mild to moderate asthma, during long-term treatment with inhaled budesonide, and compared openly the findings with those obtained from children not treated with steroids. The children were ''old'' asthmatics (mean duration of asthma 3½ years) having used β_2-agonists and only occasionally steroids. The annual increase in FEV_1 was greatest in those children whose asthma was of shortest duration when inhaled budesonide was started.

The available data seem to show that early intervention with inhaled steroid may prevent the development of irreversible airway obstruction and reduce the risk of undertreatment. More prospective clinical trials are needed, however, to confirm the observations.

VI. Treatment Guidelines

The benefits of early treatment of symptomatic asthma are obvious and several recent guidelines recommend anti-inflammatory medication, preferably with inhaled steroids, as first-line treatment to gain control of the disease as fast as possible (39–41). The guidelines recommend increasingly inhaled steroids not only in moderate and severe but in mild asthma as well. Treatment is started as soon as the functional diagnosis of asthma has been established, and the so called step-down approach is gaining popularity. Higher initial doses are followed with decreasing the dose to a level that is able to control the condition. The British guidelines (40) also use an important clinical argument for the step-down strategy: the patient's confidence is gained when symptoms are rapidly relieved.

There is some evidence from a meta-analysis to support the policy to treat also mild steroid-naive asthmatics with inhaled steroids from the very beginning (42), but more studies are needed, especially to justify the step-down strategy. Higher initial doses would probably have a better effect on the underlying inflammation and increased bronchial responsiveness—which are loosely related to each other (43)—than lower doses, which effectively abolish symptoms and increase PEF values (Fig. 5). Fahy and Boushey (44) found that 4 weeks' treatment with beclomethasone (336 µg daily) improved symptoms and lung function but did not have significant effect on markers of eosinophilic inflammation. However, van der Molen et al. (45) did not find any difference in lung function improvement in those patients treated initially with

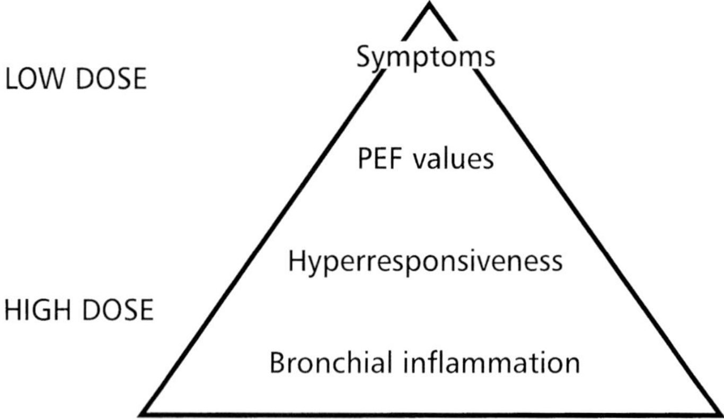

Figure 5 Hypothetical asthma pyramid. Low doses of inhaled steroids relieve symptoms and increase PEF values, but may not have much effect on underlying mechanisms.

a high dose compared to those treated with a lower dose. The subjects enrolled had persistent asthma (average duration 7 years), and it is possible that the results would be different in patients with newly acquired asthma with fully reversible lung function.

In many immunological/inflammatory diseases of long duration the concept of induction treatment is used. It could be applied to asthma treatment as well. Induction is followed by maintenance treatment and treatment of relapses.

VII. Association of Treatment and Use of Health Care Services

The two most economically important consequences of persistent asthma are hospitalizations and lost production owing to illness and retirement, and these may be reduced by improving treatment and patient education (46). In 1995 in Denmark costs for a ''well-treated patient'' were DKK 37,723 and for a ''poorly treated patient'' 48,579 per year. The costs for a patient with severe disease were DKK 171,489 and with mild disease 3180 per year. The total annual costs were estimated to be DKK 9.6 billion for an asthmatic population of 212,000. In 1996 the total costs caused by asthma in New Zealand ranged from NZ\$ 251–340 million, and the costs per treated patient were NZ\$ 796 (47).

In Finland it was estimated that 20% of those patients receiving reimbursement for the drug costs—caused by regular medication—had severe disease while 60% had mild disease. The severely ill patients are causing, however, 60–70% of the costs (Fig. 6). To reduce the costs the patients with severe asthma should be treated more effectively, but in the long run preventing escalation of asthma from becoming persistent in the patients with mild to moderate disease could be even more cost saving.

It is well known that regular use of inhaled steroids prevents exacerbations of asthma (48), fatal and near-fatal episodes of asthma (49), and accelerated loss of lung function (50). It is less well known that regular use of inhaled steroids initiated in the year following the recognition of asthma can reduce, by up to 80%, the risk of a hospitalization for asthma as compared with regular therapy with theophylline (51). From 1985 to 1993 anti-inflammatory treatment with inhaled steroids decreased the number of hospital days per year in Swedish children to less than a third (52). In a large community sample in

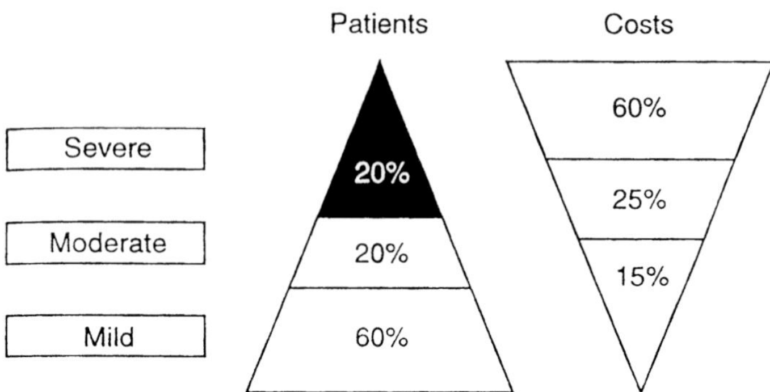

Figure 6 Distribution (%) of asthma patients and costs resulting from asthma, according to the severity of the disease (39).

eastern Massachusetts inhaled steroids halved the risk of hospitalization in each severity group (53). In contrast, overconfidence in β_2-agonist combined with suboptimal use of inhaled steroids increased the risk for hospitalization fivefold in Belgium (54).

Hospitalization for asthma is a marker of severe asthma and uncontrolled disease, and indicates an increased risk of a subsequent fatal attack (55). The cost of hospitalizations represents 25–50% of the total costs for asthma depending on whether the calculations include only direct medical costs or the additional indirect costs caused mainly by loss of production (56,57). Thus, decrease in hospitalizations would reflect improved disease control meaning less human suffering and great savings for society.

Marked undertreatment still prevails in most parts of the world. In Canada, so-called mild asthmatic patients were not so mild on a closer look (58). In France, Bousquet et al. (59) found astonishing undertreatment of severe asthma: 85% of patients living in Paris, and 60% in Montpellier were not receiving any anti-inflammatory treatment. Ferrante et al. (60) found that inhaled anti-inflammatory drugs were insufficiently utilized in Italian young men: only 16% of those who showed bronchial obstruction used inhaled steroids or cromolyn sodium. Changes in treatment practices are slow. In Denmark Gaist et al. (61) selected from a nationwide register those asthmatics who used a lot of β_2-agonists, more than 1600 inhalations per year. In 1991 33% of them did not use inhaled steroids. When the survey was repeated in

1994, the situation had not improved: 37% were still without inhaled steroids. In 1991 the new U.S. guidelines promoted earlier use of anti-inflammatory medication (62), but in Philadelphia a gap between optimal asthma drug prescribing and actual patterns widened from 1991 to 1993 (63). Underuse of inhaled steroids was closely associated with lower educational attainment. In east London Griffiths et al. (64) observed that practices prescribing lower ratios of prophylactic anti-inflammatory to bronchodilator medication had higher hospital admission rates.

Although we lack evidence that inhaled steroids, or any other pharmacological intervention, change the natural course of asthma, their invaluable short-term effects justify their introduction as soon as the diagnosis of asthma is established.

VIII. Finnish Experience

From the beginning of the 1990s much emphasis has been placed on early detection of asthma and introduction of inhaled steroids as first-line therapy

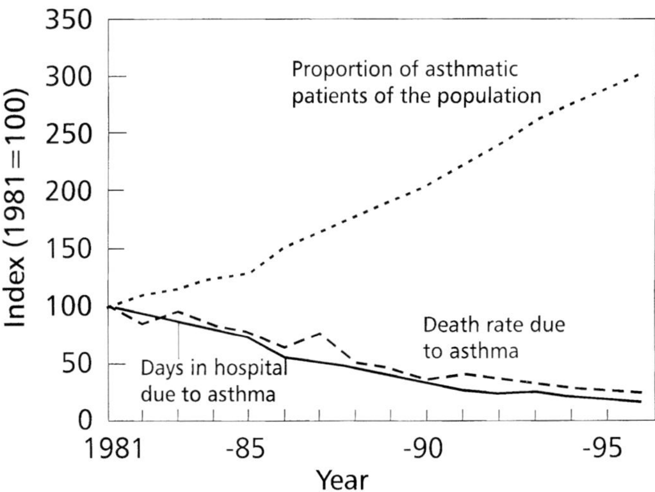

Figure 7 Asthma in Finland 1981–1996, showing the relative increase in the number of patients entitled to special reimbursement for their drug costs, and decreases of death rate and days in hospital among them (index, 1981 = 100).

for all asthmatics except perhaps small children. Simple and cost-effective self-management programs based on adjusting the dose of regular inhaled steroid according to symptoms and home monitoring of peak flow values were also developed (65,66). This policy was strengthened by the national Asthma Programme, launched in 1994 (39). The Programme was implemented efficiently at the local level, and one doctor and one nurse in each health center were appointed to take charge of the quality of asthma treatment as well as patient education.

Several indicators show that active treatment of asthma in primary care supported by specialists in secondary care has been successful, and the burden of the disease on society is decreasing in spite of an increase in occurrence. In 1981 the Finnish Social Insurance Institution recorded 49,259 asthma patients who were entitled to special reimbursement for their drug costs. In 1996 the figure had increased about threefold, to 159,105 patients (population 5.1 million). Nevertheless, days in hospital per asthmatic population were in 1996 only one-quarter of that in 1981, and mortality due to asthma showed a similar trend (67; Fig. 7). In England and Wales the asthma mortality has also dropped since the late 1980s in spite of increasing prevalence (68). The experiences in different countries vary. In the United States asthma mortality is low but still increasing. An increase has also been observed in Japan but a decrease in New Zealand. Reasons for the differences are obscure.

Table 3 Change of Prescriptions of Inhaled Steroids Compared with β_2-Agonists in Nordic Countries and Czech Republic from 1990 to 1996[a]

	Year		
	1990	1995	1996
Finland	0.56	0.96	1.02
Iceland	0.47	0.77	
Norway	0.41	0.77	
Sweden	0.37	0.77	
Denmark		0.64	
Czech Republic		0.46	

[a] In 1996 the ratio exceeded 1 in Finland meaning more prescriptions of steroids than of β_2-agonists (Nordic Statistics of Medicine, 1996).

Although several factors have probably contributed to the positive trends in Finland and in many other countries—the disease may even have become milder—early and better treatment of asthma deserves much credit for the favorable development. The consumption of short-acting β_2-agonists has been decreasing in Finland for some years, while the use of inhaled steroids continues to increase. In 1996 the ratio of prescriptions of preventive antiasthmatic medication to β_2-agonists exceeded 1.0 in Finland as the first Nordic country (69; Table 3). In the United Kingdom increased prescribing of inhaled steroids of all prescriptions has also been observed.

Persistent asthma has always had considerable impact on the patient's life and puts demands on health care. The risk factors for asthma to become persistent are poorly known but should be identified to achieve better results with various interventions.

References

1. Panhuyesen CIM, Vonk JM, Koeter GH, Schouten JP, van Altena R, Bleecker ER, Postma DS. Adult patients may outgrow their asthma. A 25-year follow-up study. Am J Respir Crit Care Med 1997; 155:1267–1272.
2. Sears MR. Growing up with asthma. Br Med J 1994; 309:72–73.
3. Rytilä P. Metso T, Heikkinen K, Saarelainen P, Haahtela T. Airway inflammation in patients with symptoms indicating asthma but with normal lung function. Allergy 1998; 53(Suppl):P336.
4. Burrows B, Lebowitz MD, Barbee RA, Cline MG. Findings before diagnoses of asthma among the elderly in a longitudinal study of a general population sample. J Allergy Clin Immunol 1991; 88:870–877.
5. Peat JK, Woolcock AJ, Cullen K. Rate of decline of lung function in subjects with asthma. Eur J Respir Dis 1987; 70:171–179.
6. Kelly WJ, Hudson I, Raven J, Phelan PD, Pain MC, Olinsky A. Childhood asthma and adult lung function. Am Rev Respir Dis 1988; 138:26–30.
7. Paganin F, Seneterre E, Chanez P, Daures JP, Bruel JM, Michel FB, Bousquet J. Computed tomography of the lungs in asthma: influence of disease severity and etiology. Am J Respir Crit Care Med 1996; 153:110–114.
8. Irwin RS, Curley FJ, French CL. Chronic cough. The spectrum and frequency of causes, key components of the diagnostic evaluation, and outcome of specific therapy. Am Rev Respir Dis 1990; 141:640–647.
9. Puolijoki H, Lahdensuo A. Chronic cough as a risk indicator of broncho-pulmonary disease. Eur J Respir Dis 1987; 71:77–85.
10. Puolijoki H, Lahdensuo A. Causes of prolonged cough in patients referred to a chest clinic. Ann Med 1989; 21:425–427.

11. Larsson L, Boethius G, Uddenfeldt M. Differences in utilisation of asthma drugs between two neighbouring Swedish provinces: relation to prevalence of obstructive airways disease. Thorax 1994; 49:41–49.

12. Siersted HC, Boldsen J, Hansen HS et al. Population based study of risk factors for underdiagnosis of asthma in adolescence: Odense schoolchild study. Br Med J 1998; 316:615–655.

13. Siponen A. Astmapotilaan käsitys sairaudestaan (in Finnish). Psychological dissertation. University of Tampere, 1996.

14. Pizzichini MMM, Popov TA, Efthimiadis A, Hussack P, Evans S, Pizzichini E, et al. Spontaneous and induced sputum to measure indices of airway inflammation in asthma. Am J Respir Crit Care Med 1996; 154:866–869.

15. Grootendorst DC, Sont JK, Willems LNA, Kluin-Nelemans JC, van Krieken JHJM, Veselic-Charmat M, et al. Comparison of inflammatory cell counts in asthma: induced sputum vs. bronchoalveolar lavage and bronchial biopsies. Clin Exp Allergy 1997; 27:769–779.

16. Laitinen LA, Laitinen A, Haahtela T. A comparative study of the effects of an inhaled corticosteroid, budesonide, and a β_2-agonist, terbutaline, on airway inflammation in newly diagnosed asthma: A randomized, double-blind, parallel-group controlled trial. J Allergy Clin Immunol 1992; 90:32–42.

17. Jeffery PK, Godfrey RW, Ädelroth E, et al. Effects of treatment on airway inflammation and thickening of basement membrane reticular collagen in asthma. Am Rev Respir Dis 1992; 145:890–899.

18. Djukanovic R, Wilson JW, Britten KM, et al. Effect of an inhaled corticosteroid on airway inflammation and symptoms in asthma. Am Rev Respir Dis 1992; 145:669–674.

19. Juniper EF, Kline PA, Vanzieleghem MA, O'Byrne PM, Hargreave FE. Reduction of budesonide after a year of increased use: a randomized controlled trial to evaluate whether improvements in airway responsiveness and clinical asthma are maintained. J Allergy Clin Immunol 1991; 87:483–489.

20. van Essen-Zandvliet EE, Hughes MD, Waalkens HJ, Duiverman EJ, Kerrebijn KF. Remission of childhood asthma after long-term treatment with an inhaled corticosteroid (budesonide): can it be achieved? Eur Respir J 1994; 7:63–68.

21. Lundgren R, Soderberg M, Horstedt P, Stenling R. Morphological studies of bronchial biopsies from asthmatics before and after ten years of treatment with inhaled steroids. Eur Respir J 1988; 1:883–889.

22. Olivieri D, Chetta A, Del Donno M, Bertorelli G, Casalini A, Pesci A, Testi R, Foresi A. Effect of short-term treatment with low-dose inhaled fluticasone propionate on airway inflammation and remodeling in mild asthma: a placebo-controlled study. Am J Respir Crit Care Med 1997; 155:1864–1871.

23. Boulet L, Belanger M, Carrier G. Airway responsiveness and bronchial wall thickness in asthma with and without fixed airflow obstruction. Am J Respir Crit Care Med 1995; 152:865–871.

24. Sont JK, Han J, van Krieken JM, Evertse CE, Hooijer R, Willems LNA, Sterk

PJ. Relationship between the inflammatory infiltrate in bronchial biopsy specimens and clinical severity of asthma in patients treated with inhaled steroids. Thorax 1996; 51:496–502.

25. Chetta A, Foresi A, Del Donno M, Consigli GF, Bertorelli G, Pesci A, Barbee R, Olivieri D. Bronchial responsiveness to distilled water and metacholine and its relationship to inflammation and remodelling of the airways in asthma. Am J Respir Crit Care Med 1996; 153:910–917.

26. Sont JK, Willems LN, Bel EH, van Krieken JH, Vandenbroucke JP, Sterk PJ. Clinical control and histopathologic outcome of asthma when using airway hyperresponsiveness as a guide to long-term treatment. Am J Respir Crit Care Med 1999; 159:1043–1051.

27. Hoshino M, Nakamura Y, Sim JJ, Yamashiro Y, Uchida K, Hosaka K, Isogai S. Inhaled corticosteroid reduced lamina reticularis of the basement membrane by modulation of insulin-like growth factor (IGF)-1 expression in bronchial asthma. Clin Exp Allergy 1998; 28:568–577.

28. Kraan J, Koeter GH, van der Mark Th W, et al. Changes in bronchial hyperactivity induced by 4 weeks of treatment with antiasthmatic drugs in patients with allergic asthma: a comparison between budesonide and terbutaline. J Allergy Clin Immunol 1985; 76:628–636.

29. Jenkins CR, Woolcock AJ. Effect of prednisone and bechlomethasone dipropionate on airway responsiveness in asthma: a comparative study. Thorax 1988; 43: 378–384.

30. Laitinen LA, Laitinen A, Heino M, Haahtela T. Eosinophilic airway inflammation during exacerbation of asthma and its treatment with inhaled corticosteroid. Am Rev Respir Dis 1992; 143:423–427.

31. Laitinen LA, Laitinen A, Haahtela T. Airway mucosal inflammation even in patients with newly diagnosed asthma. Am Rev Respir Dis 1993; 147:697–704.

32. van Schayck CP, van den Broek PJ, den Otter JJ, van Herwaarden CL, Molema J, van Weel C. Periodic treatment regimens with inhaled steroids in asthma or chronic obstructive pulmonary disease. Is it possible? JAMA 1995; 274(2):161–164.

33. Osterman K, Carlholm M, Ekelund J, Kiviloog J, Nikander K, Nilholm L, Salomonsson P, Strand V, Venge P, Zetterström O. Effect of 1 year daily treatment with 400 micrograms budesonide (Pulmicort Turbuhaler) in newly diagnosed asthmatics. Eur Respir J 1997; 10:2210–2215.

34. Simons FER. A comparison of beclomethasone, salmeterol, and placebo in children with asthma. N Engl J Med 1997; 337:1659–1665.

35. Haahtela T, Järvinen M, Kava T, Kiviranta K, Koskinen S, Lehtonen K, Nikander K, Persson T, Reinikainen K, Selroos O, Sovijärvi A, Stenius-Aarniala B, Svahn T, Tammivaara R, Laitinen LA. Comparison of a β_2-agonist, terbutaline, with an inhaled corticosteroid, budesonide, in newly detected asthma. N Engl J Med 1991; 325:388–392.

36. Haahtela T, Järvinen M, Kava T, Kiviranta K, Koskinen S, Lehtonen K, Nikander K, Persson T, Selroos O, Sovijärvi A, Stenius-Aarniala B, Svahn T, Tammivaara R, Laitinen LA. Effects of reducing or discontinuing inhaled budesonide in patients with mild asthma. N Engl J Med 1994; 331:700–705.

37. Selroos O, Pietinalho A, Löfroos A-B, Riska H. Effect of early vs late intervention with inhaled corticosteroids in asthma. Chest 1995; 108:1228–1234.

38. Agertoft L, Pedersen S. Effects of long-term treatment with an inhaled corticosteroid on growth and pulmonary function in asthmatic children. Respir Med 1994; 88:373–381.

39. Asthma Programme in Finland 1994–2004. Ministry of Social Affairs and Health. Clin Exp Allergy 1996; 26(Suppl 1):1–24.

40. British Asthma Guidelines Co-ordinating Committee. British guidelines on asthma management: 1995 review and position statement. Thorax 1997; 52:S1–24.

41. Expert Panel Report II: Guidelines for the Diagnosis and Management of Asthma Bethesda: US National Institutes of Health, 1997.

42. Hatoum HT, Schumock GT, Kendzierski DL. Meta-analysis of controlled trials of drug therapy in nild chronic asthma: the role of inhaled corticosteroids. Ann Pharmacother 1994; 28:1285–1289.

43. Brusasco V, Crimi E, Pellegrino R. Airway hyperresponsiveness in asthma: not just a matter of airway inflammation. Thorax 1998; 53:992–998.

44. Fahy JV, Boushey HA. Effect of low-dose beclomethasone dipropionate on asthma control and airway inflammation. Eur Respir J 1998; 11:1240–1247.

45. van der Molen T, De Jong BM, Mulder HH, Postma DS. Starting with a higher dose of inhaled corticosteroids in primary care asthma treatment. Am J Respir Crit Care Med 1998; 158:121–125.

46. Storensen L, Weng S, Weng SL, Wulf-Andersen L, Ostergaard D, et al. The costs of asthma in Denmark. Br J Med Econ 1997; 11:103–111.

47. Scott WG, Scott HM, Frost GD. Pharmacoeconomic evaluation of asthma treatment costs. Br J Med Econ 1997; 11:87–101.

48. Juniper EF, Kline PA, Vanzielegheim MA, Ramsdale MH, O'Byrne PM, Hargreave FE. Effect of long-term treatment with an inhaled corticosteroid (budesonide) on airway hyperresponsiveness and clinical asthma in nonsteroid-dependent asthmatics. Am Rev Respir Dis 1990; 142:832–836.

49. Ernst P, Spitzer WO, Suissa S et al. Risk of fatal asthma and near-fatal asthma in relation to inhaled corticosteroid use. JAMA 1992; 268:3462–3464.

50. Dompeling E, van Schayk CP, van Grunsven PM et al. Slowing the deterioration of asthma and chronic obstructive pulmonary disease observed during bronchodilator therapy by adding inhaled corticosteroids: a 4-year prospective study. Ann Intern Med 1993; 118:770–778.

51. Blais L, Suissa S, Boivin J-F, Ernst P. First treatment with inhaled corticosteroids and the prevention of asthma hospitalisations. Thorax 1998; 53:1025–1029.

52. Wennergren G, Kristjánsson S, Strannegård I-L. Decrease in hospitalization for

treatment of childhood asthma with increased use of antiinflammatory treatment, despite an increase in the prevalence of asthma. J Allergy Clin Immunol 1996; 97:742–748.

53. Donahue JG, Weiss ST, Livingston JM, Goetsch MA, Greineder DK, Platt R. Inhaled steroids and the risk of hospitalization for asthma. JAMA 1997; 277: 887–891.

54. Van Ganse E, Hubloue I, Vincken W, Leufkens HG, Gregoire J, Ernst P. Actual use of inhaled corticosteroids and risk of hospitalisation: a case-control study. Eur J Clin Pharmacol 1997; 51:449–454.

55. Crane J, Pearce N, Burgess C, Woodman K, Robson B, Beasley R. Markers of risk of asthma death or readmission in the 12 months following a hospital admission for asthma. Int J Epidemiol 1992; 21:737–744.

56. Weiss KB, Gergen PJ, Hodgson TA. An economic evaluation of asthma in United States. N Engl J Med 1992; 326:862–866.

57. Haahtela T, Terho EO, Hannuksela M, Vohlonen I. Allergian esiintyvyys ja kansantaloudellinen merkitys (in Finnish). Occurrence of allergy and its economical impact. In: Haahtela T, Hannuksela M, Terho EOT, eds. Allergologia. Helsinki: Duodecim, 1993:19–29.

58. O'Byrne PM, Cuddy L, Taylor DW, Birch S, Morris J, Syrotuik J. The clinical efficacy and cost benefit of inhaled corticosteroids as therapy in patients with mild asthma in primary care practice. Can Respir J 1996; 3:169–175.

59. Bousquet J, Knani J, Henry C et al. Undertreatment in a nonselected population of adult patients with asthma. J Allergy Clin Immunol 1996; 98:514–521.

60. Ferrante E, Muzzolon R, Fuso L, Corbo GM, Pistellini R, Ciappi G. Bronchial asthma: still an inadequately assessed and improperly treated disease. J Asthma 1994; 31:117–121.

61. Gaist D, Hallas J, Hansen N-CG, Gram LF. Are young adults with asthma treated sufficiently with inhaled steroids? A population-based study of prescription data from 1991 and 1994. Br J Clin Pharmacol 1996; 41:285–289.

62. Guidelines for the Diagnosis and Management of Asthma. Washington, DC: US Dept of Health and Human Services, 1991. Publication 91-3042.

63. Lang DM, Sherman MS, Polansky M. Guidelines and realities of asthma management. The Philadelphia story. Arch Intern Med 1997; 157:1193–1200.

64. Griffths C, Naish J, Sturdy P, Pereira F. Prescribing and hospital admissions for asthma in east London. Br Med J 1996; 312:481–482.

65. Lahdensuo A, Haahtela T, Herrala J, Kava T, Kiviranta K, Kuusisto P, Perämäki E, Poussa T, Saarelainen S, Svahn T. Randomised comparison of self management and traditional treatment of asthma over one year. Br Med J 1996; 312: 748–752.

66. Lahdensuo A, Haahtela T, Herrala J, Kava T, Kiviranta K, Kuusisto P, Pekurinen M, Perämäki E, Saarelainen S, Svahn T, Liljas B. A cost effectiveness analysis of guided self management of asthma in Finland. Br Med J 1998; 316:1138–1139.

67. Haahtela T, Klaukka T. Societal and health care benefits of early use of inhaled steroids. Thorax 1998; 53:1005–1006.
68. Campbell MJ, Cogman GR, Holgate ST, Johnston SL. Age specific trends in asthma mortality in England and Wales, 1983–95: results of an observational study. Br Med J 1997; 314:1439–1441.
69. Nordic Statistics on Medicines 1993–1995. NLN Publication No 43. Nordic Council on Medicines, Uppsala, 1996.

6

Signaling Mechanisms That Regulate Airway Smooth Muscle Cell Function and Growth

AILI L. LAZAAR and REYNOLD A. PANETTIERI, JR.

University of Pennsylvania Medical Center
Philadelphia, Pennsylvania

I. Introduction

Asthma, a chronic disease characterized by airway hyperreactivity, occurs in 5–8% of the U.S. population and is an extraordinarily common cause of pulmonary impairment. Despite considerable research effort, asthma mortality rates continue to rise and the primary defects that underlie airway hyperreactivity are unknown, although an intrinsic abnormality of airway smooth muscle (ASM) has been postulated (1–3). Increased smooth muscle mass in airways of patients with chronic severe asthma is a well-documented pathological finding. Studies have reported that this increased ASM mass is due to an increased number of airway myocytes (4–7). Some information is available with respect to factors that promote ASM cell proliferation; however, few studies to date have addressed cellular mechanisms that regulate ASM cell growth. Such studies are critical for an understanding of the pathogenesis of chronic severe asthma. We postulate that frequent stimulation of ASM by contractile agonists, inflammatory mediators, and growth factors induces chronic adaptive alterations in the airways that result in myocyte proliferation and airway remodeling. Such alterations may have important consequences in determining airway caliber and airway smooth muscle contractility. Proliferation of smooth muscle as described above significantly alters force generation by the muscle (8–10). Compelling evidence suggests that smooth muscle cells undergo proliferation in response to a variety of chemical and trophic stimuli, and these alterations profoundly affect the force-generation of the muscle (8–10).

Recent studies also suggest that ASM cells may modulate airway remodeling by secreting cytokines or growth factors and by expressing cell adhesion molecules (CAMs). These ASM cell functions may directly or indirectly modulate immunocyte trafficking or function. This chapter will examine the signaling pathway by which ASM cell growth is mediated as well as review the mechanism by which cytokines induce ASM cells to secrete cytokines or growth factors and to express CAMs.

II. Airway Smooth Muscle Cell Growth

Many studies have characterized the stimulation of smooth muscle proliferation in response to mitogenic agents such as polypeptide growth factors (3,11), inflammatory mediators (12,13), and cytokines (10,14). Other trophic factors, such as alterations in extracellular matrix and mechanical stress, have also been identified (15,16). In recent studies, the important observation that contractile agonists induce smooth muscle proliferation may be a critical link between the chronic stimulation of muscle contraction and myocyte proliferation (17–20). Although the mechanisms by which contractile agonists induce cell proliferation are unknown, similarities exist between signal transduction processes activated by these agents and those of known growth factors. Interestingly, these growth factors can also stimulate smooth muscle contraction (3,21). This section will review recent advances in signaling pathways regulating ASM growth and will not be an exhaustive review of all signal transduction processes modulating cell growth.

A. Cellular Signaling Pathways That Modulate Airway Smooth Muscle Growth

Some growth factors, like platelet-derived growth factor (PDGF) (17,22) and the contractile agonists serotonin (23), endothelin (12,13,24,25), and thrombin (26), appear to mediate their mitogenic effects, in part, through receptor-dependent activation of phospholipase C. Phospholipase C hydrolyzes phosphatidylinositides to inositol polyphosphates and diacylglycerol; these important second messengers increase cytosolic calcium and activate protein kinase C. Interestingly, these signaling events are neither essential nor sufficient to mediate airway smooth muscle cell proliferation (reviewed in Ref. 27). New evidence suggests that activation of cell proliferation by contractile agonists and growth factors may, in part, be mediated by activation of p60[src] and p21[ras], a small guanine nucleotide protein. The potential signal transduction pathways that mediate agonist- and growth-factor-induced proliferation of smooth muscle are summarized in Figure 1.

Despite similarities in activation of stimulatory and inhibitory signaling pathways between growth factors and contractile agonists, important disparities exist. First, cell proliferation stimulated by polypeptide growth factors is mediated by receptors with intrinsic tyrosine kinase (RTK) activity whereas G-protein-coupled receptors (GPCR) transduce signals through receptors that lack intrinsic tyrosine kinase activity. Second, mitogenesis induced by RTK activation appears to be Ras-dependent whereas that induced by GPCRs may be more diverse and use an array of small G proteins and phosphotyrosine scaffolding proteins (21,24,28–30). In addition to differences between the proliferative mechanisms of growth factors and those of GPCR agonists, there exists substantial variability in the mitogenic capacity among contractile agonists. First, some, but not all, contractile agonists stimulate smooth muscle cell proliferation, even though most of these agonists induce comparable levels of polyphosphoinositide hydrolysis and cytosolic calcium transients (26,31–33). Second, the mitogenic effects of endothelin (13,20,25) and serotonin (28) on vascular smooth muscle and thrombin on airway smooth muscle (26) appear to be coupled to pertussis-toxin-sensitive G proteins, not pertussis-toxin-insensitive G proteins, which are largely responsible for agonist-induced PI hydrolysis, cytosolic calcium release, or smooth muscle contraction. The differences in proliferative responses induced by growth factors and contractile agonists (and among contractile agonists) imply that other regulatory components are involved.

Activation of Ras and Src

The proteins encoded by *ras* genes serve as transducers of diverse physiological signals. Although the *ras* gene was first identified in transforming retroviruses (*v-ras*), the identification that retroviral oncogenes (*v-ras*) were derived from normal cellular genes (*c-ras*) has led to the recognition that Ras activa-

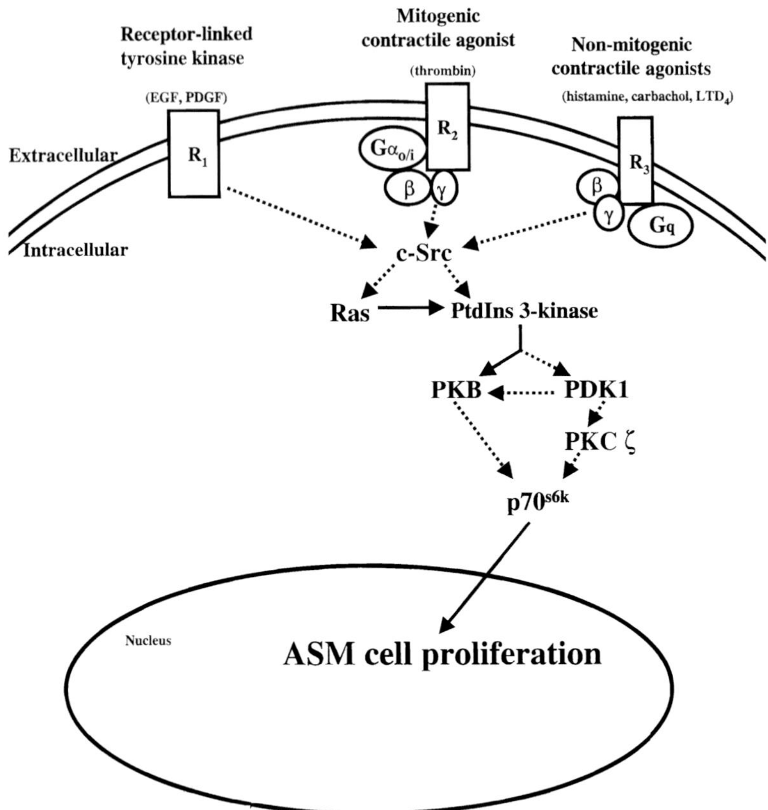

Figure 1   A model to illustrate the proposed mechanisms that regulate airway smooth muscle cell proliferation induced by contractile agonists and growth factors. R, receptor; EGF, epidermal growth factor; PDGF, platelet-derived growth factor; LTD$_4$: leukotriene D4; G proteins, guanine nucleotide binding regulatory proteins; Gα and G$\beta\gamma$, G-protein subunits; PtdIns 3-kinase, phosphatidylinositol 3-kinase; PKB, protein kinase B; PDK1, phosphoinositide-dependent kinase1; PKCζ, protein kinase ζ; p70^{s6k}, 70/85-kDa S6 protein kinases; ASM, airway smooth muscle. Signaling pathways marked with a solid line are known to modulate ASM cell proliferation induced by agonists. The dotted lines represent pathways that may modulate ASM cell growth. For ease of presentation, the signaling molecules are shown to be in the cytosol. However, most are associated with the cell membrane and not all promitogenic signaling pathways are shown (e.g., mitogen-activated protein kinases).

tion plays a critical role in mediating normal cell growth and differentiation (34,35).

Ras has served as a prototype for the superfamily of Ras-related proteins, a group of guanine-nucleotide-binding proteins that share structural homology (34–36). The discovery that Ras proteins bind guanine nucleotides (GTP and GDP) with high affinity and could hydrolyze GTP suggested a mechanism that regulated Ras activity. Ligand-bound receptors induce the active GTP-bound form of Ras by enhancing the ability of guanine-nucleotide-exchange factors to accelerate the replacement of bound GDP with GTP. Ras proteins are then deactivated by interaction with GTPase-activating proteins (GAPs) that promote GTP hydrolysis by Ras. In some cell types, activated Ras promotes cell proliferation; in others, it arrests cell division and induces the expression of differentiated phenotypes (37). Our studies suggest that Ras activation modulates ASM cell growth (38). We have shown that contractile agonists and growth factors that induce Ras activation also stimulate ASM cell growth and that Ras activation is necessary for agonist-induced ASM cell proliferation (38). Together, these studies suggest that Ras activation plays a crucial role in regulating mitogen-induced ASM proliferation.

The intermediary signaling events that link receptors to Ras activation remain controversial and appear to be cell- and receptor-specific (39,40). Recent studies suggest that RTK- and GPCR-signaling pathways may converge to activate Src, which in turn stimulates Ras (39,40). Src, the best understood member of a family of nine (nonreceptor) tyrosine kinases, regulates a variety of cellular responses to extracellular stimuli. Src-dependent cellular responses include cell growth, cell migration, cytoskeletal reorganization, and integrin-dependent cell adhesion (39,41). Although the kinase activity of Src appears critical for activation of some signaling pathways, kinase activation is not essential for all of Src's functions. In some cell types, the tyrosine kinase activity is necessary for stimulating mitogen-induced cell proliferation (39,40,42,43). In other cells, Src-dependent cell growth occurs independently of Src kinase activity but is due to Src subserving an adapter protein role (39,44,45).

The upstream activators and downstream effectors of Src remain unclear and, again, depend on the activating extracellular signal. In some cells, stimulation of GPCRs induces Src activation via release of G$\beta\gamma$ subunits (46). In the case of integrin signaling, the focal adhesion kinase as well as paxillin, vinculin, tensin, and cortactin are substrates for Src (39). In the case of growth factor signaling, downstream targets are ill-defined but a variety of proteins appear phosphorylated by v-Src including PtdIns 3-kinase, Ras-GAP, SHC, and PLC-γ (41). Interestingly, v-Src also modulates activation of p85 PtdIns 3-kinase and Ras in transformed cell lines (41). Currently, the role of Src in stimulating mitogen-induced ASM cell growth is unknown. Preliminary studies suggest that Ras is necessary for ASM cell proliferation and that Src inhibition also abrogates ASM cell proliferation, which suggests that Src serves as an upstream activator of Ras (38,47).

Downstream Targets of Phosphatidylinositol 3-Kinase (PtdIns 3-Kinase)

PtdIns 3-kinase is activated by its association with membrane phosphotyrosine residues on receptor tyrosine kinases (48). PtdIns 3-kinase phosphorylates phosphatidylinositides at the D3 position of the inositol ring, to promote formation of phosphatidylinositol 3-phosphate, phosphatidylinositol 3,4-bisphosphate, and phosphatidylinositol 3,4,5-trisphosphate (48–51). These phospholipids have been recognized as a new class of second messengers (48,49). Based on a number of studies, PtdIns 3,4,5-P_3 appears to be the critical signaling 3-phospholipid (48,51). The 3-phosphoinositides are not substrates for any known phospholipase C (48,51) and are not components of the canonical phosphoinositide turnover pathway. Further, their rapid increase upon growth factor stimulation suggests that the lipids themselves may act as second messengers mediating PtdIns 3-kinase mitogenic signals (50). New evidence suggests that PKB and PDK1, both serine/threonine kinases activated by 3-phosphoinositides, function as downstream effectors of PtdIns 3-kinase. Depending on the cell type, PKB activation is required for a variety of cellular processes including cell survival, carcinogenesis, differentiation, metabolism, and cell growth (52–54). Other studies suggest that PDK1 may activate PKB and also serves as a downstream effector of PtdIns 3-kinase (55–57). In some cells, PDK1 stimulates activation of the ζ isoform of protein kinase C (PKCζ), protein kinase A, and p70[s6k] (56). It is particularly interesting that PDK1 activates PKCζ since agonist-induced ASM cell growth is thought to be protein kinase C–dependent (58). Despite these new studies, the precise downstream effectors of PtdIns 3-kinase that modulate cell proliferation remain unknown. In human ASM cells, PtdIns 3-kinase regulates mitogen-induced ASM cell growth (33). In our studies, agonists that stimulate ASM mitogenesis activate PtdIns 3-kinase and those that are nonmitogenic do not (33). In addition, PtdIns 3-kinase is necessary and sufficient to induce ASM cell proliferation (33,59). Because new studies suggest that agonists activate PKB and that PtdIns 3-kinase inhibition abrogates agonist-induced PKB activation, PKB appears to serve as a downstream effector of PtdIns 3-kinase and may play an important role in regulating ASM cell growth induced by mitogens (59).

Upstream Activators of pp70^{s6k} Kinases

An essential step in the pathway by which growth factors trigger cellular proliferation is the induction of high levels of protein synthesis (60). This appears to be controlled by phosphorylation of the ribosomal protein S6. The 70/85-kDa S6 protein kinases, referred to collectively as p70^{s6k}, regulate phosphorylation of S6. Activation of p70^{s6k} is required for growth-factor-induced G_1 progression in transformed fibroblasts (61), hepatoma cells, and T lymphocytes (62). Although the precise signaling pathways that activate p70^{s6k} remain unknown, these pathways appear to be distinct from those that activate c-Ras, c-Raf, MEK, MAPK, and p90^{rsk} (60).

Although the regulation of p70^{s6k} appears complex, evidence suggests that sequential phosphorylation at multiple sites is required for full activation of the kinase (63,64). In vitro studies and those performed in transformed cell lines have identified many potential upstream modulators of p70^{s6k}. Evidence suggests that PKB and PDK1 (distinct from its ability to activate PKB) induce activation of S6 kinase in some but not all cell types' kinase (63,64). Other studies suggest that protein kinase Cζ modulates p70^{s6k} activation. Whether PKB, PDK1, or PKCζ modulates activation of S6 kinase in ASM remains unclear. Studies suggest that agonists that stimulate ASM growth also activate PKB and p70^{s6k} (33,59,65). In addition, activation of p70^{s6k} appears necessary for agonist-induced ASM cell proliferation (33). Based on these data, PKB, PDK1, and PKCζ appear to function upstream of p70^{s6k} to regulate ASM cell growth.

B. What Is Known About Smooth Muscle Proliferation Induced by Contractile Agonists?

Recent studies show that contractile agonists serotonin (28,66), vasopressin (30,67), and endothelin (13) induce proliferation of human vascular smooth muscle cells. To date, few studies have examined the mechanisms by which contractile agonists induce human ASM cell growth; thrombin and lysophosphatidic acid (LPA) are the only contractile agonists to date that robustly stimulate human ASM cell proliferation (26,68,69). Interestingly, histamine, LTD$_4$, endothelin-1, and carbachol alone are nonmitogenic; however, these agonists can significantly increase epidermal growth factor (EGF) and PDGF-mediated growth (19,20,65). Although the signaling events that mediate contractile agonist effects on ASM cell proliferation remain ill-defined, our studies suggest that PI-PLC–dependent increases in cytosolic calcium induced by thrombin (as well as by EGF) are not necessary for agonist-induced ASM mitogenesis (26). Based on current evidence and published studies, agonist-induced ASM cell proliferation appears dependent on Ras, PtdIns 3-kinase, and p70^{s6k} activation.

In most cell types, activation of p21^{ras} is considered essential for polypeptide growth factors to stimulate DNA synthesis (34,70). Recent studies suggest that Ras is also necessary for agonist-induced ASM cell growth (38). In addition, evidence suggests that Ras activation is either upstream or parallel to PtdIns 3-kinase activation. In some cells, Src in conjunction with G$\beta\gamma$ subunits act upstream of Ras to mediate GPCR responses (46). New studies suggest that inhibition of Src abrogates thrombin- and EGF-induced ASM cell growth (47). These data imply that Src may play an important role in the integration of mitogenic signals from receptors coupled to intrinsic tyrosine kinases and those coupled to heterotrimeric G proteins. To date, no studies have addressed the role of Src in mediating p21^{ras} dependent stimulation of smooth muscle cell growth.

In human ASM cells, PtdIns 3-kinase activation is necessary and also sufficient to stimulate mitogenesis (33). However, the precise upstream activators and downstream effectors of PtdIns 3-kinase activation remain unknown. Evidence suggests that Ras activation may lie downstream from PtdIns 3-kinase activation (71). Other studies, however, show that Ras acts upstream from, or in parallel to, PtdIns 3-kinase in modulating ASM cell growth (38). The recent identification of PKB and PDK1, which are modulated by 3-phospholipids and potentially serve as downstream effectors of PtdIns 3-kinase, may offer insight into signaling mechanisms by which PtdIns 3-kinase modulates cellular responses (55–57). In ASM cells, thrombin and EGF activate PKB and agonist-induced PKB activation is abrogated by PtdIns 3-kinase (59). These data suggest that PKB and PDK1 may act downstream of PtdIns 3-kinase to modulate ASM cell proliferation.

Activation of p70^{s6k} induces phosphorylation of the ribosomal protein S6, which is necessary for cell transit from G_1 to S phase of the cell cycle. Studies suggest that thrombin and EGF induce p70^{s6k} activation and that PtdIns 3-kinase inhibition with wortmannin or with dominant-negative PtdIns 3-kinase cDNA blocks this response (33). Based on these data and current evidence, p70^{s6k} appears to function as a downstream effector of PtdIns 3-kinase, and p70^{s6k} appears important in modulating ASM cell growth induced by growth factors. Recent evidence suggests that protein kinase Cζ as well as PDK1 and PKB may function as an upstream activator of p70^{s6k} in some but not all cell types (63). The precise events that link PtdIns 3-kinase activation to S6 kinase remain unknown. The role of PKB, PDK1, and protein kinase Cζ in modulating p70^{s6k} dependent ASM cell growth remains unknown.

In summary, signal transduction pathways that regulate cell transformation and human carcinogenesis have been investigated extensively. From these studies, it is evident that the molecular mechanisms that induce cell proliferation are cell type–and growth factor–specific. Recent studies in vascular biology have revealed that contractile agonists induce smooth muscle cell proliferation and that such proliferation is central to the pathogenesis of atherosclerosis. In ASM cells, current evidence suggests that mitogenic signals from agonists and growth factors converge to activate Ras, PtdIns 3-kinase, and pp70^{S6k}.

The chronic nature of asthma, combined with marked inflammation of the airways and repeated exposure of airway smooth muscle to contractile agonists, may induce profound increases in airway smooth muscle mass. Such alterations in smooth muscle mass may play an important role in the development of airway hyperreactivity seen in patients with chronic severe asthma. Therefore, identification of the critical cellular and molecular mechanisms by which mitogens induce airway smooth muscle cell proliferation will be necessary before the role of the ASM hyperplasia in the pathogenesis of asthma can be addressed, and therapeutic measures to prevent these alterations can be developed.

III. Cytokines Modulate Calcium Homeostasis and Cell Adhesion Molecule Expression in Airway Smooth Muscle Cells

Eosinophils, macrophages, and particularly lymphocytes residing in or infiltrating the inflamed submucosa can potentially interact with ASM cells and alter myocyte function. One mechanism by which immunocytes initiate and perpetuate the asthmatic response is through the production of proinflammatory mediators that may act directly or indirectly on ASM cells. The presence of several cytokine mRNAs and proteins has been detected within the airways of asthmatic subjects. The precise role of these cytokines in modulating ASM cell function, including the modulation of calcium homeostasis and cell adhesion molecule expression, is the focus of the remainder of this chapter.

A. Cytokines Alter Agonist-Induced Calcium Responses

ASM in vivo is either electrically quiescent or generates slow waves and some active tone, but does not generate action potentials under resting conditions or when stimulated by neurotransmitters or autocoids. Excitatory stimulation, whether neural, hormonal, or due to the release of autocoids, results in a graded depolarization and increase in tone in the muscle. Since excitatory and inhibitory stimuli are imposed on a tissue with little intrinsic contractile tone, the degree of muscle stimulation (and bronchodilation) will be the summated effect of bronchoconstrictor and bronchodilator stimuli.

Activation of an airway smooth muscle cell by a bronchoconstrictor induces a rapid rise in $[Ca^{2+}]_i$, associated with the release of intracellular calcium stores, to a peak level roughly 10-fold higher than the resting level (100 nM to greater than 1 µM at maximum agonist concentration). Following this peak, calcium falls but remains elevated as long as the contractile stimulus is present. The elevation of $[Ca^{2+}]_i$ results in the activation of the calcium/calmodulin-sensitive myosin light chain kinase, and the subsequent phosphorylation of the regulatory myosin light chain (MLC_{20}) at Ser 19. Phosphorylation of this residue by myosin ATPase activity initiates cross-bridge cycling between myosin and actin. ATP binding, hydrolysis, and ADP release continue as long as MLC_{20} is phosphorylated; dephosphorylation terminates crossbridge cycling and relaxes smooth muscle. In addition to the regulation of tension by $[Ca^{2+}]_i$, several mechanisms have been advanced to explain a lack of correlation between $[Ca^{2+}]_i$ and tension between different modes of stimulation. The G-protein-coupled regulation of myosin phosphatase may be an important mechanism by which ''sensitization'' of myosin phosphorylation occurs (72).

Evidence now suggests that TNF and IL-1β, cytokines found in the bronchoalveolar lavage of patients with allergen-induced asthma (73), may directly alter myocyte calcium homeostasis and render airway smooth muscle hyperresponsive to contractile agonists. Since ASM is an essential effector cell modulating bronchoconstriction, and since calcium regulates ASM cell contraction, interactions between cytokines, such as TNFα and IL-1β released from inflammatory cells, and calcium mobilization may represent a mechanism underlying bronchial hyperresponsiveness in asthma. Amrani et al. (74) recently investigated whether TNFα modulated cytosolic calcium responses in ASM stimulated with carbachol. Carbachol- (74,75) and thrombin-induced (76) increases in $[Ca^{2+}]_i$ were enhanced by TNFα or IL-1 in human ASM. Both phases of agonist-induced calcium levels were affected by TNFα, suggesting an increased calcium mobilization from both intracellular and extracellular stores. Activation of TNFRp55, the predominant receptor expressed in human ASM cells, and de novo protein synthesis were also found to be required for TNFα effects on calcium mobilization (75,76). The ability of TNFα to alter the $[Ca^{2+}]_i$ signals induced by a variety of different agonists suggested that this cytokine may "prime" ASM cells for an increase in agonist responsiveness. This is an interesting finding since TNFα can also induce the "primed" ASM to become more contractile to the same agonists either in vivo (77–79) or in vitro (80,81). Whether both phenomena (i.e., increased receptor-mediated calcium responses and increased smooth muscle contractility) are linked remains to be determined. However, the ability of IL-1β to also induce bronchial hyperresponsiveness (81) in a similar manner to that of TNFα (76) strongly suggests that cytokines may modulate calcium homeostasis induced by agonists and, therefore, may represent a potential mechanism underlying bronchial hyperresponsiveness in asthma (Fig. 2).

B. Potential Intracellular Mechanisms Altered by Cytokines

G-Protein-Mediated Signal Transduction

Since TNFα alone did not stimulate either a calcium response or phosphoinositide hydrolysis in human ASM, TNFα likely augments agonist-induced increases in $[Ca^{2+}]_i$ by directly affecting the coupling process of agonist receptors to downstream signaling events. In human ASM, such receptors are known to be coupled to phospholipase C, which catalyzes the hydrolysis of phosphotidylinositol 4,5 bisphosphate, yielding inositol trisphosphate and diacylglycerol (reviewed in Refs. 82 and 83). Recent studies suggest that TNFα significantly enhanced phosphoinositide accumulation in response to bradykinin in human ASM and epidermoid carcinoma cells (76,84). In addition, G-protein-induced activation of adenylyl cyclase by isoproterenol or G-protein-mediated arachidonic acid metabolism by bradykinin was also shown to be enhanced by TNFα (85,86). In ASM, however, TNFα as well as IL-1β has been reported to inhibit isoproterenol-stimulated activation of adenylyl cyclase (87,88).

Cytokines have also been reported to modulate expression of G-proteins. TNFα increases the amount, as well as the activity, of G-proteins in several cell types including ASM (86,89–92). The finding that TNFα enhances calcium mobilization in response to NaF (76), an agent that bypasses membrane receptors and directly activates G-proteins (93,94), supports the notion that TNFα acts directly at the level of G-proteins rather than modifying the expression of contractile agonists receptors. This observation supports previous find-

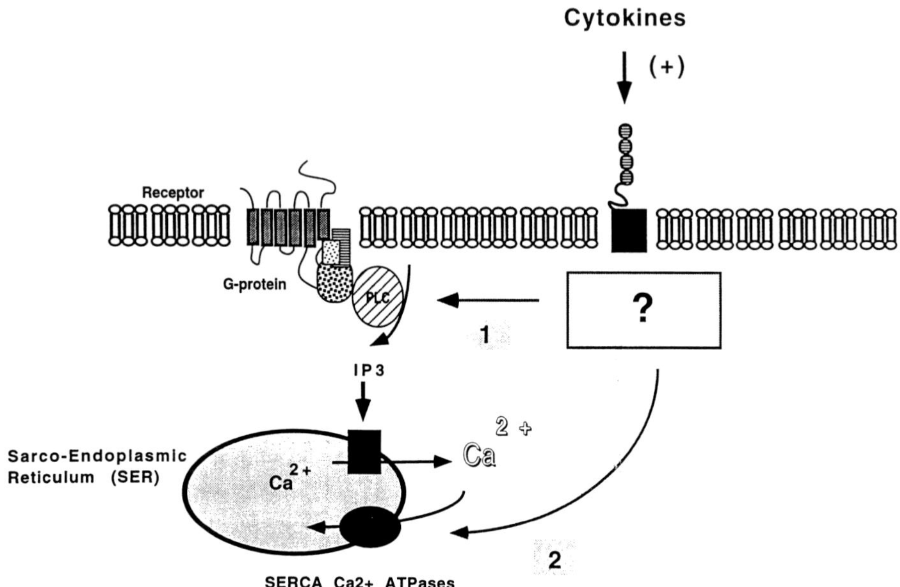

Figure 2   Potential sites for cytokine-induced alterations in calcium homeostasis in human ASM cells. This involves 1) the receptor/G-protein/effector system and 2) the calcium regulatory proteins such as SERCA-type calcium pumps, which function by pumping calcium from the cytosol to the internal stores. IP3, inositol-1,4,5 trisphosphate; PLC, phospholipase C.

ings that, despite increased calcium signals to carbachol, TNFα did not increase muscarinic receptor numbers (74). Finally, TNFα may also alter phospholipase C activity, as has been shown in a mouse fibrosarcoma cell line (95). Taken, together, these studies show that cytokines modulate ASM functions not only by activating specific cytokine receptors, but also by dramatically amplifying the ability of other agonists to induce increases in $[Ca^{2+}]_i$.

Intracellular Calcium Stores

In many cell types, the activation of calcium pumps directly regulates the calcium ion concentration both in the cytosol and in intracellular stores, either by extruding calcium from the cell via plasma membrane Ca^{2+}-ATPases

(96,97) or by sequestering calcium into intracellular calcium stores by the SERCA-type Ca^{2+}-ATPases (98–103). A variety of SERCA isotypes (Sarco-Endoplasmic Reticulum Calcium-ATPase) are expressed in different tissues and are the products of both distinct genes and alternative mRNA splicing. For the SERCA-type Ca^{2+}-ATPases, three genes have been identified: $SERCA_1$, expressed in fast skeletal muscle (104), $SERCA_2$, which gives rise to $SERCA_{2a}$ and $SERCA_{2b}$ isoforms (98,101) mainly expressed in cardiac and smooth muscle, respectively; and $SERCA_3$, which is a nonmuscle isoform (98).

Thapsigargin, a specific inhibitor of SERCA (105–107), has been useful in defining the role of SERCA-associated calcium pools in activating cellular signal transduction pathways. Thapsigargin-sensitive calcium stores not only provide a source of calcium following bronchoconstrictor stimulation (102,103) but also appear to exert a profound control over cell proliferation and progression through the cell cycle (108,109). Calcium responses to thapsigargin, which triggers calcium signals by directly releasing intracellular stores, are potentiated by pretreating cells with $TNF\alpha$ (75,110). This effect may be due to an increased release of calcium, to an increase in calcium content, or to an increase in the number of SERCA-type calcium-ATPases sensitive to thapsigargin. Alternatively, cytokines may directly affect $[Ca^{2+}]_i$ by altering the type of SERCA associated with the calcium stores. Interestingly, $SERCA_{2a}$ protein and mRNA content are increased in a time-dependent manner by $TNF\alpha$ (111). Several reports have also shown a modulation of SERCA-type Ca^{2+}-ATPase expression in pathological conditions such as hyperthyroidism and hypertension (112–115). In other studies, thyroid hormone (112), platelet-derived growth factor (116), and insulin growth factor (117) upregulated transcription of the $SERCA_2$ and $SERCA_1$ gene. Taken together, these studies suggest that calcium pumps that regulate intracellular calcium stores may also be altered by cytokines and growth factors and may represent another pathway by which cytokines alter agonist-induced calcium responses or modulate cell growth.

Characterization of the cellular and biochemical events that are involved in activation of ASM is likely to be the major consideration in the design of future therapies for asthma. Because calcium is an essential regulatory element for cell growth and cell contraction, it is likely that alterations in calcium mobilization may, in part, play a role in creating an ASM phenotype that is hyperresponsive to contractile agonists. Further studies will be required to determine the precise mechanisms involved in cytokine modulation of calcium homeostasis in ASM.

IV. Cytokines Induce Cell Adhesion Molecule Expression in Airway Smooth Muscle Cells

A. Role of CAMs in Leukocyte Recruitment

Recruitment and activation of T cells, eosinophils, and mast cells are critical for initiation of the inflammatory response. Cell adhesion molecules (CAMs) mediate leukocyte endothelial cell interactions during the process of cell recruitment and homing (118). The expression and activation of a cascade of CAMs that include selectins, integrins, and members of the immunoglobulin superfamily (such as ICAM-1, VCAM-1, and PECAM), as well as the local production of chemoattractants, lead to leukocyte adhesion and transmigration into lymph nodes and sites of inflammation involving nonlymphoid tissues. Most studies have emphasized the mechanisms that regulate extravasation of leukocytes from the circulation during the establishment of a local inflammatory response. However, the subsequent interactions of the infiltrating leukocytes with other cell types in the bronchial submucosa or with the extracellular matrix may also be important for sustaining the inflammatory response and are less well defined.

Recent attention has focused on the role of CAMs in mediating the asthmatic response (119). Numerous descriptive studies of CAM expression in asthmatic tissue have confirmed the upregulation of ICAM-1 and E-selectin, and, in some populations, VCAM-1, on endothelial and bronchial epithelial cells (120–122). Increased concentrations of soluble sICAM-1 and sE-selectin have also been found in bronchoalveolar lavage fluid of asthmatics (123,124). To determine a more mechanistic role for CAMs, many investigators have used blocking antibodies in animal models of airway inflammation and airway hyperresponsiveness (AHR). Wegner et al. (125) demonstrated that antibodies against ICAM-1 decreased eosinophil infiltration and attenuated bronchial hyperresponsiveness in a primate model of asthma. ICAM-1-deficient mice also demonstrate a significant decrease in airway eosinophilia and bronchial hyperresponsiveness (126,127). Studies utilizing anti-VLA-4 antibodies have also demonstrated significant inhibition of both leukocyte recruitment and bronchial hyperreactivity (128–130) in antigen-sensitized animals. VCAM-1-hypomorphic mice have significantly reduced airway eosinophilia (131). Failure to induce VCAM-1 in IL-4 knockout mice results in the inability to recruit TH2-type T cells to the airway following antigen challenge (132).

The role of CAMs as ''gatekeepers,'' however, may be too simplistic. Several investigators have now shown that treatment with antibodies to CAMs can block AHR without affecting eosinophil and lymphocyte recruitment

(130,133–135). These data suggest that persistent AHR following antigen challenge cannot be totally accounted for by inhibition of leukocyte recruitment. Despite the attempt to link airway hyperreactivity to leukocyte recruitment, these data suggest that CAMs may modulate cell–cell or cell–matrix interactions apart from those promoting leukocyte infiltration.

B. CAMs Mediate Cell–Cell and Cell–Matrix Interactions in Inflammation

ASM cell activation is regulated by cell–cell interactions through CAMs, adherence to extracellular matrix proteins, and by exposure to soluble cytokines and growth factors. ASM is known to express CAMs, which are inducible by a wide range of inflammatory mediators (136). This has been demonstrated both in vitro and in an in situ bronchial xenograft model in SCID mice. Contractile agonists such as bradykinin and histamine, on the other hand, have no effect on ASM CAM expression (136). Lazaar et al. (136) have demonstrated that activated T lymphocytes adhere via LFA-1 and VLA-4 to cytokine-induced ICAM-1 and VCAM-1 on cultured human ASM cells. Moreover, an integrin-independent component of lymphocyte–smooth muscle cell adhesion appeared to be mediated by CD44-hyaluronan interactions. In a companion study, BAL-derived T cells obtained from allergic asthmatic subjects following segmental antigen challenge also adhered to ASM. Furthermore, cytokines secreted by in vitro activated or BAL-derived T cells induced smooth muscle cell expression of ICAM-1 and HLA-DR (137).

One well-established function of CAMs is to function as accessory molecules for leukocyte activation (118,138,139). Although SMC have not previously been identified as participants in the immune response, recent studies suggest, in some instances, that MHC class II–expressing vascular smooth muscle (VSM) induces T-cell activation (140,141). Other recent studies in both VSM and ASM found that these cells, in fact, were not able to present alloantigen to CD4[+] T cells, despite the the expression of MHC class II and costimulatory molecules such as CAMs (137,142). Whether this is because of a lack of other necessary costimulatory molecules or secretion of an inhibitory substance by the smooth muscle cells has yet to be determined. Functionally, however, adhesion of stimulated CD4[+] T cells *can* induce smooth muscle cell DNA synthesis (136). This appears to require direct cell-cell contact and cannot be mimicked by treatment of the cells with T-cell-conditioned medium. In this sense, ASM differs from vascular smooth muscle (143). One could postulate, therefore, that CAM-mediated T-cell adhesion to smooth muscle may induce smooth muscle cell growth and thereby contribute to the airway remodeling that occurs in asthmatics as shown in Figure 3.

Finally, CAMs may also contribute to the development of airway reactivity by their ability to act as receptors for common respiratory viruses. For example, rhinovirus is known to bind to ICAM-1 on the cell surface (144). Interestingly, rhinovirus has been shown to increase expression of its own receptor by an NF-κB-dependent mechanism (145), which may result in further leukocyte recruitment and inflammation. Recent data also suggest that infection of ASM with rhinovirus increases smooth muscle cell contractility and autocrine secretion of the proinflammatory cytokine, IL-1β (146).

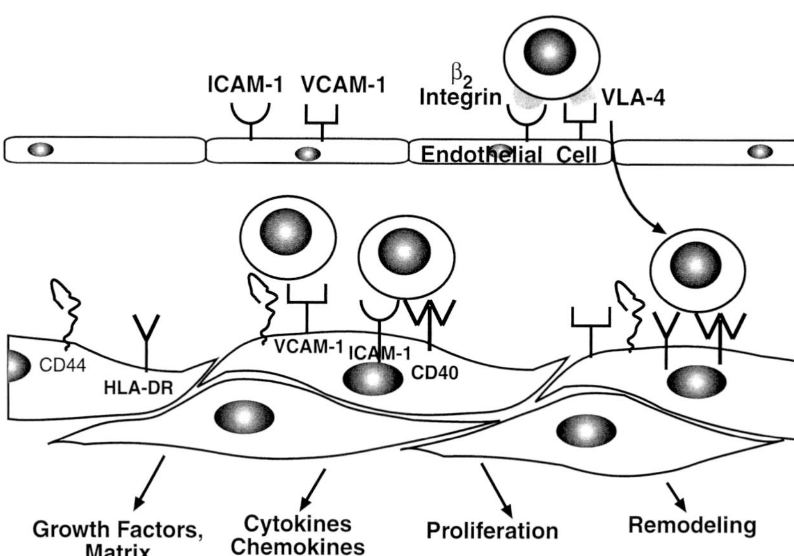

Figure 3   A proposed model for amplification loops in airway inflammation. T lymphocytes adhere to activated endothelial cells, transmigrate into the submucosa, and then adhere to cytokine-activated ASM via cell adhesion molecules. T-cell-derived cytokines further upregulate ICAM-1 and VCAM-1 and MHC class II on ASM. Activated smooth muscle cells secrete cytokines, chemokines, and growth factors, and increase production of matrix proteins. T cell–smooth muscle cell interactions may also stimulate smooth muscle cell proliferation and airway remodeling: ICAM-1, intercellular adhesion molecule 1; VCAM-1, vascular cell adhesion molecule 1; ASM, airway smooth muscle.

C. Intracellular Signaling and CAM Expression in ASM Cells

The intracellular signals by which agents such as TNFα regulate adhesion molecule expression remain unknown, although recent data suggest that generation of sphingosine 1-phosphate, as well as activation of Raf and Ras, may be involved (147,148). In human ASM cells, investigators reported the effects of activation of cAMP-dependent protein kinase A (A-kinase) on ICAM-1 and VCAM-1 expression in airway myocytes treated with TNFα. As determined by cell surface expression, cells pretreated with forskolin, a direct stimulator of adenylyl cyclase, prior to stimulation with TNFα, had markedly reduced ICAM-1 expression, while VCAM-1 expression was less affected, compared with those cells that were treated with TNFα alone (149). Corresponding T-cell adhesion was also reduced by forskolin pretreatment compared to TNFα alone. These studies suggest that signaling pathways that increase cAMP and activate A-kinase appear to inhibit cytokine-induced expression of ICAM-1 and VCAM-1 in human ASM cells. On the other hand, TNFα-induced activation of the transcription factor NF-κB and subsequent expression of ICAM-1 in human ASM cells were *not* inhibited by pretreatment of the cells with dexamethasone (150). This differs from the conventional understanding of corticosteroids as anti-inflammatory agents with effects on nuclear transcription and cytokine gene expression (reviewed in Ref. 151). These studies highlight the need for understanding the impact of specific cytokines on both the expression and function of airway CAMs and for defining the genetic regulation of these molecules. This knowledge will facilitate the development of rational therapeutic strategies for modulating CAM function in airway inflammation.

D. Cytokine Secretion by ASM

The variety of cell types that reside in or infiltrate the inflamed submucosa present the potential for many important cell–cell interactions. Eosinophils, macrophages, and lymphocytes are critical in the initiation and perpetuation of airway inflammation. One mechanism by which immunocytes exert their effects is by the production of proinflammatory mediators. Exposure of airway smooth muscle to cytokines or growth factors is known to result in SMC hypertrophy and hyperplasia (152–154). The presence of an ever-expanding number of cytokine mRNAs or secreted proteins has been detected within the airways of asthmatic subjects, including TNFα, IL-1, IL-3, IL-4, IL-5, IL-6, IL-10, IL-12, IL-13, IL-16, eotaxin, TGF-β, and GM-CSF (73,155–165).

More recent data have shown that ASM cells themselves can secrete a number of cytokines and chemoattractants (Table 1). Several reports (166–168) have demonstrated the expression and release of both C-C (MIP-1α, RANTES, eotaxin) and C-X-C (IL-8) chemokines. Studies of bronchial biopsies in mild asthmatics revealed constitutive staining for RANTES in ASM (169). IL-1 and TGF-β were found to induce secretion of the proinflammatory cytokine IL-6 by ASM (170). In addition, ligation of CD40, a member of the TNF receptor superfamily, also induced ASM expression of IL-6 (171). Interestingly, transgenic expression of IL-6 in the murine lung resulted in a peribronchiolar inflammatory infiltrate along with airway *hypo*responsiveness, suggesting an intriguing role for IL-6 in controlling local inflammation and regulating airway reactivity (172).

Infection of ASM with respiratory syncitial virus or parainfluenza virus type 3 specifically stimulated secretion of IL-11 (170). This cytokine may be important for the inflammatory response in the airway as targeted overexpression of IL-11 in the lung resulted in airway remodeling, subepithelial fibrosis,

Table 1 Synthetic Function of Human Airway Smooth Muscle Cells

Cytokine	IL-6 (170,171)
	IL-11 (170)
	LIF (170,176)
	GM-CSF (177–179)
	IL-1β (146)
	IL-5 (179)
	IL-2 (179)
	IL-12 (179)
	IFN-γ (179)
Chemokine	IL-8 (166,168,180)
	ENA-78 (166)
	RANTES (168,169)
	MIP-1α (166)
	MIP-1β (166)
	MCP-1 (181)
	Eotaxin (182,183)
Other	PDGF (153)
	MMP-1 (174,175)
	TIMP-1,-2 (184)
	Gelatinase B (184)

and increased bronchial hyperreactivity to methacholine (173). Additional studies have shown that cytokine-activated ASM cells can secrete growth factors and matrix metalloproteinases (153,174,175). These data support a role for ASM as effector cells in perpetuating airway inflammation and in contributing to airway remodeling.

V. Summary

Asthma, as well as bronchiolitis obliterans and chronic bronchitis, are chronic lung diseases characterized by airflow obstruction. Despite considerable research effort, primary defects that underlie airway obstruction remain unknown although an intrinsic abnormality of airway smooth muscle has been postulated.

Although asthma typically induces reversible airway obstruction, in some asthmatics airflow obstruction can become irreversible. Such obstruction may be a consequence of persistent structural changes in the airway wall due to the frequent stimulation of airway smooth muscle by contractile agonists, inflammatory mediators, and growth factors. Increased smooth muscle mass, which has been attributed to increases in myocyte number, is a well-documented pathological finding in the airways of patients with chronic severe asthma.

Although the mechanisms by which mitogens induce cell proliferation are unknown, similarities exist between signal transduction processes activated by these agents and those of known growth factors. Diverse extracellular stimuli induce cell growth, in part, by activating common intracellular signal transduction pathways.

Airway inflammation, a hallmark of asthma, appears to be mediated by the secretion of cytokines. Cytokines have been recognized as molecules critically important in altering the function of mast cells, lymphocytes, and eosinophils, which play important roles in modulating airway function. Recent studies suggest that cytokines may directly alter ASM function and induce a myocyte phenotype that manifests hyperresponsiveness to most bronchoconstrictors. The "cytokine priming" of ASM likely occurs at multiple sites downstream from the agonist receptors and involves calcium homeostasis. Other studies have revealed that ASM may also secrete cytokines and thereby modulate the inflammatory response in the airways of asthmatics.

Recent studies have also determined that ASM cells may directly interact with infiltrating immunocytes. The functional consequences of immunocyte-myocyte adherence may modulate inflammatory responses in the asthmatic airway. Studies have shown that activated T lymphocytes can adhere to cultured ASM. In addition, airway myocytes upregulated expression of ICAM-1 and VCAM-1 in response to inflammatory cytokines, in both in vitro and in situ models of transplanted human bronchial tissue into SCID mice. Further, ASM constitutively expresses another CAM, CD44, and blocking antibodies to ICAM-1, VCAM-1, and CD44 in combination completely abolished adhesion of activated T cells to ASM. Finally, adherence of activated T cells to ASM induces DNA synthesis in quiescent myocytes. The identification of the critical regulatory sites that mediate ASM cell proliferation or modulate CAM expression on airway myocytes may provide new therapeutic approaches to alter the airway remodeling seen in patients with chronic airflow obstruction.

References

1. Boushey HA, Holtzman MJ, Sheller JR, Nadel JA. State of the art: Bronchial hyperreactivity. Am Rev Respirat Dis 1980; 121:389–413.
2. Woolcock AJ. Asthma—what are the important experiments? State of the art/ conference summary. Am Rev Respir Dis 1988; 138:730–744.
3. Panettieri RA, Jr., Grunstein MM. Airway smooth muscle hyperplasia and hypertrophy. In: Barnes PJ, Grunstein MM, Leff AR, Woolcock AJ, eds. Asthma. New York: Lippincott-Raven Publishers, 1997:823–842.
4. Dunnill MS. The pathology of asthma, with special reference to the changes in the bronchial mucosa. J Clin Pathol 1960; 13:27–33.
5. Dunnill MS, Massarella GR, Anderson JA. A comparison of the quantitative anatomy of the bronchi in normal subject, in status asthmaticus, in chronic bronchitis and in emphysema. Thorax 1969; 24:176–179.
6. Hossain S. Quantitative measurement of bronchial muscle in asthma. Am Rev Respir Dis 1973; 107:99–109.
7. Ebina M, Takahashi T, Chiba T, Motomiya M. Cellular hypertrohy and hyperplasia of ASM underlying bronchial asthma. Am Rev Respir Dis 1993; 148: 720–726.
8. Malmqvist U, Amer A. Contractile properties during development of hypertrophy of the smooth muscle in the rat portal vein. Acta Physiol Scand 1988; 133: 49–61.
9. Gabella G. Hypertrophic smooth muscle. I. Size and shape of cells, occurrence of mitoses. Cell Tissue Res 1979; 201:63–78.
10. Owens GK, Geisterfer AAT, Wei-Hwa Yang Y, Komoriya A. Transforming growth factor-β-induced growth inhibition and cellular hypertrophy in cultured vascular smooth muscle cells. J Cell Biol 1988; 107:771–780.

11. Alexander RW, Griendling KK. Signal transduction in vascular smooth muscle. J Hypertens 1996; 14:S51–S54.

12. Bobik A, Grooms A, Millar JA, Mitchell A, Grinpukel S. Growth factor activity of endothelin on vascular smooth muscle. Am J Physiol: Cell Physiol 1990; 258/27:C408–C415.

13. Komuro I, Kurihara H, Sugiyama T, Takaku F, Yazaki Y. Endothelin stimulates c-fos and c-myc expression and proliferation of vascular smooth muscle cells. FEBS Lett 1988; 238:249–252.

14. Owens GK, Schwartz SM, McCanna M. Evaluation of medial hypertrophy in resistance vessels of spontaneously hypertensive rats. Hypertension 1988; 11: 198–207.

15. Westermark B, Heldin C-H, Ek B, et al. Biochemistry and biology of platelet-derived growth factor. In: Guroff G, ed. Growth and Maturation Factors, 1. New York: Wiley, 1983:73–115.

16. Smith PG, Moreno R, Ikebe M. Strain increases airway smooth muscle contractile and cytoskeletal proteins in vitro. Am J Physiol (Lung Cell Mol Physiol) 1997; 272:L20–L27.

17. Berk BC, Alexander RW, Brock TA, Gimbrone J, MA, Webb RC. Vasoconstriction: A new activity for platelet-derived growth factor. Science 1986; 232: 87–90.

18. Panettieri RA, Jr., Krymskaya V, Scott P, et al. Thrombin induces human airway smooth muscle (ASM) cell proliferation by activation of a novel signaling pathway. Am J Respir Crit Care Med 1996; 153:A742.

19. Panettieri RA, Jr., Tan EML, Ciocca V, Luttmann MA, Leonard TB, Hay DWP. Effects of LTD_4 on human airways smooth muscle cell proliferation, matrix expression, and contraction in vitro: differential sensitivity to cysteinyl leukotriene receptor antagonists. Am J Respir Cell Mol Biol 1998; 19:453–461.

20. Panettieri RA, Jr., Goldie RG, Rigby P, Eszterhas AJ, Hay DWP. Endothelin-1-induced potentiation of human airway smooth muscle proliferation: an ET_A receptor-mediated phenomenon. Br J Pharmacol 1996; 118:191–197.

21. Berk BC, Brock TA, Webb RC, et al. Epidermal growth factor, a vascular smooth muscle mitogen, induces rat aortic contraction. J Clin Invest 1985; 75: 1083–1086.

22. Glenn K, Bowen-Pope DF, Ross R. Platelet-derived growth factor. III. Identification of a platelet-derived growth factor receptor by affinity labeling. J Biol Chem 1982; 257:5172–5176.

23. Kelleher MD, Abe MK, Chao T-SO, et al. Role of MAP kinase activation in bovine tracheal smooth muscle mitogenesis. Am J Physiol (Lung Cell Mol Physiol) 1995; 268/12:L894–L901.

24. Rozengurt E. Growth factors and cell proliferation. Curr Opin Cell Biol 1992; 4:161–165.

25. Noveral JP, Rosenberg SM, Anbar RA, Pawlowski NA, Grunstein MM. Role of

endothelin-1 in regulating proliferation of cultured rabbit airway smooth muscle cells. Am J Physiol (Lung Cell Mol Physiol) 1992; 263/7:L317–L324.

26. Panettieri RA, Jr., Hall IP, Maki CS, Murray RK. α-Thrombin increases cytosolic calcium and induces human airway smooth muscle cell proliferation. Am J Respir Cell Mol Biol 1995; 13:205–216.

27. Panettieri RA, Jr., Kotlikoff MI. Cellular and molecular mechanisms regulating airway smooth muscle cell physiology and pharmacology. In: Fishman AP, Elias JA, Fishman JA, Grippi MA, Kaiser LR, Senior RM, eds. Pulmonary Diseases and Disorders, 3rd ed. New York: McGraw-Hill, 1998:107–117.

28. Kavanaugh WM, Williams LT, Ives HE, Coughlin SR. Serotonin-induced deoxyribonucleic acid synthesis in vascular smooth muscle cells involves a novel, pertussis toxin-sensitive pathway. Mol Endocrinol 1988; 123:599–605.

29. Chambard JC, Paris S, L'Allemain G, Pouyssegur J. Two growth factor signaling pathways in fibroblasts distinguished by pertussis toxin. Nature (Lond) 1987;326:800–803.

30. Vicentini LM, Villereal ML. Serum, bradykinin and vasopressin stimulate release of inositol phosphates from human fibroblasts. Biochem Biophys Res Commun 1984; 123:663–670.

31. Panettieri RA, Jr., Murray RK, DePalo LR, Yadvish PA, Kotlikoff MI. A human airway smooth muscle cell line that retains physiological responsiveness. Am J Physiol: Cell Physiol 1989; 256/25:C329–C335.

32. Wolf M, Cuatrecasas P, Sahyoun N. Interaction of protein kinase C with membranes is regulated by Ca^{2+}, phorbol esters, and ATP. J Biol Chem 1985; 260: 15718–15722.

33. Krymskaya VP, Penn RB, Orsini MJ, et al. Phosphatidylinositol 3-kinase mediates mitogen-induced human airways smooth muscle cell proliferation. Am J Physiol (Lung Cell Mol Physiol) 1999; 277/21:L65–L78.

34. Lowy DR, Willumsen BM. Function and regulation of ras. Annu Rev Biochem 1993; 62:851–891.

35. Feig LA, Schaffhausen B. The hunt for ras targets. Nature 1994; 370:508–509.

36. Monia BP, Johnston JF, Ecker DJ, Zounes MA, Lima WF, Freier SM. Selective inhibition of mutant Ha-ras mRNA expression by antisense oligonucleotides. J Biol Chem 1992; 267:19954–19962.

37. Brass LF, Manning DR, Williams A, Woolkalis MJ, Poncz M. Receptor and G protein–mediated responses to thrombin in HEL cells. J Biol Chem 1991; 266:958–965.

38. Ammit AJ, Kane SA, Panettieri RA Jr. Activation of K-p21ras and N-p21ras, but not H-p21ras, is necessary for mitogen-induced human airway smooth muscle proliferation. Am J Respir Cell Mol Biol. In press.

39. Schwartzberg PL. The many faces of Src: multiple functions of a prototypical tyrosine kinase. Oncogene 1998; 17:1463–1468.

40. Schieffer B, Drexler H, Ling BN, Marrero MB. G protein-coupled receptors

control vascular smooth muscle cell proliferation via pp60[c-src] and p21[ras]. Am J Physiol: Cell Physiol 1997; 272/41:C2019–C2030.

41. Brown MT, Cooper JA. Regulation, substrates and functions of src. Biochim Biophys Acta 1996; 1287:121–149.

42. Schieffer B, Paxton WG, Chai Q, Marrero MB, Bernstein KE. Angiotensin II controls p21[ras] activity via pp60[c-src]. J Biol Chem 1996; 271:10329–10333.

43. Gutkind JS. Cell growth control by G protein-coupled receptors: from signal transduction to signal integration. Oncogene 1998; 17:1331–1342.

44. Valius M, Kkazlauskas A. Phospholipase C-gamma 1 and phosphatidylinositol 3 kinase are the downstream mediators of the PDGF receptor's mitogenic signal. Cell 1993;73:321–334.

45. Barone MV, Courtneidge S. Myc but not Fos rescue of PDGF signalling block caused by kinase inactive Src. Nature 1995; 378:509–512.

46. Ushio-Fukai M, Alexander RW, Akers M, Lyons PR, Lassegue B, Griendling KK. Angotensin II receptor coupling to phospholipase D is mediated by the $\beta\gamma$ subunits of heterotrimeric G proteins in vascular smooth muscle cells. Mol Pharmacol 1999; 55:142–149.

47. Krymskaya VP, Penn RB, Hoffman R, Eszterhas A, Panettieri RA Jr. Phosphatidylinositol 3-kinase (PI3K) modulates human airway smooth muscle (HASM) cell mitogenesis by activating p70S6 kinase (p70S6K). Am J Respir Crit Care Med 1999; 159:A533.

48. Rameh LE, Cantley LC. The role of phosphoinositide 3-kinase lipid products in cell function. J Biol Chem 1999; 274:8347–8350.

49. Stephens LT, Cooke FT, Walters R, et al. Characterization of a phosphatidylinositol-specific phosphoinositide 3-kinase from mammalian cells. Curr Biol 1994; 4:203–214.

50. Kapeller R, Cantley LC. Phosphatidylinositol 3-kinase. BioEssays 1994; 16:565–576.

51. Fry MJ. Structure, regulation and function of phosphoinositide 3-kinases. Biochim Biophys Acta 1994; 1226:237–268.

52. Coffer PJ, Jin J, Woodgett JR. Protein kinase B (c-Akt): a multifunctional mediator of phosphatidylinositol 3-kinase activation. Biochem J 1998; 335:1–13.

53. Aoki M, Batista O, Bellacosa A, Tsichlis P, Vogt PK. The Akt kinase: molecular determinants of oncogenicity. Proc Natl Acad Sci USA 1998; 95:14950–14955.

54. Burgering BMT, Coffer PJ. Protein kinase B (c-Akt) in phosphatidylinositol-3-OH kinase signal transduction. Nature 1995; 376:599–602.

55. Belham C, Wu S, Avruch J. Intracellular signalling: PDK1—a kinase at the hub of things. Curr Biol 1999; 9:R93–R96.

56. Dong LQ, Zhang R, Langlais P, et al. Primary structure, tissue distribution, and expression of mouse phosphoinositide-dependent protein kinase-1, a protein kinase that phosphorylates and activates protein kinase Cζ. J Biol Chem 1999; 274:8117–8122.

57. Le Good JA, Ziegler WH, Parekh DB, Alessi DR, Cohen P, Parker PJ. Protein kinase C isotypes controlled by phosphoinositide 3-kinase through the protein kinase PDK1. Science 1998; 281:2042–2045.

58. Nakarish H, Brewer KA, Exton JH. Activation of the zeta isoenzyme of protein kinase C by phosphotidylinositol 3,4,5-trisphosphate. J Biol Chem 1993; 268: 13–16.

59. Walker TR, Moore SM, Lawson MF, Panettieri RA, Jr., Chilvers ER. Platelet-derived growth factor-BB and thrombin activate phosphoinositide 3-kinase and protein kinase B: role in mediating airway smooth muscle proliferation. Mol Pharmacol 1998; 54:1007–1015.

60. Blenis J. Signal transduction via the MAP kinases: proceed at your own RSK. Proc Nat Acad Sci USA 1993; 90:5889–5892.

61. Lane TA, Lamkin GE, Wancewicz EV. Modulation of endothelial cell expression of intercellular adhesion molecule 1 by protein kinase C activation. Biochem Biophys Res Commun 1989; 161:945–952.

62. Monfar M, Lemon KP, Grammer TC, et al. Activation of pp70/85 S6 kinases in interleukin-2-responsive lymphoid cells is mediated by phosphatidylinositol 3-kinase and inhibited by cyclic AMP. Mol Cell Biol 1995; 15:326–337.

63. Peterson RT, Schreiber SL. Translation control: connecting mitogens and the ribosome. Curr Biol 1998; 8:R248–R250.

64. Romanelli A, Martin KA, Toker A, Blenis J. p70 S6 kinase is regulated by protein kinase Cζ and participates in a phosphoinositide 3-kinase-regulated signalling complex. Mol Cell Biol 1999; 19:2921–2928.

65. Krymskaya VP, Orsini MJ, Eszterhas AJ, Benovic JL, Panettieri RA Jr., Penn RB. Potentiation of human airway smooth muscle proliferation by receptor tyrosine kinase and G protein-coupled receptor activation. J Biol Chem.

66. Nemecek GM, Coughlin SR, Handley DA, Moskowitz MA. Stimulation of aortic smooth muscle cell mitogenesis by serotonin. Proc Nat Acad Sci USA 1986; 83:674–678.

67. Nambi P, Watt R, Whitman M, et al. Induction of c-fos protein by activation of vasopressin receptors in smooth muscle cells. FEBS Lett 1989; 245:61–64.

68. Stewart AG, Fernandes D, Tomlinson PR. The effect of glucocorticoids on proliferation of human cultured airway smooth muscle. Br J Pharmacol 1995; 116:3219–3226.

69. Cerutis DR, Nogami M, Anderson JL, et al. Lysophosphatidic acid and EGF stimulate mitogenesis in human airway smooth muscle cells. Am J Physiol (Lung Cell Mol Physiol) 1997; 273:L10–L15.

70. van Corven EJ, Hordijk PL, Medema RH, Bos JL, Moolenaar WH. Pertussis toxin–sensitive activation of p21^{ras} by G protein-coupled receptor agonists in fibroblasts. Proc Nat Acad Sci USA 1993; 90:1257–1261.

71. Roche S, Koegl M, Courtneidge SA. The phosphatidylinositol 3-kinase is required for DNA synthesis induced by some, but not all, growth factors. Proc Nat Acad Sci USA 1994; 91:9185–9189.

72. Panettieri RA, Jr. Cellular and molecular mechanisms regulating airway smooth muscle cell proliferation and cell adhesion molecule expression. Am J Respir Crit Care Med 1998; 158:S133–S140.

73. Broide DH, Lotz M, Cuomo AJ, Coburn DA, Federman EC, Wasserman SI. Cytokines in symptomatic asthma airways. J Allergy Clin Immunol 1992; 89: 958–967.

74. Amrani Y, Martinet N, Bronner C. Potentiation by tumour necrosis factor-α of calcium signals induced by bradykinin and carbachol in human tracheal smooth muscle cells. Br J Pharmacol 1995; 114:4–5.

75. Amrani Y, Penettieri RA, Jr., Frossard N, Bronner C. Activation of the TNFα-p55 receptor induces myocyte proliferation and modulates agonist-evoked calcium transients in cultured human tracheal smooth muscle cells. Am J Respir Cell Mol Biol 1996; 15:55–63.

76. Amrani Y, Krymskaya V, Maki C, Panettieri RA, Jr. Mechanisms underlying TNFα effects on agonist-mediated calcium homeostasis in human airway smooth muscle cells. Am J Physiol (Lung Cell Mol Physiol) 1997; 273/17: L1020–L1028.

77. Kips JC, Tavernier JH, Pauwels RA. Tumor necrosis factor (TNF) causes bronchial hyperresponsiveness in rats. Am Rev Respir Dis 1992; 145:332–336.

78. Wheeler AP, Hardie WD, Bernard GR. The role of cyclooxygenase products in lung injury induced by tumor necrosis factor in sheep. Am Rev Respir Dis 1992; 145:632–639.

79. Thomas PS, Yates DH, Barnes JP. Tumor necrosis factor-alpha increases airway responsiveness and sputum neutrophilia in normal human subjects. Am J Respir Crit Care Med 1995; 152:76–80.

80. Pennings HJ, Kramer K, Bast A, Buurman W, Wouters E. Tumour necrosis factor causes hyperresponsiveness in tracheal smooth muscle of the guinea-pig model in vitro. Eur Respir J 1993; 70:325s.

81. Souhrada M, Souhrada JF. Potentiation of electrical and contractile response of sensitized airway smooth muscle to a specific antigen by interleukin-1β. Am Rev Respir Dis 1993; 147:A52.

82. Coburn RF, Baron CB. Coupling mechanisms in airway smooth muscle. Am J Physiol (Lung Cell Mol Physiol) 1990; 258:L119–L133.

83. Giembycz MA, Raeburn D. Current concepts on mechanisms of force generation and maintenance in airway smooth muscle. Pulm Pharmacol 1992; 5:279–297.

84. Sawutz DG, Singh SS, Tiberio L, Koszewski E, Johnson CG, Johnson CL. The effect of TNFα on bradykinin receptor binding, phosphotidylinositol turnover and cell growth in human A431 epidermoid carcinoma cells. Immunopharmacology 1992; 24:1–10.

85. Burch RM, Tiffany CW. Tumor necrosis factor causes amplification of arachidonic acid metabolism in response to interleukin-1, bradykinin, and other agonists. J Cell Physiol 1989; 141:85–89.

86. Klein JB, Scherzer JA, Harding G, Jacobs AA, Mcleish KR. TNF-α stimulates increased plasma membrane guanine nucleotide binding protein activity in polymorphonuclear leukocytes. J Leuko Biol 1995; 57:500–506.

87. Emala CW, Kuhl J, Hungerford CL, Hirshman CA. TNFα inhibits isoproterenol-stimulated adenylyl cyclase activity in cultured airway smooth muscle cells. Am J Physiol (Lung Cell Mol Physiol) 1997; 272:L644–L650.

88. Shore SA, Laporte J, Hall IP, Hardy E, Panettieri RA, Jr. Effect of IL-1β on responses of cultured human airway smooth muscle cells to bronchodilator agonists. Am J Respir Cell Mol Biol 1997; 16:702–712.

89. Reithmann C, Gierschik P, Werdan K, Jacobs KH. Tumor necrosis factor-α up-regulates Giα and Gβ proteins and adenylyl cyclase responsive in rat cardiomyocytes. Eur J Pharmacol 1991; 206:53–60.

90. Scherzer JA, Lin Y, McLeich KR, Klein JB. TNF translationally modulates the expression of G protein α_{i2} subunits in human polymorphonuclear leukocytes. J Immunol 1997; 158:913–918.

91. Hakonarson H, Herrick DJ, Grunstein MM. Mechanism of impaired β-adrenoceptor responsiveness in atopic sensitized airway smooth muscle. Am J Physiol (Lung Cell Mol Physiol) 1995; 269:L645–L652.

92. Hotta K, Emala CW, Hirshman CA. TNF-α upregulates $G_i\alpha$ and $G_q\alpha$ protein expression and function in human airway smooth muscle cells. Am J Physiol (Lung Cell Mol Physiol) 1999; 276/20:L405–L411.

93. Hall IP, Donaldson J, Hill SJ. Modulation of fluoroaluminate-induced inositol phosphate formation by increases in tissue cyclic AMP content in bovine tracheal smooth muscle. Br J Pharmacol 1990; 100:646–650.

94. Hardy E, Farahani M, Hall IP. Regulation of histamine H1 receptor coupling by dexamethasone in human cultured airway smooth muscle. Br J Pharmacol 1996; 118:1079–1084.

95. Machleidt T, Kramer B, Adam D, et al. Function of the p55 tumor necrosis factor receptor "death domain" mediated by phosphatidylcholine-specific phospholipase C. J Exp Med 1996; 184:725–733.

96. Greeb J, Shull GE. Molecular cloning of the third isoform of the calmodulin-sensitive plasma membrane Ca^{2+}-transporting ATPase that is expressed predominantly in brain and skeletal muscle. J Biol Chem 1988; 264:18569–18576.

97. De Jaegere S, Wuytack F, Eggermont JA, Verboomen H, Casteel R. Molecular cloning and sequencing of the plasma-membrane Ca^{2+} pumps of pig smooth muscle. Biochem J 1990; 271:655–660.

98. Lytton J, Maclennan DH. Molecular cloning of cDNAs from human kidney coding for two alternatively spliced products of the cardiac Ca^{2+}-ATPase gene. J Biol Chem 1988; 263:15024–15031.

99. Burk SE, Lytton J, MacLennan DH, Shull GE. cDNA cloning, functional expression, and mRNA tissue distribution of a third organellar Ca^{2+} pump. J Biol Chem 1989; 264:18561–18568.

100. Eggermont JA, Wuytack F, Verbist J, Casteels R. Expression of endoplasmic-

reticulum Ca^{2+} pump isoforms and of phospholamban in pig smooth muscle tissues. Biochem J 1990; 266:901–907.

101. Zarain-Herzberg A, MacLennan DH, Periasamy M. Characterization of rabbit cardiac sarco(endo)plasmic reticulum Ca^{2+}-ATPase gene. J Biol Chem 1990; 265:4670–4677.

102. Amrani Y, Da Silva A, Kassel O, Bronner C. Biphasic increase in cytosolic free calcium induced by bradykinin and histamine in cultured tracheal smooth muscle cells: is the sustained phase artifactual? Naunyn-Schmied Arch Pharmacol 1994; 350:662–668.

103. Amrani Y, Magnier C, Wuytack F, Enouf J, Bronner C. Ca^{2+} increase and Ca^{2+} influx in human tracheal smooth muscle cells: Role of Ca^{2+} pools controlled by sarco-endoplasmic reticulum Ca^{2+}-ATPase 2 isoforms. Br J Pharmacol 1995; 115:1204–1210.

104. Arai M, Otsu K, MacLennan DH, Periasamy M. Regulation of sarcoplasmic reticulum gene expression during cardiac and skeletal muscle development. Am J Physiol: Cell Physiol 1992; 262:C614–C630.

105. Thastrup O. Role of Ca^{2+}-ATPases in regulation of cellular Ca^{2+} signalling, as studied with the selective microsomal Ca^{2+}-ATPase inhibitor, thapsigargin. Agents Actions 1990; 29:8–15.

106. Thastrup O, Cullen PJ, Drobak BK, Hanley MR, Dawson AP. Thapsigargin, a tumor promoter, discharges intracellular Ca^{2+} stores by specific inhibition of the endoplasmic reticulum Ca^{2+}-ATPase. Proc Natl Acad Sci USA 1990; 87: 2466–2470.

107. Takemura H, Ohshika H, Yokosawa N, Oguma K, Thastrup O. The thapsigargin-sensitive intracellular Ca^{2+} pool is more important in plasma membrane Ca^{2+} entry than the IP3-sensitive intracellular Ca^{2+}-pool in neuronal cell lines. Biochem Biophys Res Commun 1991; 180:1518–1526.

108. Short AD, Bian J, Ghosh TK, Waldrom RT, Rybak SL, Gill DL. Intracellular Ca^{2+} pool content is linked to control of cell growth. J Biol Chem 1993; 90: 4986–4990.

109. Graber MN, Alfonso A, Gill DL. Ca^{2+} pools and cell growth: Arachidonic acid induces recovery of cells growth-arrested by Ca^{2+} pool depletion. J Biol Chem 1996; 271:883–888.

110. Peiretti F, Fossat C, Anfosso F, et al. Increase in cytosolic calcium upregulates the synthesis of type I plasminogen activator inhibitor in the human histiocytic cell line U937. Blood 1996; 87:162–173.

111. Amrani Y, Bobe R, Enouf J, Aubier M, Bronner C. TNFα activates the transcription of SERCA$_{2a}$ gene in cultured human tracheal smooth muscle cells. Am J Respir Crit Care Med 1996; 153:A164.

112. Nagai R, Zarain-Herzberg A, Brandl CJ, et al. Regulation of myocardial Ca^{2+}-ATPase and phospholamban mRNA expression in response to pressure overload and thyroid hormone. Proc Natl Acad Sci USA 1989; 86:2966–2970.

113. Levitsky DO, Clergue M, Lambert F, et al. Sarcoplasmic reticulum calcium

transport and Ca^{2+}-ATPase gene expression in thoracic and abdominal aortas of normotensive and spontaneously hypertensive rats. J Biol Chem 1993; 268: 8325–8331.

114. Papp B, Corvazier E, Magnier C, et al. Spontaneously hypertensive rats and platelet Ca^{2+}-ATPases: Specific up-regulation of the 97 kDa isoform. Biochem J 1993; 295:685–690.

115. Bobe R, Bredoux R, Wuytack F, et al. The rat platelet 97-kDa Ca^{2+}-ATPase isoform is the sarcoendoplasmic reticulum Ca2+ATPase 3 protein. J Biol Chem 1994; 269:1417–1424.

116. Magnier C, Papp B, Corvazier E, et al. Regulation of sarco-plasmic reticulum Ca^{2+}-ATPases during platelet-derived growth factor-induced smooth muscle proliferation. J Biol Chem 1992; 267:15808–15815.

117. Thelen MHM, Muller A, Zuidwijk MJ, Van Der Linden GC, Simonides WS, Van Hardeveld C. Differential regulation of the expression of fast-type sarco-plasmic-reticulum Ca^{2+}-ATPase by thyroid hormone and insulin-like growth factor-1 in the L6 muscle cell line. Biochem J 1994; 303:467–474.

118. Springer TA. Adhesion receptors of the immune system. Nature 1990; 346: 425–434.

119. Smith CH, Barker JNWN, Lee TH. Adhesion molecules in allergic inflammation. Am Rev Respir Dis 1993; 148:S75–S78.

120. Gundel RH, Wegner CD, Torcellini CA, et al. Endothelial leukocyte adhesion molecule-1 mediates antigen-induced acute airway inflammation and late-phase airway obstruction in monkeys. J Clin Invest 1991; 88:1407–1411.

121. Montefort S, Roche WR, Howarth PH, et al. Intercellular adhesion molecule-1 (ICAM-1) and endothelial leukocyte adhesion molecule-1 (ELAM-1) expression in the bronchial mucosa of normal and asthmatic patients. Eur Respir J 1992; 5:815–823.

122. Ohkawara Y, Yamauchi K, Maruyama N, et al. In situ expression of the cell adhesion molecules in bronchial tissues from asthmatics with air flow limitation: in vivo evidence of VCAM-1/VLA-4 interaction in selective eosinophil infiltration. Am J Respir Cell Mol Biol 1995; 12:4–12.

123. Georas SN, Liu MC, Newman W, Beall LD, Stealey BA, Bochner BS. Altered adhesion molecule expression and endothelial cell activation accompany the recruitment of human granulocytes to the lung after segmental antigen challenge. Am J Respir Cell Mol Biol 1992; 7:261–269.

124. Takahashi N, Liu MC, Proud D, Yu XY, Hasegawa S, Spannhake EW. Soluble intracellular adhesion molecule 1 in bronchoalveolar lavage fluid of allergic subjects following segmental antigen challenge. Am J Respir Crit Care Med 1994; 150:704–709.

125. Wegner CD, Gundel RH, Reilly P, Haynes N, Letts LG, Rothlein R. Intercellular adhesion molecule-1 (ICAM-1) in the pathogenesis of asthma. Science 1990; 247:456–459.

126. Wolyniec WW, DeSanctis GT, Nabozny G, et al. Reduction of antigen-induced

airway hyperreactivity and eosinophilia in ICAM-1-deficient mice. Am J Respir Cell Mol Biol 1998; 18:777–785.

127. Broide DH, Sullivan S, Gifford T, Sriramarao P. Inhibition of pulmonary eosinophilia in P-selectin- and ICAM-1-deficient mice. Am J Respir Cell Mol Biol 1998; 18:218–225.

128. Nakajima H, Sano H, Nishimura T, Yoshida S, Iwamoto I. Role of vascular cell adhesion molecule 1/very late activation antigen 4 and intercellular adhesion molecule 1/lymphocyte function-associated antigen 1 interactions in antigen-induced eosinophil and T cell recruitment into the tissue. J Exp Med 1994; 179: 1145–1154.

129. Pretolani M, Ruffie C, Silva JR, Joseph D, Lobb RR, Vargaftig BB. Antibody to very late activation antigen 4 prevents antigen-induced bronchial hyperreactivity and cellular infiltration in the guinea pig airways. J Exp Med 1994; 180: 795–805.

130. Henderson WR Jr., Chi EY, Albert RK, et al. Blockade of CD49d (α4 integrin) on intrapulmonary but not circulating leukocytes inhibits airway inflammation and hyperresponsiveness in a mouse model of asthma. J Clin Invest 1997; 100: 3083–3092.

131. Gonzalo JA, Lloyd CM, Kremer L, et al. Eosinophil recruitment to the lung in a murine model of allergic inflammation. The role of T cells, chemokines, and adhesion receptors. J Clin Invest 1996; 98:2332–2345.

132. Cohn L, Homer RJ, Marinov A, Rankin J, Bottomly K. Induction of airway mucus production by T helper 2 (Th2) cells: A critical role for interleukin 4 in cell recruitment but not mucus production. J Exp Med 1997; 186:1737–1747.

133. Abraham WM, Sielczak MW, Ahmed A, et al. α4-integrins mediate antigen-induced late bronchial responses and prolonged airway hyperresponsiveness in sheep. J Clin Invest 1994; 93:776–787.

134. Rabb HA, Olivenstein R, Issekutz TB, Renzi PM, Martin JG. The role of leukocyte adhesion molecules VLA-4, LFA-1, and Mac-1 in allergic airway responses in the rat. Am J Respir Crit Care Med 1994; 149:1186–1191.

135. Nagase T, Fukuchi Y, Matsuse T, Sudo E, Matsui H, Orimo H. Antagonism of ICAM-1 attenuates airway and tissue responses to antigen in sensitized rats. Am J Respir Crit Care Med 1995; 151:1244–1249.

136. Lazaar AL, Albelda SM, Pilewski JM, Brennan B, Pure E, Panettieri RA, Jr. T lymphocytes adhere to airway smooth muscle cells via integrins and CD44 and induce smooth muscle cell DNA synthesis. J Exp Med 1994; 180:807–816.

137. Lazaar AL, Reitz HE, Panettieri RA, Jr., Peters SP, Pure E. Antigen receptor-stimulated peripheral blood and bronchoalveolar lavage-derived T cells induce MHC class II and ICAM-1 expression on human airway smooth muscle. Am J Respir Cell Mol Biol 1997; 16:38–45.

138. Dustin ML, Springer TA. Role of lymphocyte adhesion receptors in transient interactions and cell locomotion. Annu Rev Immunol 1991; 9:27–66.

139. van Seventer GA, Shimuzu Y, Shaw S. Roles of multiple accessory molecules in T-cell activation. Curr Opin Immunol 1991; 3:294–303.

140. Fabry Z, Waldschmidt MM, Moore SA, Hart MN. Antigen presentation by brain microvessel smooth muscle and endothelium. J Neuroimmunol 1990; 28: 63–71.

141. Fabry Z, Waldschmidt MM, Van Dyk L, Moore SA, Hart MN. Activation of CD4+ lymphocytes by syngeneic brain microvascular smooth muscle cells. J Immunol 1990; 145:1099–1104.

142. Murray AG, Libby P, Pober JS. Human vascular smooth muscle cells poorly co-stimulate and actively inhibit allogeneic CD4+ T cell proliferation in vitro. J Immunol 1995; 154:151–161.

143. Rolfe BE, Campbell JH, Smith NJ, Cheong MW, Campbell GR. T lymphocytes affect smooth muscle cell phenotype and proliferation. Arterioscler Thromb Vasc Biol 1995; 15:1204–1210.

144. Greve JM, Davis G, Meyer AM, et al. The major human rhinovirus receptor is ICAM-1. Cell 1989; 56:839–847.

145. Papi A, Johnston SL. Rhinovirus infection induces expression of its own receptor intercellular adhesion molecule 1 (ICAM-1) via increased NF-κB-mediated transcription. J Biol Chem 1999; 274:9707–9720.

146. Hakonarson H, Carter C, Maskeri N, Hodinka R, Grunstein MM. Rhinovirus-mediated changes in airway smooth muscle responsiveness: induced autocrine role of interleukin-1β. Am J Physiol (Lung Cell Mol Physiol) 1999; 277/21: L13–L21.

147. Xia P, Gamble JR, Rye K-A, et al. Tumor necrosis factor-α induces adhesion molecule expression through the sphingosine kinase pathway. Proc Natl Acad Sci USA 1998; 95:14196–14201.

148. Xu XS, Vanderziel C, Bennett CF, Monia BP. A role for c-raf kinase and Ha-ras in cytokine-mediated induction of cell adhesion molecules. J Biol Chem 1998; 273:33230–33238.

149. Panettieri RA, Jr., Lazaar AL, Pure E, Albelda SM. Activation of cAMP-dependent pathways in human airway smooth muscle cells inhibits TNF-α-induced ICAM-1 and VCAM-1 expression and T lymphocyte adhesion. J Immunol 1995; 154:2358–2365.

150. Amrani Y, Lazaar AL, Panettieri RA, Jr. Up-regulation of ICAM-1 by cytokines in human tracheal smooth muscle cells involves an NF-κB-dependent signaling pathway that is only partially sensitive to dexamethasone. J Immunol 1999; 163:2128–2134.

151. Baldwin AS, Jr. The NF-κB and IκB proteins: New discoveries and insights. Annu Rev Immunol 1996; 14:649–681.

152. Hirst SJ, Barnes PJ, Twort CHC. Quantifying proliferation of cultured human and rabbit airway smooth muscle cells in response to serum and platelet-derived growth factor. Am J Respir Cell Mol Biol 1992; 7:574–581.

153. De S, Zelazny ET, Souhrada JF, Souhrada M. Interleukin-1β stimulates the

proliferation of cultured airway smooth muscle cells via platelet-derived growth factor. Am J Respir Cell Mol Biol 1993; 9:645–651.

154. De S, Zelazny ET, Souhrada JF, Souhrada M. IL-1β and IL-6 induce hyperplasia and hypertrophy of cultured guinea pig airway smooth muscle cells. J Appl Physiol 1995; 78:1555–1563.

155. Gosset P, Tsicopoulos A, Wallaert B, et al. Increased secretion of tumor necrosis factor alpha and interleukin-6 by alveolar macrophages consecutive to the development of the late asthmatic reaction. J Allergy Clin Immunol 1991; 88: 561–571.

156. Hamid Q, Azzawi M, Ying S, et al. Expression of mRNA for interleukin-5 in mucosal bronchial biopsies from asthma. J Clin Invest 1991; 87:1541–1546.

157. Robinson DS, Hamid Q, Ying S, et al. Predominant TH2-like bronchoalveolar T-lymphocyte population in atopic asthma. N Engl J Med 1992; 326:298–304.

158. Krishnaswamy G, Liu MC, Su S-N, et al. Analysis of cytokine transcripts in the bronchoalveolar lavage cells of patients with asthma. Am J Respir Cell Mol Biol 1993; 9:279–286.

159. Bradding P, Roberts JA, Britten KM, et al. Interleukin-4, -5, and -6 and tumor necrosis factor-alpha in normal and asthmatic airways: evidence for the human mast cell as a source of these cytokines. Am J Respir Cell Mol Biol 1994; 10: 471–480.

160. Robinson DS, Tsicopoulos A, Meng Q, Durham S, Kay AB, Hamid Q. Increased interleukin-10 messenger RNA expression in atopic allergy and asthma. Am J Respir Cell Mol Biol 1996; 14:113–117.

161. Naseer T, Minshall EM, Leung DY, et al. Expression of IL-12 and IL-13 mRNA in asthma and their modulation in response to steroid therapy. Am J Respir Crit Care Med 1997; 155:845–851.

162. Humbert M, Durham SR, Kimmitt P, et al. Elevated expression of messenger ribonucleic acid encoding IL-13 in the bronchial mucosa of atopic and non-atopic subjects with asthma. J Allergy Clin Immunol 1997; 99:657–665.

163. Laberge S, Ernst P, Ghaffar O, et al. Increased expression of interleukin-16 in bronchial mucosa of subjects with atopic asthma. Am J Respir Cell Mol Biol 1997; 17:193–202.

164. Minshall EM, Leung DY, Martin RJ, et al. Eosinophil-associated TGF-β1 mRNA expression and airways fibrosis in bronchial asthma. Am J Respir Cell Mol Biol 1997; 17:326–333.

165. Lamkhioued B, Renzi PM, Abi-Younes S, et al. Increased expression of eotaxin in bronchoalveolar lavage and airways of asthmatics contributes to the chemotaxis of eosinophils to the site of inflammation. J Immunol 1997; 159:4593–4601.

166. Lukacs NW, Kunkel SL, Allen R, et al. Stimulus and cell-specific expression of C-X-C and C-C chemokines by pulmonary stromal cell populations. Am J Physiol (Lung Cell Mol Physiol) 1995; 268/5:L856–L861.

167. John M, Hirst SJ, Jose PJ, et al. Human airway smooth muscle cells express

and release RANTES in response to T helper 1 cytokines. Regulation by T helper 2 cytokines and corticosteroids. J Immunol 1997; 158:1841–1847.

168. John M, Au B-T, Jose PJ, et al. Expression and release of interleukin-8 by human airway smooth muscle cells: Inhibition by Th-2 cytokines and corticosteroids. Am J Respir Cell Mol Biol 1998; 18:84–90.

169. Berkman N, Krishnan VL, Gilbey T, et al. Expression of RANTES mRNA and protein in airways of patients with mild asthma. Am J Respir Crit Care Med 1996; 154:1804–1811.

170. Elias JA, Wu Y, Zheng T, Panettieri RA, Jr. Cytokine- and virus-stimulated airway smooth muscle cells produce IL-11 and other IL-6-type cytokines. Am J Physiol (Lung Cell Mol Physiol) 1997; 273/17:L648–L655.

171. Lazaar AL, Amrani Y, Hsu J, et al. CD40-mediated signal transduction in human airway smooth muscle. J Immunol 1998; 161:3120–3127.

172. DiCosmo BF, Geba GP, Picarella D, et al. Airway epithelial cell expression of interleukin-6 in transgenic mice. Uncoupling of airway inflammation and bronchial hyperreactivity. J Clin Invest 1994; 94:2028–2035.

173. Tang W, Geba GP, Zheng T, et al. Targeted expression of IL-11 in the murine airway causes lymphocytic inflammation, bronchial remodeling, and airways obstruction. J Clin Invest 1996; 98:2845–2853.

174. Rajah R, Nunn S, Herrick D, Grunstein MM, Cohen P. LTD-4 induces matrix metalloproteinase-1 which functions as an IGFBP protease in airway smooth muscle cells. Am J Physiol (Lung Cell Mol Physiol) 1996; 271:L1014–L1022.

175. Rajah R, Nachajon RV, Collins MH, Hakonarson H, Grunstein MM, Cohen P. Elevated levels of the IGF-binding protein protease MMP-1 in asthmatic airway smooth muscle. Am J Respir Cell Mol Biol 1999; 20:199–208.

176. Knight DA, Lydell CP, Zhou D, Weir TD, Schellenberg RR, Bai TR. Leukemia inhibitory factor (LIF) and LIF receptor in human lung: distribution and regulation of LIF release. Am J Respir Cell Mol Biol 1999; 20:834–841.

177. Hallsworth MP, Soh CPC, Twort CHC, Lee TH, Hirst SJ. Cultured human airway smooth muscle cells stimulated by interleukin-1β enhance eosinophil survival. Am J Respir Cell Mol Biol 1998; 19:910–919.

178. Saunders MA, Mitchell JA, Seldon PM, et al. Release of granulocyte-macrophage colony stimulating factor by human cultured airway smooth muscle cells: suppression by dexamethasone. Br J Pharmacol 1997; 120:545–546.

179. Hakonarson H, Maskeri N, Carter C, Grunstein MM. Regulation of TH1- and TH2-type cytokine expression and action in atopic asthmatic sensitized airway smooth muscle. J Clin Invest 1999; 103:1077–1087.

180. Pang L, Knox AJ. Bradykinin stimulates IL-8 production in cultured human airway smooth muscle cells: role of cyclooxygenase products. J Immunol 1998; 161:2509–2515.

181. Sousa AR, Lane SJ, Nakhosteen JA, Yoshimura T, Lee TH, Poston RN. Increased expression of the monocyte chemoattractant protein-1 in bronchial tissue from asthmatic subjects. Am J Respir Cell Mol Biol 1994; 10:142–147.

182. Ghaffar O, Hamid Q, Renzi PM, et al. Constitutive and cytokine-stimulated expression of eotaxin by human airway smooth muscle cells. Am J Respir Crit Care Med 1999; 159:1933–1942.

183. Chung KF, Patel HJ, Fadlon EJ, et al. Induction of eotaxin expression and release from human airway smooth muscle cells by IL-1β and TNFα: effects of IL-10 and corticosteroids. Br J Pharmacol 1999; 127:1145–1150.

184. Foda HD, George S, Rollo E, et al. Regulation of gelatinases in human airway smooth muscle cells: Mechanism of progelatinase A activation. Am J Physiol (Lung Cell Mol Physiol) 1999; 277/21:L174–L182.

7

The Bronchial Vessels in Airway Remodeling

JOHN W. WILSON and XUN LI

The Alfred Campus
Monash University
Prahran, Australia

I. Introduction

Airway wall remodeling in asthma is now recognized to be the product of long-standing bronchial inflammation. Inflammatory mediators and growth factors produced by this process have the capacity to cause cell infiltration, epithelial injury, collagen deposition, matrix restructuring, smooth muscle hypertrophy/hyperplasia, and increased bronchial vascularity. The bronchial vasculature may contribute to an increase in wall thickness and change in bronchial wall compliance through increased vessel caliber (vasodilatation), increased vessel numbers (angioneogenesis), and the formation of interstitial edema within the airway wall (microvascular leakage). Indirectly, vessels increase airway wall thickness by acting as portals of entry for inflammatory cells, by local upregulation of adhesion glycoproteins. Major advances in the study of vascular function and revascularization after tissue injury, combined with recent observations concerning the immunology of the asthmatic airway, have highlighted the importance of the vasculature in airway remodeling, now identifiable with specific stains (see Fig. 1).

The blood supply of the airway comprises a superficial peribronchial capillary bed and a deeper submucosal plexus, joined by perforating vessels passing through smooth muscle and cartilage (1,2). The more superficial, subepithelial capillary bed is ideally placed, therefore, to cause tissue swelling, internal to layers of increased scar-type collagen seen in asthma (3), thereby adding to obstruction of the lumen during periods of active inflammation (see Fig. 2).

Other than supplying nutrients to the superficial epithelium and bronchial wall, the likely role of the bronchial circulation is to humidify incoming air and to allow thermoregulation through heat loss to inspired gas. Tracheal blood flow at 7 mL/min in the heat-stressed dog (4,5) is indeed greater than maximum flow in cardiac muscle (4 mL/min), skeletal muscle (1 mL/min), or rested steady renal perfusion (4 mL/min) (6). The high-flow, superficial capillary beds connect to larger-capacitance vessels deeper in the airway wall (2,6). These capacitance vessels may have smooth muscle in their walls that

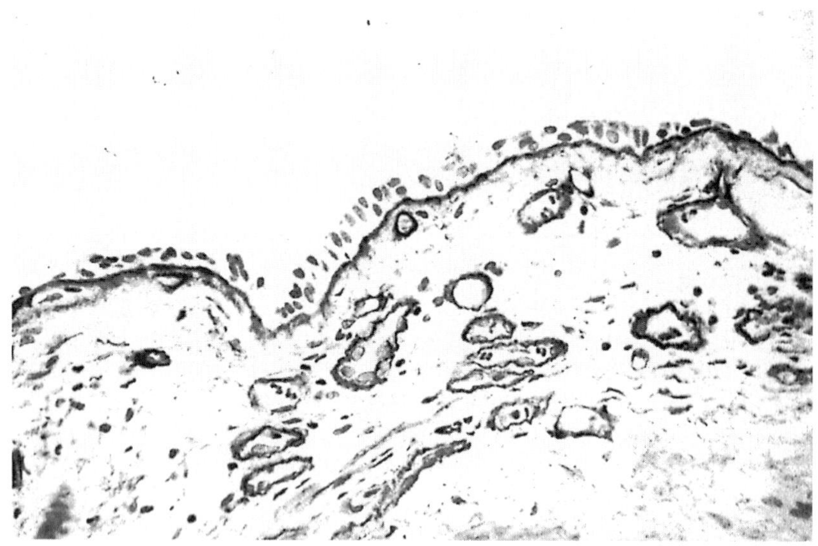

Figure 1   Bronchial biopsy from an asthmatic subject, stained with anticollagen type IV. Basement membranes of the epithelium and vessels are identified. Superficial vessels show adherent inflammatory cells attached to endothelium.

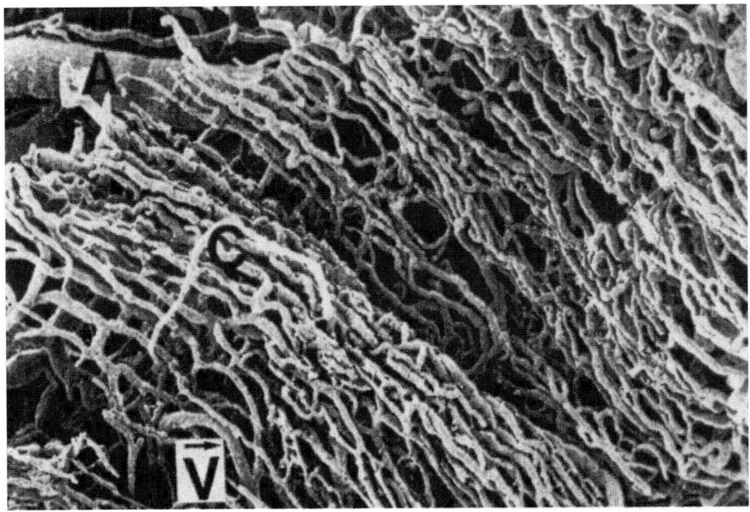

Figure 2 Digestion preparation of airway submucosa, showing the dense capillary plexus (C), afferent arteriole (A), and efferent venule (V). (Scanning electromicrograph by Dr. John Widdicombe (13), with permission of *Thorax*.)

appear similar to venules (2). Increased pressure in this system, associated with vasodilatation, may cause substantial mucosal thickening (7). The implication of this finding is important, indicating some ''reserve'' that may act after provocation to increase vasodilatation. The effect of vascular congestion within the mucosa on airflow will therefore depend on 1) the site of any enhanced vascular response within the airway (depth within the wall, as well as airway caliber), 2) the number and density of vessels at that site, 3) underlying bronchial smooth muscle tone, and 4) preexisting mucosal thickening. In addition to impairment of airflow, there may be reduced compliance of the airway wall (2).

Gross anatomical and microscopic studies of the blood supply to the conducting airways have been reviewed extensively (8–13). Airway vessels have been studied using a number of techniques, including anatomical dissection (14), light and electron microscopy (12,15), angiography (11), silver nitrate staining (16), vascular casts (12,17), and monoclonal antibody staining (18,19). Although much information has been gained regarding the bronchial circulation from animal studies, many animal models show major differences from the structure of human airways. For example, rats and guinea pigs provide ideal models for the study of airway inflammation (12,20) and airflow obstruction (20). For the study of airway vasculature, however, they are limited because of the formation of a single plexus vessels within the mucosa rather than a system of separate capillary beds connected by capacitance vessels characteristic of the human airway. Much of the evidence described in pharmacological responses of the bronchial vasculature to date comes from studies in dog, guinea pig, and rat models, for which comparative studies are not yet available in humans.

II. Quantitation of Bronchial Vasculature in Asthma

The airway in human asthma is accessible for study from only three sources. Postmortem material has the advantages of being potentially well characterized on clinical grounds and available in sufficient amounts for detailed studies (21–26). Specimens from lung resection also have the advantage of being available in reasonable quantities for study; however, they are available infrequently and may be complicated by other factors such as cigarette smoking injury (18). The use of fiberoptic bronchoscopy has allowed repeated interventions in well-characterized asthmatic volunteers, as well as the study of immunological challenge and pharmacological intervention (27–31). Fiberoptic bronchoscopy has also allowed the study of relatively well-characterized, mild asthmatics. Early studies attempted to quantitate vascularity using nonspecific stains. Beasley and colleagues (32) used an azure II–methylene blue–basic fuchsin method and found 123 vessels/mm² in controls, and 142 vessels/mm² in subjects with mild asthma (see Table 1). There was no difference between groups and neither total vascularity nor vessel size was measured. Kuwano and co-workers used an antibody to Factor VIII antigen to study vessel numbers and vascularity in asthmatic and control airways from resected lung and postmortem specimens (18). They found an airway vascularity of 3.3% in asthma and 0.6% in control subjects. A valid conclusion from this study would be that airway vascularity alone was unlikely to have contributed significantly to airflow obstruction in asthma.

In a detailed study of postmortem material from fatal asthma, nonfatal asthma, and controls, Carroll and colleagues also used a monoclonal antibody to Factor VIII antigen to measure vessels and their size (25). They found an increase in the number of larger blood vessels in patients with fatal asthma, suggesting that vascular congestion associated with an acute severe asthma attack may cause distended blood vessels. The finding that there were similar

Table 1 Comparison of Studies Quantifying Large Airway Vascularity in Asthma

Ref.	Tissue	Stain	Control		Asthma	
			Vascularity	Vessels/mm^2	Vascularity	Vessels/mm^2
Beasley et al. (32)	Bronchoscopic biopsy	Azure II methy-lene blue basic fushsin		123		142
Kuwano et al. (18)	Post mortem/re-sected lung	Anti-Factor VIII Ag	0.6	320	3.3	465
Carroll et al. (25)	Post mortem	Anti-Factor VIII Ag	6.6	155	10.2	231
Li and Wilson (19)	Bronchoscopic biopsy	Anticollagen type IV	10.3	539	17.2	738
Orsida et al. (31)	Bronchoscopic biopsy	Anticollagen type IV	10.1	329	5.6	485

numbers of vessels in controls (280/mm^2), nonfatal asthma (260/mm^2), and fatal asthma (250/mm^2) led to the conclusion that increased vessel numbers in asthma must therefore be a reflection of the increased wall thickness, rather than a causative factor.

While examining the distribution of scar-type collagen in the asthmatic airway (collagen I, III, V), it became clear that collagen type IV (a component of true epithelial basement membrane) was clearly capable of identifying vessels in the airway submucosa (19) (see Figs. 3 and 4). By comparison to previous studies using Factor VIII antigen, significantly more vessels were detected in both groups. Asthmatics have an increase in density of vessels (738/mm^2) compared to controls (539/mm^2). Airway vascularity was also increased in asthma (16.8%) compared to controls (10.3%) (see Table 1). These findings indicate that the method of vessel identification is crucial to determination of airway vascularity and the likelihood of vessel proliferation in asthma. A number of comparisons can be made between the studies on postmortem and the

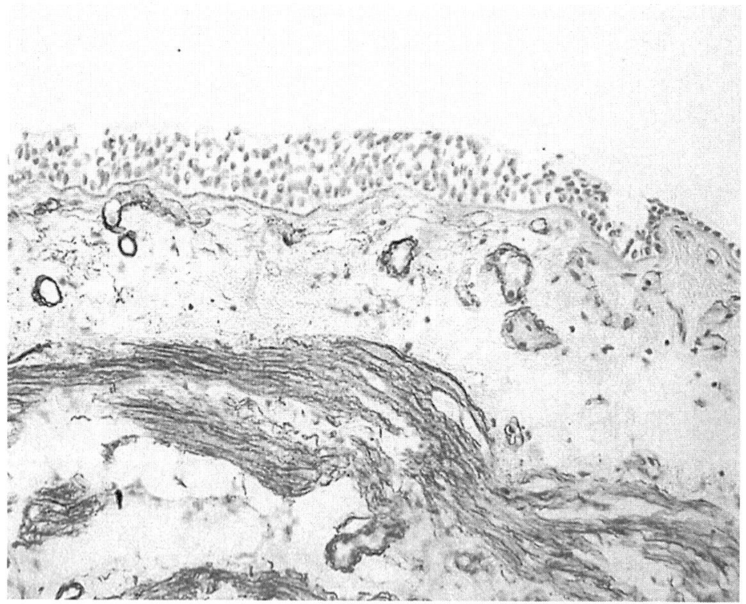

Figure 3 Bronchial biopsy from a control subject, stained with anticollagen type IV. Basement membranes of the epithelium and vessels are identified between the muscularis and the true basement membrane.

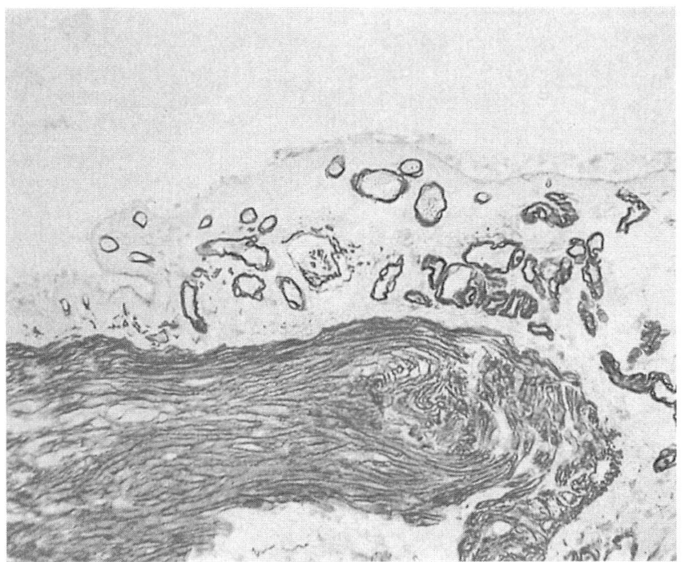

Figure 4 Bronchial biopsy from an asthmatic subject, stained with anticollagen type IV. In addition to staining of basement membranes, increased smooth muscle fibers are surrounded by collagen IV.

resected lung using Factor VIII antigen to determine vessel numbers and size. In neither study were specimens perfused and in both proximal airways were examined. There is little concordance between estimates of vascularity (as percent of section) and vessel density per square millimeter. In the fiberoptic bronchoscopy study (19), smaller pieces of proximal airway were obtained, but fixed and embedded by a similar means. More detailed studies are therefore required to identify the vessels as capillaries, venules, or lymphatics in the superficial submucosa. Considerable difficulties still remain in trying to identify the nature of specific vessels, particularly the subgroup accounting for the apparent increase in asthma. Immunohistochemical techniques using monoclonal antibodies to platelet-endothelial cell adhesion molecule-I (PECAM-1, CD31) may detect a high proportion of the vessels in the microcirculation (33,34). Selective staining of blood vessels but not lymphatics can be achieved using the specific monoclonal antibody PAL-E (35). Using a combined approach, the determination of lymphatic vessel density may be possible in microcirculatory beds (36). Possibly, vessels not detected by staining with Factor

VIII antigen may be either lymphatics or capillaries detectable with anti-PECAM-1. The term "angiogenesis" must be used cautiously in this setting, as the two-dimensional section may be unable to distinguish between elongation and folding of vessels, endothelial proliferation with vessel expansion, and true capillary budding in a three-dimensional sense.

III. Airway Inflammation and Increased Vascularity

A large body of work now exists describing the characteristics changes of airway injury and its inflammatory response in asthma. The capillary bed of the bronchial wall may respond to inflammatory products including soluble mediators and growth factors through a combination of vasodilatation, angiogenesis, and microvascular leakage.

A wide range of vasoactive mediators, cytokines, and physical factors are known to induce a vascular response, many of which are directly relevant to the airway wall in active asthma (see Table 2). Major difficulties exist in the interpretation of the specific role of many of these factors, given that original descriptions apply to animal models, in vitro conditions, tissues other than the

Table 2 Growth Factors and Inflammatory Mediators Capable of Stimulating a Vascular Response

Angiogenesis	Vasodilation	Microvascular leakage
Histamine	Histamine	O_2^-
NO	Tryptase	Adenosine
LTC2	Heparin	Histamine
PGD2	Angiogenin	Bradykinin
PG12	TNFα	SP
PAF	TGFα	CGRP
NK1	TGFβ	NK1
VIP	VEGF	LTB4
CGRP	bFGF	LTC4
TNFα	aFGF	LTD4
IL-1	IL-4	PAF
IL-6	EGF	TNFα
	EC matrix	VEGF/VPF
		ET-1

airway, and often in isolation from important synergistic influences that may be relevant to human asthma. The major preformed mast cell mediator histamine may exert potent effects on the airway wall including contraction of bronchial smooth muscle, increased mucous production, vasodilatation, and increased vascular permeability (37). The vasoactive role of histamine assumes importance because of the close proximity of mast cells to vessels in the airway microcirculation. Possibly, mast cells have migrated from vessels during active inflammation; however, their degranulation in the proximity of vessels releasing histamine may act either directly or indirectly through a neural axon reflex to induce tissue swelling through vasodilation or enhanced capillary leakage. The potential for tissue expansion attributable to histamine is well demonstrated by the dermal response seen after the use of histamine as a positive control in skin prick testing for allergen responsiveness.

Nitric oxide may potentially be produced by three enzymes, the nitric oxide synthases (NOS). NOS I is primarily produced by neural tissue, inducible NOS II is produced by inflammatory cells, and constitutive NOS III by vascular endothelium (38). Hence, ongoing inflammation and involvement of the endothelium itself may lead to autoregulation of vascular tone (39). It is now accepted that exhaled nitric oxide levels are increased in asthma and may be a surrogate marker of activity for the inflammatory response in the airway (40).

Of the newly generated prostanoid mediators produced by mast cells after allergen challenge, PGI_2, PGD_2, and LTC_4 are all known to be capable of causing vasodilatation. They are potent contributors to the classic type I response to allergen in the asthmatic airway through multiple mechanisms (37,41). Platelet acting factor has a wide range of biological actions relevant to asthma, including eosinophil chemotaxis (42), bronchoconstriction (43), as well as increased vascular permeability and mucosal edema (44). Although not considered a major mediator in asthma, partly because of a relative lack of potency of PAF antagonists, its potent vasodilator properties and its potential elaboration by eosinophils suggest a role in active asthma (45). The proinflammatory cytokines IL-1, IL-6, and TNFα are produced by stimulated monocyte/macrophages and are associated with an acute-phase response to infection (46). Increased production of these factors in the asthmatic airway (47,48) and the production of IL-6 and TNFα by mast cells (48) in stable asthma may indicate a more long-term role in the asthmatic response involving regulation of cell function and structural remodeling, rather than the accepted classic early and late asthmatic responses (EAR and LAR) alone.

IV. Angiogenesis

The finding of increased numbers of vessels in the airway in asthma (19) is not surprising, given the presence of replicating endothelial cells in vessels in asthma (see Fig. 5). For some time, histamine has been thought to be capable of stimulating new vessel growth following studies of the chick cornea (49). This has been confirmed more recently, and has been shown to act through both H_1 and H_2 receptors (50).

Evidence has accumulated over some years that heparin, the major glycosaminoglycan constituent of mast cell granules, may be angiogenic (51,52). Because of its action in regulating the binding of specific growth factors to basement membranes and glycosaminoglycan matrix, it has not yet been determined whether heparin acts predominantly in a direct or indirect manner to stimulate endothelial cell growth.

The major human mast cell protease tryptase, which binds to protease-activated receptors (PAR) on cells in a variety of tissues, may also be angiogenic. Many other growth factors recently found to be present in asthma have

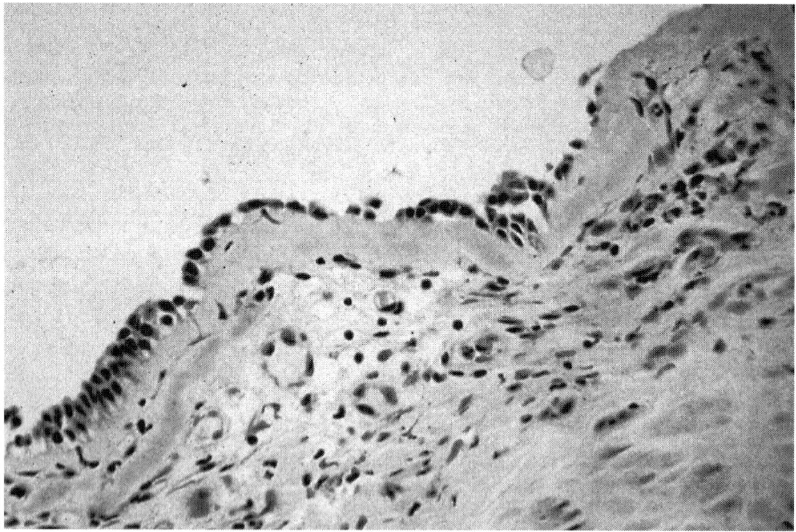

Figure 5 Bronchial biopsy from an asthmatic subject, stained with antibody to proliferating cell nuclear antigen (PCNA). Note positive epithelium, subepithelial myofibroblasts, and endothelial cells in vessel walls.

angiogenic potential (53). Fibroblast growth factors (acidic aFGF and basic bFGF) are potent angiogenic agents (54). Interestingly, bFGF may be sequested and localized by extracellular matrix at specific sites (55). This apparent localization of an angiogenic factor may promote growth of the dense subepithelial plexus of vessels seen in asthma (19).

Vascular endothelial growth factor (VEGF) is a heparin-binding protein that is relatively specific for the stimulation of endothelial cells (56). In addition, VEGF may regulate cell adhesion molecule expression on endothelial cells, thereby influencing transendothelial migration of inflammatory cells. It exhibits high-level homology with vascular permeability factor (VPF), suggesting a mechanistic link between microvascular leakage and angiogenesis related by components with structural identity (57). Transforming growth factor-β (TGF-β) has multiple actions of relevance to airway wall remodeling in asthma (58). The TGF-β family (β1, β2, and β3) have various actions depending on the influence of serine protease inhibitors (59,60).

Interleukin-4 (IL-4) is of specific interest, other than being in the cluster of Th_2 cytokines characteristic of the allergic-type inflammatory response in the asthmatic airway (61). It has been shown to play an important role in regulating TNFα-dependent expression of endothelial cell adhesion molecules. In addition, IL-4 enhances endothelial cell proliferation in capillaries (62). Possibly, a dominance of the Th_2-type phenotype may predispose to vascular remodeling in the airway wall. Many of the matrix molecules present in the airway wall are capable of inducing endothelial growth migration and differentiation (53). Laminin, as well as collagens III and IV, are proliferative stimuli for endothelial cells (64).

Physical factors, including mechanical stress, applied to vessels may act either directly to enhance vessel growth or indirectly through the release of growth factors to enhance endothelial cell replication (65,66). The airway wall in asthma is subjected to stress and sheer forces associated with mucosal swelling and smooth muscle contraction. These forces, above those present in the normal airway, may well be a stimulus for vessel proliferation.

V. Microvascular Leakage

Despite early descriptions of airway wall edema in fatal asthma (21), this aspect of airway inflammation remains one of the most important yet most difficult to study. Much information gained from observational studies of the airway in asthma is based on cell, molecule, or vessel concentration per square millimeter. Should tissue expansion occur because of capillary leakage, the denominator may show considerable variation. Values derived may indeed be underrepresentative because of airway wall swelling. Mast cell mediators including histamine (acting through H_1 and H_2 receptors) may cause capillary leakage. Newly generated eicosanoids, including LTB_4, C_4, and LTD_4 are also implicated (67). Endothelial cells may be capable of autoregulation, through the production of leukotrienes (68). Although unable to produce LTA_4 because of an inability to express 5-lipoxygenase, they may, however, metabolize LTA_4 produced by other cells (69). Downstream metabolic products, particularly LTC_4, are potent inducers of vascular permeability. In addition to a vasodilatory action, PAF is also shown to cause mucosal edema (44). Of the neurokinins, NKA and substance P (SP) can cause capillary leakage through axonal stimulation (70). Vascular permeability factor (VPF), which is identical to VEGF apart from a 24-amino-acid insert, is a member of the platelet-derived growth factor family (PDGF) (57). It is tempting to speculate that capillary leakage is followed by angiogenesis when VPF is cleaved to form VEGF.

McDonald and co-workers have provided some insight into the relationship between inflammation and capillary leakage in the airway using the rat model (71,72). In a review of microvascular leakage within the airway, they identify a range of methods for assessing plasma leakage, including labeling with Evans blue (73), iodine [131]I (74), fluorescine (75), Monastral blue (71), India ink (76), and fluorescent microspheres (72). Identification of leakage in human asthma is more difficult, being less able to rely on tracer substances for quantitation.

Rather than identify the presence of edema in human tissues, its occurrence is assumed, based on the observed presence of intercellular gaps (32,77,78). Qualitative assessment of tissue spaces has found little difference between mucosal edema in asthma, chronic bronchitis, or normal subjects (28,79).

The leakage of plasma into the airway wall occurs with the opening of intercellular endothelial gaps, predominantly in postcapillary venules (71,80). Gaps that occur in capillaries are indeed small in relation to endothelial cell area, occupying less than 3% of the total endothelium (81). The formation of endothelial gaps is mediated through a rise in intracellular calcium and actin-myosin-dependent contractility (82). Factors regulating endothelial leakage are reviewed in detail elsewhere (83). Given the significant number of inflammatory mediators associated with microvascular leakage, it will be reasonable to propose that vessels in contact with activated leukocytes would be most susceptible to leakage. Baluk and co-workers used allergen-sensitized rats to study early- and late-phase plasma leakage. They found that capillaries and arterioles did not leak and that endothelial gap formation occurred predominantly in venules. Only 6% of gaps were associated with leukocyte adhesion and most leakage apparently occurred in small vessels upstream to adherent leukocytes (84).

Microvascular leakage results in increased local hydrostatic pressure, under the influence of Starling equilibrium forces. Of importance for the role of inflammation in the airway wall is the eventual resolution of airway wall edema. Minimal inflammatory lesions of the airway result in significant microvascular leakage with eventual exudation into the airway lumen of larger airways (85,86). This effect may possibly be confined to large but not small airways (87). Indeed, measurable levels of mediators, cytokines, and plasma proteins (including albumin) in bronchial lavage fluid are, to a large part, dependent on diffusion from the submucosa across the epithelial basement membrane and into the airway lumen. It is tempting to speculate that measurable levels of albumin may act as an index for microvascular leakage. Widdicombe (2) has drawn attention to this point, indicating that albumin may be actively transported across the airway epithelium, thereby complicating interpretation of results (88,89). The estimation of true capillary leakage in the airway wall remains problematic, but may be addressed by the identification of macromolecules (such as α_2-macroglobulin) or the use of fluorscein as a tracer substance.

In examining the overall importance of the contribution of microvasculature to airflow obstruction in asthma, the contribution from vessel number and size may be of little importance compared to the increase in wall thickness attributable to edema and the site of mucosal thickening.

VI. Airflow and Bronchial Vasculature

Bronchial microcirculation may influence airflow through mechanisms of bronchial wall thickening (vasodilatation, angiogenesis, microvascular leakage) and through the production of inflammatory mediators and cytokines. In addition, the bronchial circulation has an indirect role by acting as the portal of entry of inflammatory cells to the submucosa during the inflammatory response. Evidence for the role of the bronchial circulation in airflow obstruction has come from histopathological studies in asthmatics, animal models, and the example of left ventricular failure. The specific importance of the vasculature in airflow obstruction may depend on 1) stimulus for bronchoconstriction, and 2) the site of microvascular dilatation or leakage.

The observation of bronchial vascular swelling in severe asthma has been documented in postmortem studies and at bronchoscopy (19,21,25,90–92). The interpretation of these observations, taking into account recent experimental studies, has led to various interpretations of the way airway wall thickening contributes to airflow obstruction (93–98). Initial comparison with vascular mechanisms applicable to the nasal mucosa illustrates the potential for lumenal occlusion. However, structural differences limit the value of this comparison (98). Vascular engorgement may occur within the confine of a poorly distensible airway (99), a denser submucosal collagen network (3), and a thickened muscularis (100). Indeed, whether the tissue expansion attributable to edema in the airway wall leads to an *outward* expansion or an *inward* expansion obstructing the lumen is highly dependent on the initial size of the airway (with smaller airways being less vascular) and the degree of surrounding airway remodeling (101). As few bronchially active substances are capable of acting on airways with muscle alone without affecting bronchial vascular tone, the use of specific pharmacological challenges has been of little use in dissecting the proportional contribution of the way smooth muscle and bronchial vascular tone change in acute bronchoconstriction. Indirectly, airway smooth muscle contraction may result in bronchial mucosal hyperaemia with capillary congestion and secondary vascular swelling.

The phenomenon of airflow obstruction in left ventricular failure is an example of the potential role of bronchial circulation in airflow obstruction (102). In addition to airflow obstruction, the bronchial wall has been shown to be radiologically thicker in left ventricular failure (103). In addition, airway reactivity to methacholine is known to be enhanced in left ventricular failure (104). Interestingly, the associated increased bronchial reactivity was abolished by methoxamine (an α-adrenergic antagonist), suggesting that subsequent bronchial vasoconstriction prevented the phenomenon. Additional work examining airflow and bronchial responsiveness after fluid loading has found a causal relationship. Although this circumstantial evidence is helpful, there are no direct measurements of tracheobronchial blood flow in humans to date. Observation at bronchoscopy has provided relatively gross descriptions of blanching followed by hyperemia after allergen exposure (105).

Well-developed animal models have investigated the role of fluid loading, bronchial provocation, and pharmacological intervention. Animal studies ideally relate bronchial blood flow and airflow in vivo (97,98). Studies in sheep found that histamine-induced airflow obstruction and bronchial vasodilatation were prevented by chlorpheniramine (H_1 antagonism) and metiamide (H_2 antagonism), indicating independent mechanisms (106). Similar studies in pigs have found abolition of bronchial obstruction with histamine by terfenadine (H_1 antagonism), while vasodilatation was reduced only partly by the addition of cimetidine (H_2 antagonism) (107). It was subsequently suggested that bronchial blood flow changes during the acute asthmatic response were related to inflammatory mediator release (106). It is tempting, therefore, to speculate a relationship between tracheobronchial vasodilators such as histamine and acetylcholine and airflow obstruction. However, both are constrictors of airway smooth muscle in vitro (108). Again, the independent contributions of smooth muscle and vascular responses become impossible to fully distinguish. Detailed studies of distribution of blood flow in histamine-provoked sheep indicated a selective increase in mucosal and submucosal blood flow, up to 15 times above baseline (109).

Of interest is the finding that either saline or blood infusion could cause vascular congestion and exudation, leading to increased airway wall thickness (98) (see Fig. 6). Saline caused considerably more airway wall thickening than blood, presumably because of a component of edema formation associated with crystalloid infusion. In a series of important studies, Wagner and Mitzner have examined airflow and responsiveness to methacholine and correlated them with lumenal area and airway wall thickness using high-resolution CT scanning (110–113). Although hyperperfusion of the bronchial circulation re-

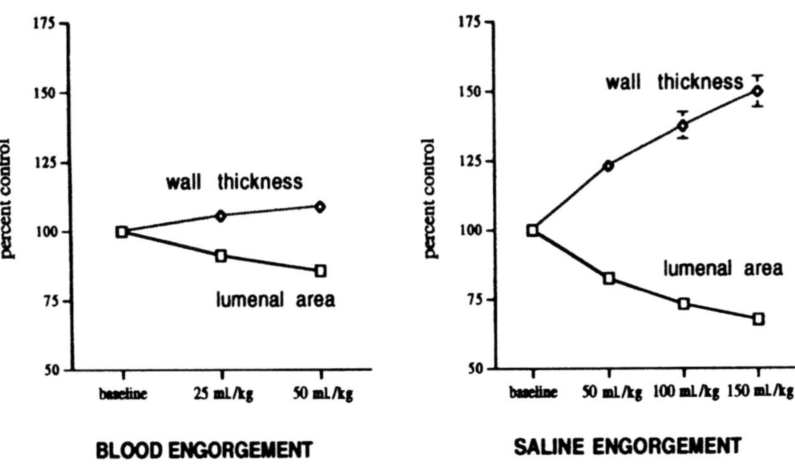

Figure 6 The relationship between fluid loading and airway wall thickness after either saline or blood. (From Ref. 98.)

sulted in no change in baseline airway resistance or methacholine responsiveness, there were considerable reductions in airway lumenal area associated with increasing airway wall thickness (see Fig. 7). With these results, it is tempting to speculate that airway wall thickness secondary to vascular engorgement is a significant cause of airflow obstruction. It is clear however, that vascular responses alone do not account for asthma (98). In addition to wall thickness, other factors including distribution of airflow (longitudinal and cross-sectional), activation of sensory nerve endings, structural changes in the airway wall, as well as clearance of inflammatory mediators are confounding factors likely to act in concert with vascular changes (97).

Vascular remodeling may increase airway wall thickness by the process of angiogenesis, dilatation, or permeability (see Fig. 8). Current techniques of investigation of the airway in asthmatic volunteers have not allowed an accurate estimation of the contribution of the airway circulation in acute or chronic airflow obstruction. However, given that adequate circumstantial evidence exists for a role in asthma, it is possible that future studies will link the immunological stimuli for vascular remodeling with bronchial wall thickening and clinical asthma.

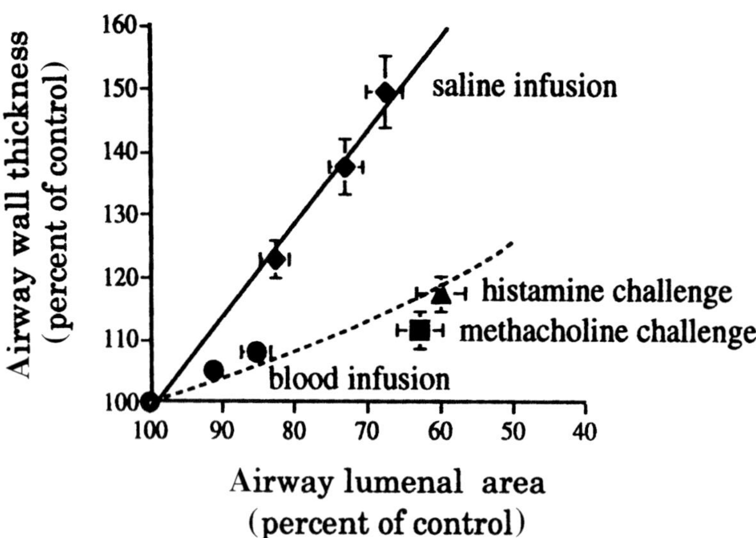

Figure 7 The relationship between wall thickness and lumenal narrowing in fluid-loaded sheep. (From Ref. 98.)

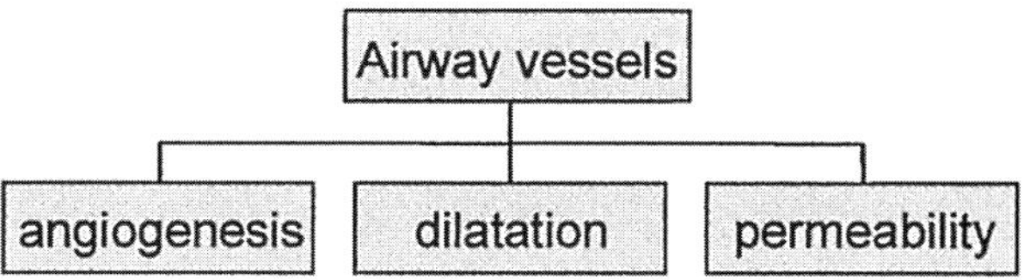

Figure 8 The role of vessels in airway remodeling.

Acknowledgments

The authors wish to thank Ms. Barbara Welton for assistance with the manuscript and Ms. Tiffany Bamford for technical assistance. Work was supported by grants from the NHMRC and Government Employees Medical Research Fund.

References

1. Magno M, Fishman AP. Origin, distribution, and blood flow of bronchial circulation in anesthetised sheep. J Appl Physiol 1982; 53:272–279.
2. Widdicombe J. Physiologic control: anatomy and physiology of the airway circulation. Am Rev Respir Dis 1992; 146:S3–S7.
3. Wilson JW, Li X. The measurement of reticular basement membrane and submucosal collagen in the asthmatic airway. Clin Exp Allergy 1997; 27:363–371.
4. Baile EM, Guillemi S, Paré PD. Tracheobronchial and upper airway blood flow in dogs during thermally-induced panting. J Appl Physiol 1987; 63:2240–2246.
5. Baile EM, Paré PD. Methods of measuring bronchial blood flow. In: Butler J, ed. The Bronchial Circulation. New York: Marcel Dekker, 1992:101–180.
6. Schindt RF, Thews T. Human Physiology, 2nd ed. Berlin: Springer, 1987:506.
7. Corfield DR, Hanafi Z, Webber SE, Widdicombe JG. Changes in tracheal mucosa thickness and blood flow in sheep. J Appl Physiol 1991; 71:1282–1288.
8. Aviado DM. The bronchial circulation. In: Aviado DM, ed. The Lung Circulation. Oxford: Pergamon Press, 1965:185–254.
9. Cudkowicz L. Bronchial arterial circulation in man. In: Moser KM, ed. Pulmonary Vascular Diseases. New York: Marcel Dekker, 1979:111–232.
10. Butler J, ed. The Bronchial Circulation. New York: Marcel Dekker, 1991.
11. Berry JL, Brailsford JF, Daly IDB. The bronchial vascular system in the dog. Proc R Soc Lond 1931; 109:214–228.
12. McDonald DM. The ultrastructure and permeability of tracheobronchial blood vessels in health and disease. Eur Respir J 1990; 3(Suppl 12):572s–585s.

13.   Widdicombe J. Why are the airways so vascular? Thorax 1993; 48:290–295.

14.   Nagaishi C. Functional Anatomy and Histology of the Lung. Baltimore: University Park Press, 1972.

15.   Laitinen A, Laitinen LA. Vascular beds in the airways of normal subjects and asthmatics. Eur Respir J 1990; 3:658s–662s.

16.   McDonald DM. Endothelial gaps and permeability of venules in rat tracheas exposed to inflammatory stimuli. Am J Physiol 1994; 266:L61–L83.

17.   Laitinen A, Laitinen LA, Widdicombe JG. Organisation and structure of the tracheal and bronchial blood vessels in the dog. J Anat 1989; 165:133–140.

18.   Kuwano K, Bosken CH, Paré PD, Bai TR, Wiggs BR, Hogg JC. Small airways dimensions in asthma and in chronic obstructive pulmonary disease. Am Rev Respir Dis 1993; 149:1220–1225.

19.   Li X, Wilson JW. Increased vascularity of the bronchial mucosa in mild asthma. Am J Respir Crit Care Med 1997; 156:229–233.

20.   Hutson PA, Church MK, Clay TP, Miller P, Holgate ST. Early and late-phase bronchosconstriction after allergen challenge of nonanesthetised guinea pigs. I. The association of disordered airway physiology to leukocyte infiltration. Am Rev Respir Dis 1988; 137:548–557.

21.   Dunnill MS. The pathology of asthma, with special reference to the bronchial mucosa. J Clin Pathol 1960; 13:27–33.

22.   Dunnill MS, Massarella GR, Anderson JA. A comparison of the quantitative anatomy of the bronchi in normal subjects, in status asthmaticus, in chronic bronchitis and in emphysema. Thorax 1969; 24:176–179.

23.   Jeffery PK. Pathology of asthma. Br Med Bull 1992; 48:23–39.

24.   Hogg JC. Pathology of asthma. J Allergy Clin Immunol 993; 92:1–5.

25.   Carroll NG, Cooke C, James AL. Bronchial blood vessel dimensions in asthma. Am J Respir Crit Care Med 1997; 155:689–695.

26.   Carroll N, Elliot J, Morton A, James A. The structure of large and small airways in nonfatal and fatal asthma. Am Rev Respir Dis 1993; 147:405–410.

27.   Djukanovic R, Wilson JW, Lai CKW, et al. The safety aspects of fiberoptic bronchoscopy, bronchoalveolar lavage and endobronchial biopsy in asthma. Am Rev Respir Dis 1991; 143:772–777.

28.   Jeffery PK, Wardlaw AJ, Nelson FC, Collins JV, Kay AB. Bronchial biopsies in asthma: An ultrastructural, quantitative study and correlation with hyperreactivity. Am Rev Respir Dis 1989; 140:1745–1753.

29.   Djukanovic R, Wilson JW, Britten DM, et al. Effect of an inhaled corticosteroid on airway inflammation and symptoms in asthma. Am Rev Respir Dis 1992; 145:669–674.

30.   Wilson JW, Djukanovic R, Howarth PH, Holgate ST. Lymphocyte activation in BAL and peripheral blood in atopic asthmatics. Am Rev Respir Dis 1992; 145:958–960.

31.   Orsida B, Li X, Hickey B, Thien F, Wilson JW, Walters EH. Increase in subepithelial vessels in moderate asthma and the effect of inhaled glucocorticoid therapy on vascularity. Thorax 1999; 54:289–295.

32. Beasley R, Roche WR, Roberts JA, Holgate ST. Cellular events in the bronchi in mild asthma and after bronchial provocation. Am Rev Respir Dis 1989; 139: 906–817.

33. Newman PJ, Berndt MC, Gorski J, White GC II, Lyman S, Paddock C, Muller WA. PECAM-1 (CD31) cloning and relation to adhesion molecules of the immunoglobulin gene superfamily. Science 1990; 247:1219–1222.

34. Erhard H, Rietveld FJR, Bröcker eB, de Waal RMW, Ruiter DJ. Penotype of normal cutaneous microvasculature. J Invest Dermatol 1996; 106:135–140.

35. Schlingemann RO, Dingjan GM, Emeis JJ, Blok J, Warnaar SO, Ruiter DJ. Monoclonal antibody PAL-E specific for endothelium. Lab Invest 1985; 52: 71–76.

36. de Waal RM, van Altena MC, Erhard H, Weidle UH, Nooijen PTGA, Ruiter DJ. Lack of lymphangiogenesis in human primary cutaneous melanoma. Consequences for the mechanism of lymphatic dissemination. Am J Pathol 1997; 150: 1951–1957.

37. Bradding P, Walls AF, Church MK. The role of mast cells and basophils in asthma. In: Holgate ST, ed. Immunopharmacology of the Respiratory System. London: Academic Press, 1995:147–168.

38. Schmidt HHHW, Walter U. NO at work. Cell 1994; 78:919–925.

39. Dinh-Xuan AT. Endothelial modulation of pulmonary vascular tone. Eur Respir J 1992; 5:757–762.

40. Texeroux J, Nguyen-Huu L, Dinh-Xuan AT. Role of NO in asthma. Rev Pneumol Clin 1998; 54 (Suppl 1):S9–S10.

41. Holgate ST, Djukanovic R, Wilson J, Roche W, Britten K, Howarth PH. Allergic inflammation and its pharmacological modulation in asthma. Int Arch Allergy Appl Immunol 1991; 94:210–217.

42. Wardlaw AJ, Moqbel R, Cromwell O, Kay AB. Platelet activating factor. A potent chemotactic and chemokinetic factor for human eosinophils. J Clin Invest 1986; 78:1701–1706.

43. Rubin AE, Smith LJ, Patterson R. The bronchoconstrictor properties of platelet-activating factor in human. Am Rev Respir Dis 1987; 136:1145–1151.

44. Evans TW, Chung K, Rogers DF, Barnes PJ. Effects of platelet-activating factor on airway vascular permeability: possible mechanisms. J Appl Physiol 1987; 63:479–484.

45. Spry CJ, Kay AB, Gleich GJ. Eosinophils 1992. Immuunol Today 1992; 13: 384–387.

46. Lovett D, Kozan B, Hadam M, Resch K, Gemsa D. Macrophage cytotoxicity: interleukin 1 as a mediator of tumor cytostasis. J Immunol 1986; 136:340–347.

47. Mattoli S, Mattoso VL, Soloperto M, Allegra L, Fasoli A. Cellular and biochemical characteristics of bronchoalveolar lavage fluid in symptomatic nonallergic asthma. J Allergy Clin Immunol 1991; 84:794–803.

48. Bradding P, Roberts JA, Britten KA, Montefort S, Djukanovic R, Mueller R, Huesser CH, Howarth PH, Holgate ST. Interleukin-4, -5 and -6 and tumor necrosis factor-α in normal and asthmatic airways: evidence of the human mast

cell as a source for these cytokines. Am J Respir Cell Mol Biol 1994; 10:471–480.

49. Marks RM, Roche WR, Czerniecki M, Penny R, Nelson DS. Mast cell granules cause proliferation of human microvascular endothelial cells. Lab Invest 1986; 55:289–294.

50. Sorbo J, Jakobsson A, Norrby K. Mast-cell histamine is angiogenic through receptors for histamine$_1$ and histamine$_2$. Int J Exp Pathol 1994; 75:343–350.

51. Azizkhan RG, Azizkhan JC, Zetter BR, Folkman J. Mast cell heparin stimulates migration of capillary endothelial cells in vitro. J Exp Med 1980; 152:931–944.

52. Roche WR. Mast cells and tumour angiogenesis: the tumor-mediated release of an endothelial growth factor from mast cells. Int J Cancer 1985; 36:721–728.

53. D'Amore PA. Mechanisms of endothelial growth control. Am J Respir Cell Mol Biol 1992; 6:1–8.

54. Klagsbrun M, D'Amore PA. Regulators of angiogenesis. Annu Rev Physiol 1991; 53:217–239.

55. Folkman J, Klagsbrun M, Sasse J, Wadzinski M, Ingber D, Vlodavsky I. A heparin-binding angiogenic protein—basic fibroblast growth factor—is stored within basement membrane. Am J Pathol 1988; 130:393–400.

56. Ferrara N, Henzel WJ. Pituitary follicular cells secrete a novel heparin-binding growth factor specific for vascular endothelial cells. Biochem Biophys Res Commun 1989; 161:851–855.

57. Connolly DT, Heuvelman DM, Nelson R, et al. Tumor vascular permeability factor stimulates endothelial cell growth and angiogenesis. J Clin Invest 1989; 84:1478–1489.

58. Roberts AB, Sporn MB. Transforming growth factor-betas. In: Sporn MB, Robers AB, eds. Handbook of Experimental Pharmacology. Heidelberg: Springer-Verlag, 1990:419–472.

59. Jennings JC, Mohan S, Linkhart TA, Widstrom R, Baylink DJ. Comparison of the biological actions of TGF beta-1 and TGF beta-2: differential activity in endothelial cells. J Cell Biol 1988; 137:167–172.

60. Sato Y, Tsuboi R, Lyons R, Moses H, Rifkin DB. Characterisation of the activation of latent TGF-β by co-cultures of endothelial cells and pericytes or smooth muscle cells: a self-regulating system. J Cell Biol 1990; 111:757–763.

61. Robinson DS, Hamid Q, Ying S, et al. Predominant TH2-like bronchoalveolar T-lymphocyte population in atopic asthma. N Engl J Med 1992; 326:298–304.

62. Toi M, Harris AL, Bicknell R. Interleukin-4 is a potent mitogen for capillary endothelium. Biochem Biophys Res Commun 1991; 174:1287–1293.

63. Ingber DE, Folkman J. How does extracellular matrix control capillary morphogenesis? Cell 1989; 58:803–805.

64. Ingber DE, Madri JA, Folkman J. Endothelial growth factors and extracellular matrix regulate DNA synthesis through modulation of cell and nuclear expansion. In Vitro Cell Dev Biol 1987; 23:387–394.

65. Sumpio BE, Barnes AJ, Levin LG, Johnson G. Mechanical stress stimulates aortic endothelial cells to proliferate. J Vasc Surg 1987; 6:252–256.

66. Tozzi CA, Poiani GJ, Harangozo AM, Boyd CD, Riley DJ. Pressure-induced connective tissue synthesis in pulmonary artery segments is dependent on intact endothelium. J Clin Invest 1989; 84:1005–1012.

67. Brain SD, Williams TJ. Leukotrienes and inflammation. Pharmacol Ther 1990; 46:57–66.

68. Feinmark SJ. The role of the endothelial cell in leukotriene biosynthesis. Am Rev Respir Dis 1992; 146:S51–S55.

69. Feinmark SJ, Cannon PJ. Endothelial cell leukotriene C_4 snythesis results from intercellular transfer of leukotriene A_4 synthesized by polymorphonuclear leukocytes. J Biol Chem 1986; 261:16466–16472.

70. Bertrand C, Geppetti P, Baker J, Yamawaki I, Nadel JA. Role of neurogenic inflammation in antigen-induced vascular extravasation in guinea-pig trachea. J Immunol 1993; 150:1497–1485.

71. McDonald DM. Neurogenic inflammation in the rat trachea. I. Changes in venules, leukocytes and epithelial cells. J Neurocytol 1988; 17:583–603.

72. McDonald DM, Mitchell RA, Gabella G, Haskell A. Neurogenic inflammation in the rat trachea. II. Identity and distribution of nerves mediating the increase in vascular permeability. J Neurocytol 1988; 17:605–628.

73. Saria A, Lundberg JM. Evans blue fluorescence: quantitative and morphological evaluation of vascular permeability in animal tissues. J Neurosci Meth 1983; 8:41–49.

74. Persson CGA. The role of plasma exudation in asthma. Lancet 1986; 42:1126–1128.

75. Hulstrom D, Svensjö E. Intravital and electron microscopic study of bradykinin induced vascular permeability changes using FITC-dextran as a tracer. J Pathol 1979; 129:125–133.

76. Cotran RS, Suter ER, Majno G. The use of colloidal carbon as a tracer for vascular injury. Vasc Dis 1967; 4:107–125.

77. Laitinen LA, Laitinen A. Mucosal inflammation and bronchial hyperreactivity. Eur Respir J 1988; 1:488–489.

78. McDonald DM. The concept of neurogenic inflammation in the respiratory tract. In: Kaliner M, Barnes P, Kunkel G, Baraniuk J, eds. Neuropeptides in the Respiratory Medicine. New York: Marcel Dekker, 1994:321–349.

79. Salvato G. Some histological changes in chronic bronchitis and asthma. Thorax 1968; 23:168–172.

80. Fox J, Galey F, Wayland H. Action of histamine on the mesenteric microvasculature. Microvasc Res 1980; 81:673–676.

81. McDonald DM. Endothelial gaps and permeability of venules in rat tracheas exposed to inflammatory stimuli. Am J Physiol (Lung Cell Mol Physiol) 1994b; 266:L61–L83.

82. Schnittler H-J, Wilke A, Gress T, Suttorp N, Drenck-Hahn D. Role of actin and myosin in the control of paracellular permeability in pig, rat and human vascular endothelium. J Physiol (Lond) 1990; 431:379–401.

83. Bowden JJ, McDonald DM. The microvasculature as a participant in inflammation. In: Holgate ST, ed. Immunopharmacology of the Respiratory System. London: Academic Press, 1995:147–168.

84. Baluk P, Hirata A, Thurston G, McDonald DM. Endothelial gaps and adherent leukocytes in allergen-induced early- and late-phase plasma leakage in rate airways. Am J Pathol 1998; 152:1463–1476.

85. Persson CGA, Erjefalt I, Gustafsson B, Luts A. Subepithelial hydrostatic pressure may regulate plasma exudation across the mucosa. Int Arch Allergy Appl Immunol 1990; 92:148–153.

86. Kondo M, Finkbeiner WE, Widdicombe JH. Changes in permeability of dog tracheal epithelium in response to hydrostatic pressure. Am J Physiol 1992; 262:176–182.

87. Yager D, Kamm RD, Drazen JM. Airway wall liquid. Sources and role as an amplifier of bronchoconstriction. Chest 1995; 107 (Suppl):105S–110S.

88. Webber SE, Widdicombe JG. The transport of albumin across the ferret in vitro whole trachea. J Physiol 1989; 408:457–472.

89. Price AM, Webber SE, Widdibombe JG. Transport of albumin by the rabbit trachea in vitro. J Appl Physiol 1990; 68:726–730.

90. De Burgh Daly I. Interference of intrinsic pulmonary mechanisms as a potential cause of asthma. Edinburgh Med J 1935; 43:139–142.

91. Renault P, Paley PY, Lenegre J, Carouso H. Les alterations bronchiques des cardiaques. J Fr Med Chir Thorac 1943; 3:141–149.

92. Vallery-Radot P, Halpern BN, Dubois de Montreynaud JM, Pean V. Les bronches au cours de la crise d'asthme. Etude experimentale, bronchoscopique et anatomopathologique. Presse Med 1950; 58:661–664.

93. Hogg JC, Paré PD, Moreno R. The effect of submucosal edema in airways resistance. Am Rev Respir Dis 1987; 135:S54–S56.

94. Wiggs BR, Moreno R, Hogg JC, et al. A model of the mechanics of airway narrowing. J Appl Physiol 1990; 69:849–860.

95. Wiggs BR, Bosken C, Paré PD. et al. A model of airway narrowing in asthma and in chronic obstructive pulmonary disease. Am Rev Respir Dis 1992; 145:1251–1258.

96. Lambert RK, Wiggs BR, Kuwano K, et al. Functional significance of increased airway smooth muscle in asthma and COPD. J Appl Physiol 1993; 74:2771–2781.

97. Lockhart A, Dinh-Xuan AT, Regnard J, Cabanes L, Matran R. Effect of airway blood flow on airflow. Am Rev Respir Dis 1992; 146:S19–S23.

98. Mitzner W, Wagner E, Brown RH. Is asthma a vascular disorder? Chest 1995; 107(Suppl):97S–101S.

99. Wilson JW, Li X, Pain MC. The lack of distensibility of asthmatic airways. Am Rev Respir Dis 1993; 148:806–809.

100. Ebina M, Takahashi T, Chiba T, Motomiya M. Cellular hypertrophy and hyperplasia of airway smooth muscle underlying bronchial asthma. Am Rev Respir Dis 1993; 148:720.

101. Smith JC, Mitzner W. Elastic characteristics of the lung perivascular interstital space. J Appl Physiol 1983; 54:1717–1725.

102. Rushmer FJ. Cardiovascular Dynamics, 2nd ed. Philadelphia: Saunders, 1961: 470–471.

103. Gleason DC, Steiner RE. The lateral roentgenogram in pulmonary edema. Am J Roentgenol 1966; 98:279–290.

104. Cabanes LR, Weber SN, Matran R, et al. Bronchial hyperresponsiveness to methacholine in patients with impaired left ventricular function. N Engl J Med 1989; 320:1317–1322.

105. Metzger WJ, Zavala D, Richerson HB, et al. Local allergen and local airway inflammation. Am Rev Respir Dis 1987; 135:433–440.

106. Long WM, Yerger LD, Martinez H, et al. Modification of bronchial blood flow during allergic airway responses. J Appl Physiol 1988; 65:272–282.

107. Alving K. Airways vasodilatation in the immediate allergic reaction: involvement of inflammatory mediators and sensory nerves. Acta Physiol Scand 1991; 141(Suppl):1–64.

108. Laitinen LA, Robinson NP, Laitinen A, Widdicombe JG. Relationship between tracheal mucosal thickness and vascular resistance in dogs. J Appl Physiol 1986; 61:2186–2193.

109. Kramer GG, Lindsey C, Wu CH, Mertens S, Russell LA, Cross CE. Airway blood flow distribution and lung edema after histamine infusion in awake sheep. J Appl Physiol 1988; 65:1847–1854.

110. Wagner EM, Mitzner W. Effect of left atrial pressure on bronchial vascular hemodynamics. J Appl Physiol 1990; 69:837–842.

111. Brown RH, Herold CJ, Hirshman CA, et al. In vivo measurements of airway reactivity using high-resolution computed tomography. Am Rev Respir Dis 1991; 144:208–212.

112. Brown RH, Herold CJ, Hirshman CA, et al. Individual airway constrictor response heterogeneity to histamine assessedy by high resolution computed tomography. J Appl Physiol 1993; 74:2615–2620.

113. Blosser S, Mitzner W, Wagner EM. Effects of increased bronchial blood flow on airway morphometry, resistance and reactivity. J Appl Physiol 1994; 76: 1624–1629.

8

The Extracellular Matrix of the Airways and Bronchial Asthma

WILLIAM R. ROCHE

University of Southampton
and Southampton General Hospital
Southampton, England

Cellular changes in the conducting airways are now recognized as central to the pathogenesis of bronchial asthma. The application of cell and tissue harvesting methods, facilitated by fiberoptic bronchoscopy, has allowed significant advances to be made in the understanding of the mechanisms of airflow obstruction in bronchial asthma. Inflammatory events were the initial focus of this change in research and clinical emphasis but even in early publications, changes in the extracellular matrix were highlighted (1). Increasing awareness of the long-term loss of airway function in patients with asthma (2) has led to attention being focused on the role of changes in the structure of the airways in the production of the characteristic spirometric abnormalities. Computer modeling has shown that thickening of the airway walls is sufficient to explain the exaggerated provocant response and the loss of the plateau in the provocant dose-response curve in patients with asthma (3).

The walls of the airways are composed of a variety of differentiated epithelial and mesenchymal cells, including basal, ciliated and secretory epithelial cells, fibroblasts, myofibroblasts and smooth muscle cells, vascular endothelium, smooth muscle and pericytes, neural and perineural cells, and chondrocytes. The extension of the scope of research efforts from inflammatory events has led to more recent focusing on the responses of the bronchial epithelium and smooth muscle to inflammatory insults and soluble cytokines (4). The extracellular matrix has tended to be ignored in these studies, both in terms of the capacity to the normal extracellular matrix to modulate cellular responses and in terms of the functional consequences of the matrix alterations seen in bronchial asthma.

The extracellular matrix is not an inert filler substance between the functioning cells of an organ but is a variable and dynamic element of the tissues that contributes to both structure and function. These diverse functions are provided by molecules from a range of families, the members of which interact to form composite biological materials. Different members of the collagen family have characteristic distribution patterns in extracellular matrices and are convenient immunohistochemical markers for different forms of matrix (Fig. 1). Fibrillar collagens, such as collagen I and collagen III, provide tensile strength in tissues. Collagen I is found in tissues that experience high tensile stress such as tendons and ligaments while collagen III is distributed in more

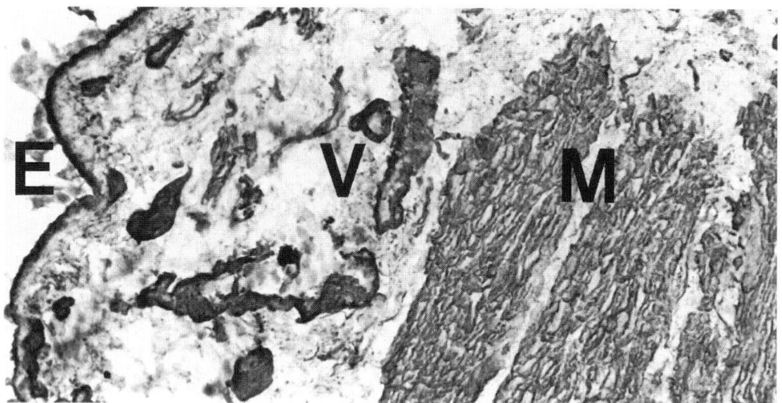

Figure 1 Collagen IV distribution in the bronchial wall. Immunohistochemistry demonstrates collagen IV in the basement membrane beneath the epithelium (E), in vascular basal laminae (V), and around smooth muscle (M). Immunoperoxidase, magnification ×360.

loosely structured connective tissue. Nonfibrillar collagens retain their globular terminal peptides and can contribute to the formation of more open meshworks, such as collagen IV in basement membranes (5). Elastin proteins contribute to the mechanical deformability and recoil of the tissues. Other proteins that contribute to flexible protein networks include the laminins, fibronectin, tenascin, and entactin. These proteins are binding sites for other matrix molecules and also for epithelial and mesenchymal cells. Thus, complex meshworks are formed by the aggregation of multiple species of extracellular matrix molecules in the assembly of specific zones in the extracellular matrix, such as basement membranes (5).

The Functions of the Extracellular Matrix
Provision of mechanical properties of tissues
Cell anchorage
Substrate for cell migration
Signals for cell survival
Site-specific differentiation signals
Growth regulation
Reservoir for cytokines and growth factors
Distribution of tissue water and electrolytes
Filtration
Repair material

The proteoglycans of the extracellular matrix have protein backbones and variable lengths of side chains composed of covalently linked disaccharides. The sugar molecules bear carboxyl and sulfate groups, which contribute the majority of the electrical charge of the matrix. The electrical charge of the extracellular matrix is a major determinant of its affinity for ions and water and hence its filtration capacity. The charges on the matrix molecules are also important in the sequestration of nonmatrix proteins. In inflammatory airways diseases, the most important group of functional proteins to be stored in the matrix are the cytokines and growth factors. Practically all the critical protein mediators of allergic inflammation and tissue remodeling can be encrypted in the extracellular matrix. This alters the time and concentration kinetics of their biological availability to such an extent that cytokines are increasingly, and correctly, regarded as matrix-bound rather than soluble mediators of cellular interactions. Beneath the bronchial epithelium, heparan sulfates of the epithelial basement membrane bind fibroblast-growth factor-2 while the proteoglycan decorin binds transforming growth factor-β in the underlying connective tissue (6).

The physical anchorage of cells to the extracellular matrix is mediated by transmembrane cell adhesion molecules, particularly the dimeric integrins. These molecules are composed of α and β chains. There are fewer different β-chain molecules that determine the major integrin families while the combination of α and β chains confers the specificity of the cell adhesion to individual motifs in matrix molecules. These molecules also have important functions in signal transduction, acting through adhesion complex–associated intracellular kinases (7). The signals sensed by these adhesion molecules and their differential adhesion to components of the extracellular matrix determine many aspects of cellular function. Thus the pericellular matrix can determine the survival, proliferation, or differentiation of the cell populations contained within it. Changes in the matrix, such as associated with wounding of the tissue, can alter the ligands available to the cell and, together with alterations in cell-surface integrins, facilitate processes such as cell migration (8).

In contrast to the information concerning airway inflammation that can be obtained from endoscopic biopsies, investigations of remodeling of the airway wall and the involvement of the extracellular matrix are almost totally dependent on autopsy studies. Although such studies potentially allow for assessment of the full thickness of the airways wall, the findings may be confounded by other variables, including sampling, uncertainty about the diagnosis and treatment of asthma, and postmortem changes. Neither biopsy nor autopsy studies can address the water content of the extracellular matrix of the airways in asthma. Although edema of the airways is described histologically (9), current technology does not allow quantitation of the water content and the effects of treatment. Nevertheless, it is likely that this edema has major effects on the abnormal airways physiology in asthma. The production of a protein-rich exudate in response to inflammatory mediators also suffuses the extracellular matrix with molecules such as plasma fibronectin and fibrinogen, which may become incorporated into the matrix, providing provisional matrices in wound healing (10). The polymerization of fibrin to form fibrinogen also contributes to plugging of the airways lumen in acute severe asthma.

The most obvious change seen in the extracellular matrix in bronchial asthma involves the zone just beneath the epithelial basement membrane of the airways. The matrix immediately beneath the epithelium is formed of distinctive components such as collagen IV, laminin, entactin, and proteoglycans. The heterogeneous complex formed by these molecules constitutes the true epithelial basement membrane, which can be resolved by electron microscopy into two layers, the lamina rara and the lamina densa (Fig. 2). Beneath the lamina densa there is a zone composed of condensed fibrillar collagens and glycoproteins, called the lamina reticularis. The overlying laminae of the basement membrane are anchored to the lamina reticularis by strands of collagen VII (11). Conventional histological preparations reveal a dense eosinophilic band of extracellular matrix beneath the epithelium of the larger conducting airways in asthma. This was initially regarded as representing a thickening of the true epithelial basement membrane but ultrastructural and immunohistochemical studies have demonstrated that this appearance is due to increased depth and density of the lamina reticularis (12). This band contains collagens III, V, and I, tenascin, and fibronectin but none of the components of the true epithelial basement membrane. This phenomenon has been reported in all forms of asthma and it is present early in the disease.

Qualitative changes in the extracellular matrix have also been described in asthma. Tensacin is a branched glycoprotein that is associated with tissue modeling in embryogenesis and is also unregulated in wound healing in adults (13). Tenascin may modulate cell adhesion and allow cell migration in the presence of other highly adhesive glycoproteins, such as fibronectin. The ten-

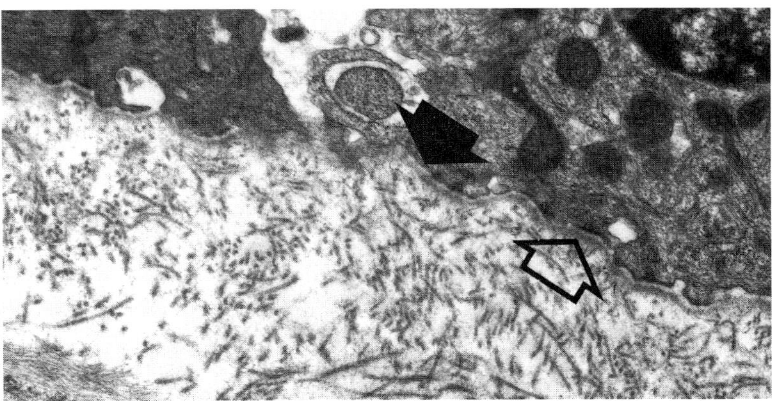

Figure 2 Ultrastructure of the epithelial basement membrane in the bronchus. Beneath the basal aspect of the epithelial cells there is a basal lamina, consisting of a lamina rara (solid arrow) and lamina densa (open arrow). Electron microscopy, uranyl acetate and lead citrate, magnification ×20,000.

ascin immunoreactivity of the bronchial lamina reticularis is reported to be increased in asthma and to decline in response to inhaled corticosteroids (14). Fetal laminins have also been described to reappear in the airway basement membrane in asthma (15). It is presently unclear whether these changes simply reflect epithelial cell injury and repair or in themselves produce alterations in the bronchial epithelial cell phenotype, through altered integrin-mediated signaling.

The pathophysiological significance of the alterations in the bronchial lamina reticularis in asthma is unclear. While the thickening of the lamina reticularis in itself may contribute little to reduction of the caliber of the airways, the stiffening effect of these changes may cause buckling of the mucosal outline when the airway smooth muscle is contracted. It more important that these changes are recognized as evidence of a disequilibrium in the normal regulatory networks acting between the epithelium and the underlying mesenchyme and may thus reflect remodeling changes throughout the airway wall. Such mesenchymal alterations are likely to be the mechanism of the progressive and irreversible loss of airway function that is seen in asthma.

The presence of an increased amount of interstitial collagen beneath the epithelial basement membrane in the airways in asthma led to a search for the cells responsible for the deposition of this material. Careful sequential sectioning and examination of mucosal biopsies at the ultrastructural level (Fig. 3) resulted in the description of a population of specialized mesenchymal cells immediately beneath the lamina reticularis (16). These cells have both the synthetic apparatus of fibroblasts in the form of rough endoplasmic reticulum and contractile thick and thin fibers, indicative of the actin-myosin complexes seen in smooth muscle. This combination of features identifies these cells as myofibroblasts. Myofibroblasts were initially described as a cell population involved in wound healing (17), where the combination of their synthetic and contractile functions plays an important role in contraction of repair tissue and the deposition of scar tissue. Subsequently, it was recognized that there are populations of cells with the constitutive phenotype of myofibroblasts in diverse anatomical locations such as Wharton's jelly of the umbilical cord, the pericryptal zone of the intestine, and the pulmonary interstitium (18).

The functional significance of the contractile apparatus of the bronchial subepithelial myofibroblasts is uncertain. While these cells may possibly perform isotonic contractions, it is unlikely that they contribute directly to the intermittent alterations in the caliber of the airway lumen in bronchial asthma. The cytoplasm of these cells extends from the central location of the nuclei

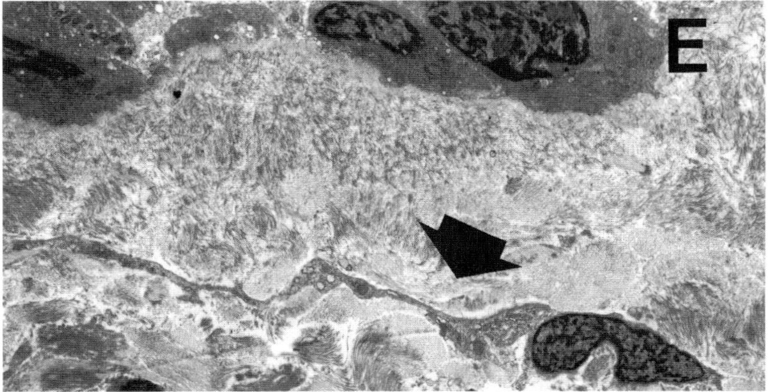

Figure 3 Elongated bronchial myofibroblast (solid arrow) in the lamina reticularis beneath the bronchial epithelium (E) in a patient with asthma. Electron microscopy, uranyl acetate and lead citrate, magnification ×5000.

to form a thin discontinuous sheet of cell processes beneath the lamina reticularis. In this location, these cells can interact with inflammatory cells as they traverse the mucosa and migrate into the epithelium. Cultured myofibroblasts secrete trophic cytokines, such as granulocyte-macrophage colony-stimulating factor in coculture with eosinophil leukocytes (19,20). The synthesis of trophic cytokines by myofibroblasts is stimulated by low levels of cytokines, such as tumor necrosis factor-α secreted by eosinophils and by cell–cell contact between eosinophils and myofibroblasts (20). This regulatory function requires that the myofibroblasts maintain their cellular outline to provide a discontinuous but extensive array of cytoplasmic processes beneath the epithelium so as to interact with any inflammatory cells migrating toward the epithelium. The maintenance of the shape of this extended cytoplasmic profile probably requires the mechanical forces generated by the actin-myosin complexes in the cytoplasm of the subepithelial myofibroblasts.

The anatomical location of these cells beneath the lamina reticularis, the presence of rough endoplasmic reticulum in their cytoplasm, and the increase in their number in association with bronchial asthma are all indirect evidence that these cells are responsible for the deposition of the increased amount of collagen in the lamina reticularis in bronchial asthma. More recently, it has been shown in tissue culture experiments that these cells proliferate in response to damage to cultured bronchial epithelial cells (21). This proliferation is induced by the release of cytokines by epithelial cells in response to either chemical or physical damage. The pattern and kinetics of cytokine release by the epithelial cells is such that proliferative cytokines, such as insulin-like growth factor-1, endothelin-1, and fibroblast-growth factor, are allowed to act in the first 24 hr after injury, driving cell proliferation. This is followed by the gradual accumulation of TGF, which can stimulate collagen synthesis by the newly proliferated cells.

The characteristic changes seen in the lamina reticularis in asthma may have limited physiological significance but if they are evidence of tissue remodeling elsewhere in the airways, their appearance in early disease has profound implications for airways function. The airway smooth muscle forms interlacing helices composed of bundles of smooth muscle cells surrounded by basal lamina. Alterations in the size and number of smooth muscle cells (22) and increased rigidity of the airways (23) are clearly important in reduction of airway function in association with bronchial asthma. Studies based on cultured smooth muscle cells have demonstrated the capacity of a range of cytokine growth factors to induce smooth muscle cell proliferation (24). However, smooth muscle cells cultured under these conditions assume a synthetic phenotype with loss of their specialized contractile apparatus (25,26). It is uncertain as to how smooth muscle hyperplasia occurs in vivo. The specialized extracellular matrix surrounding differentiated contractile smooth muscle cells in vivo contains laminin and proteoglycan molecules that may contribute to the maintenance of the contractile phenotype and prevent cell division. The increased cell number of smooth muscle cells in asthma may result from accretion of postmitotic cells from the surrounding interstitial fibroblasts and acquisition of the smooth muscle cell phenotype. Alternatively, smooth muscle cells may dissolve their surrounding matrix, dedifferentiate, divide, and redifferentiate with restoration of their surrounding basal lamina. It is essential for an understanding of the biology of the airways and of the changes in airways disease that this issue is resolved and the role of the extracellular matrix in muscle division is clarified.

The extracellular matrix has dual roles in the pathogenesis of bronchial asthma. First, changes to the matrix alter the physical properties of the airways with resultant effects on mechanics. Second, all the events involved in remodeling the airways occur in a context of the variety of structural and functional molecules contained within the airway extracellular matrix. Greater understanding of the complexity of the interactions within the airway microenvironments is fundamental to the development of therapeutic approaches targeted to prevention of the long-term morbidity of bronchial asthma.

References

1. Djukanovic R, Roche WR, Wilson JW, Beasley CRW, Twentyman OP, Holgate ST. State of the Art Review: Mucosal inflammation in asthma. Am Rev Respir Dis 1990; 142:434–457.
2. Lange P, Parner J, Vestbo J, Schnohr P, Jensen G. A 15 year follow-up study of ventilatory function in adults with asthma. N Engl J Med 1998; 339:1194–1200.
3. Wiggs BR, Bosken C, Pare PD, James A, Hogg JC. A model of airway narrowing in asthma and in chronic obstructive pulmonary disease. Am Rev Respir Dis 1992; 145:1251–1258.
4. Elias JA, Zhu Z, Chupp G, Homer RJ. Airway remodeling in asthma. J Clin Invest 1999; 104:1001–1006.
5. Timpl R. Macromolecular organization of basement membranes. Curr Opin Cell Biol 1996; 8:618–624.
6. Redington AE, Roche WR, Holgate S, Howarth PH. Co-localization of immuno-reactive transforming growth factor-beta 1 and decorin in bronchial biopsies from normal and asthmatic subjects. J Pathol 1998; 186:410–415.
7. Hemler ME. Integrin associated proteins. Curr Opin Cell Biol 1998; 10:578–585.
8. Juhasz I, Murphy GF, Yan H-C, Herlyn M, Albelda SM. Regulation of extracellular matrix proteins and integrin cell substratum adhesion receptors on epithelium during cutaneous human wound healing in vivo. Am J Pathol 1993; 143:1458–1469.
9. Dunnill MS. The pathology of asthma with specific reference to changes in the bronchial mucosa. J Clin Pathol 1960; 13:27–33.
10. Kodolova IM. Functional-morphological changes in the lungs in bronchial asthma. Arkh-Patol 1976; 38(5):60–66.
11. Wetzels RHW, Robben HCM, Leigh IM, Schaafsura HE, Vooijs GP, Ramaekers FCS. Distribution pattern of type VII collagen in normal and malignant human tissues. Am J Pathol 1991; 139:451–459.
12. Roche WR, Beasley R, Williams JH, Holgate ST. Subepithelial fibrosis in the bronchi of asthmatics. Lancet 1989; 1:520–524.
13. Koukoulis GK, Gould VE, Bhattacharya A, Gould JE, Howeedy AA, Virtanen I. Tenascin in normal, reactive, hyperplastic, and neoplastic tissues: biologic and pathologic implications. Hum Pathol 1991; 22:636–643.
14. Laitinen A, Altraja A, Kämpe M, Linden M, Virtanen I, Laitinen LA. Tenascin

is increased in airway basement membrane of asthmatics and decreased by an inhaled steroid. Am J Respir Crit Care Med 1997; 156:951–958.

15. Altraja A, Laitinen A, Virtanen I, Kämpe M, Simonsson BG, et al. Expression of laminins in the airways in various types of asthmatic patients: a morphometric study. Am J Respir Cell Mol Biol 1996; 15:482–488.

16. Brewster CEP, Howarth PH, Djukanovic R, Wilson JW, Holgate ST, Roche WR. Myofibroblasts and subepithelial fibrosis in bronchial asthma. Am J Respir Cell Mol Biol 1990; 3:507–511.

17. Gabbiani G, Ryan GB, Majuo G. Presence of modified fibroblasts in granulation tissue and their possible role in wound contraction. Experientia 1971; 27:549–550.

18. Adler KB, Low RB, Leslie KO, Mitchell LJ, Evans JN. Contractile cells in normal and fibrotic lung. Lab Invest 1989; 60:473–485.

19. Zhang S, Howarth PH, Roche WR. Cytokine production by cell cultures from bronchial subepithelial myofibroblasts. J Pathol 1996; 180:95–101.

20. Zhang S, Mohammed Q, Burbidge A, Morland CM, Roche WR. Cell cultures from bronchial subepithelial myofibroblasts enhance eosinophil survival in vitro. Eur Respir J 1996; 9:1839–1846.

21. Zhang SL, Smartt H, Holgate ST, Roche WR. Growth factors secreted by bronchial epithelial cells control myofibroblast proliferation: an in vitro co-culture model of airway remodeling in asthma. Lab Invest 1999; 79:395–405.

22. Ebina M, Takakashi T, Chiba T, Motomiya M. Cellular hypertrophy and hyperplasia of airway smooth muscles underlying bronchial asthma. Am Rev Respir Dis 1993; 148:720–726.

23. Wilson JW, Li X, Pain MCF. The lack of distensibility of asthmatic airways. Am Rev Respir Dis 1993; 148:806–809.

24. Panettieri RA Jr. Cellular and molecular mechanisms regulating airway smooth muscle proliferation and cell adhesion molecule expression. Am J Respir Crit Care Med 1998; 158:S133–140.

25. Stephens NL, Halayko AJ. Airway smooth muscle contractile, regulatory and cytoskeletal protein expression in health and disease. Comp Biochem Physiol Biochem Mol Biol 1998; 119:415–424.

26. Ma X; Wang Y; Stephens NL. Serum deprivation induces a unique hypercontractile phenotype of cultured smooth muscle cells. Am J Physiol 1998; 274:C1206–1214.

9

Role of the Airway Nervous System in Airway Remodeling

TONY R. BAI

University of British Columbia
and St. Paul's Hospital
Vancouver, British Columbia, Canada

DARRYL A. KNIGHT

University of Western Australia
Perth, Western Australia, Australia

I.   Introduction

Conceptually, we envision two major pathways by which the airway nervous system may participate in airway inflammation and, as a consequence of inflammation, remodeling. One hypothesis is that neural pathways could play a key *initiating* role in the airway inflammatory cascade that leads to remodeling. An alternate hypothesis is that airway inflammation, initiated by other means, induces changes in the behavior of airway nerves and/or receptors for products released by nerves that could contribute to the persistence (chronicity) of airway inflammation and thereby amplify the remodeling process. For the purposes of our discussion, we define remodeling as structural changes in the airways that result in measurable increases in the thickness of the airway, an alteration in the extracellular matrix components of the wall, and both hyperplasia and hypertrophy of resident cells such as smooth muscle cells (1). This is an active process and involves cell growth, cell death, cell migration,

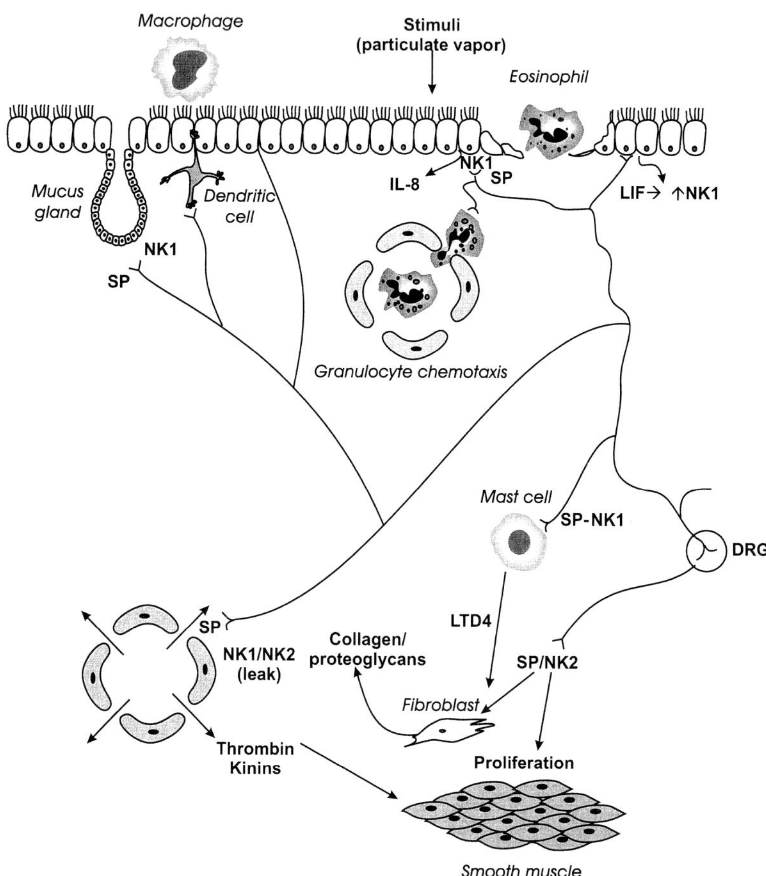

Figure 1 Diagrammatic demonstration of multiple potential sites of interactions between neurons and other cells leading to inflammation/remodeling in the airways. NK1, neurokinen 1 receptor; SP, substance P; IL-8, interleuken 8; LIF, leukemia inhibitory factor; DRG, dorsal root ganglion; LTD4, leukotriene D4.

and production or degradation of extracellular matrix. A schematic of our proposal is shown in Figure 1.

II. Airway Innervation

The human respiratory tract is innervated by nerves functionally and anatomically separated into a sensory afferent component and an autonomic efferent pathway. Both afferent and efferent nerve endings contain numerous products in addition to the classical efferent neurotransmitters acetylcholine (parasympathetic cholinergic) and noradrenaline (sympathetic). Thus airway parasympathetic nerves also contain vasoactive intestinal peptide (VIP), peptide histidine isoleucine/methionine (PHI/PHM), pituitary adenylate cyclase activating peptide (PACAP), helospectins, galanin, and nitric oxide. Afferent nerves contain glutamate, substance P, neurokinin A, calcitonin gene-related peptide (CGRP), galanin, and cholecysytokinin-octapeptide. Sympathetic nerves may release neuropeptide Y and enkephalins in addition to noradrenaline. Although the functions of some of these cotransmitters remain unclear, in general they have either facilitatory or antagonistic effects on target cells or may modulate the release of the primary neurotransmitter. There are very few efferent sympathetic nerves directly innervating human airways smooth muscle, although there is innervation of peribronchial ganglia (2). Pulmonary/mediastinal lymph nodes are also innervated (3), enhancing the potential for neuroimmune interactions to occur. Such interactions will be discussed later.

Although there are probably undiscovered neurochemicals in human airways, of the known substances the most relevant to inflammation/remodeling are the tachykinin neuropeptides.

III. Tachykinins and Sensory Neurons in the Lung

Substance P (SP), an 11-amino-acid residue, and neurokinin A (NKA), a nine-amino-acid residue, are the principal peptides of the family of tachykinin (= *quick acting*) neuropeptides found in the central and peripheral nervous system. These products are also found in low abundance in some nonneural cells such as airway epithelial cells, alveolar macrophages, and possibly eosinophils (2,4,5).

The effects of tachykinins on target cells are mediated by specific receptors. To date, three human tachykinin receptors have been cloned and sequenced. Functional data suggest that subclasses of these receptors may also exist (6). The NK-1R gene shows multiple regulatory elements, suggesting that it is inducible (7). Each tachykinin preferentially activates a distinct G-protein-coupled receptor, the NK-1R being preferentially activated by SP, the NK-2R by NKA, and NK-3R by NKB. Each ligand can, however, bind to each of the other receptors with varying affinities. At high concentrations of ligand, non-receptor-mediated effects of SP via the peptides' N-terminal have also been reported (8).

Biological responses known to be mediated by tachykinins, such as transmission of painful stimuli, chemotaxis, increases in vascular permeability and blood flow, smooth muscle contraction, stimulation of secretion from mast cells, eosinophils, and mucous glands, and epithelial/mesenchymal cell proliferation, are transduced primarily by NK-1 or 2 receptors. In contrast, NK-3 receptors may be important in modulating neurotransmission in the central nervous system and at peripheral ganglia (9). Ligand binding generates a transduction cascade involving diacylglycerol and inositol triphospate, with subsequent activation of PKC, which leads to intracellular calcium release. Activation of NK-1R also activates release of arachidonic acid (AA), although the predominant products of SP-induced AA release in specific cell types are unknown (7).

In the lung, SP along with NKA and calcitonin gene-related peptide (CGRP) are contained in sensory vagal axons (afferent nociceptive sensory or C fibers) ending as varicosities at the base of the bronchial epithelial cell layer. An example from our laboratory of an SP-containing neuron in a human, a segmental bronchus (resected lung for pulmonary nodule), is shown in Figure 2. Released tachykinins act on the various NK-1R- and/or NK-2R-bearing cells in adjacent areas. The density of tachykinin-containing neurons is species specific, with less density in the human airway compared with in rodents (10). However, our studies have shown that the concentrations of NK-1R mRNA and SP in human lung are similar to those in rodents' lung (6), and suggest nerve density should not be interpreted in the absence of data on receptor levels. Consideration should also be given to artifacts induced in human tissues by factors such as concomitant diseases, therapy, and postmortem, biopsy, or resection delays prior to neuropeptide evaluation.

Stimulation of sensory nerves following mucosal injury, trauma, or mediator release causes depolarization. Depolarization of a single peripheral axon branch leads to depolarization of the entire extensively arborized sensory neuron and neuropeptide release (axon reflexes), as well as central depolarization along the thin, unmyelinated central axon to the central nervous system (11). However, tachykinin release is not necessarily depolarization dependent, in-

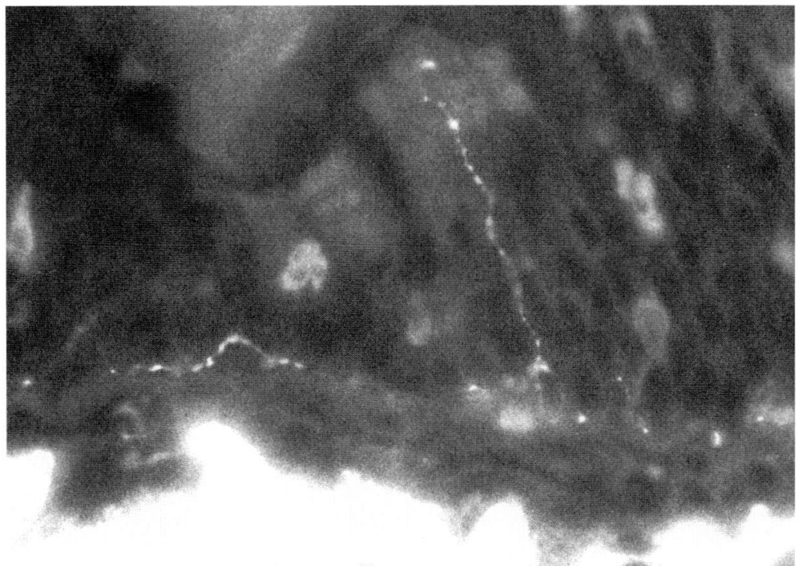

Figure 2 SP/NKA localized using a fluorescent-labeled polyclonal antibody to sensory vagal axons (afferent nociceptive sensory or C fibers) ending as varicosities at the base of the bronchial epithelial cell layer. The SP-containing fiber also runs between epithelial cells toward the lumen. An example from our laboratory using a human segmental bronchus from a surgical specimen.

stead sometimes involving stimuli such as polycations, for example major basic protein released from eosinophils (12–14). In this context, it is interesting that eosinophils tend to accumulate near sensory nerve terminals during asthmatic inflammation (15). Evidence for axon reflex release of tachykinins has been obtained in both upper and lower human airways (16,17). The sensory neuropeptides are often released in the same varicosity and yet have different effects in different tissues (2,4), suggesting that the tissue distributions of specific receptors are crucial in determining the effects of tachykinins.

Studies from several laboratories including our own (6) show that the tachykinin receptors are localized to the epithelium and lamina propria, airway smooth muscle, fibroblasts, and bronchial vascular endothelium. High-affinity tachykinin receptors (primarily NK1) have also been identified on dendritic cells, lymphocytes, macrophages, neutrophils, and mucosal-type mast cells, suggesting that tachykinins are significantly involved in neuroimmune interactions. Such interactions include macrophage, dendritic cell, eosinophil, and neutrophil chemotaxis (18,19). In addition, mast cell degranulation and increased immunoglobulin production following stimulation by tachykinins has been shown in respiratory tissue (20). Mast cells, eosinophils, and nerve terminals are found in close apposition both in the airway submucosa and within smooth muscle bundles (15,21). *Bidirectional* neuroimmune interactions are well established (22–25), which take on greater significance during inflamed airway conditions. A direct involvement of tachykinins in remodeling repair processes is suggested by the potent stimulation of human lung epithelial and fibroblast proliferation in response to SP that we and others have documented (26–29). By inducing plasma leak, triggering release of kinins, thrombins, and growth-inducing cytokines, tachykinins can also *indirectly* lead to proliferation and remodeling. There is evidence that the effects of kinins thought to be of importance in the pathogenesis of asthma, such as bradykinin, are mediated through the release of tachykinins (10). Moreover, sensory nerves in asthmatic airways may be primed to release neuropeptides as a result of exposure to inflammatory mediators such as leukotrienes and histamine (30).

Model 1: Inflammation induces changes in airway nerves and/or neuropeptide receptors that contribute to the persistence of airway inflammation and hence remodeling.

Repeated antigen stimulation and/or chronic inflammation induced by other means, such as persistent infection, may lead to phenotypic changes in the pattern of innervation through the release of neurotrophic (''neuropoietic'') factors from adjacent inflammatory cells as well as nerves and perineural cells themselves. In addition, other mediators released from inflammatory cells, for example leukotrienes (30), have been demonstrated to enhance neuronal activity.

Several investigators have addressed the question of altered nerve density in inflamed airways versus normals, with conflicting results. Tachykinin-containing nerve density has been reported to be increased in asthmatic airways and the airways of individuals with chronic cough (31,32). In a morphometric study of inflamed human airways, the density of pulmonary neuroendocrine cells increased markedly with disease severity, usually within areas of metaplastic epithelium, and was associated with a dense network of SP containing nerve fibers beneath these regions (33). Our data in asthmatic trachea suggest the density of airway nerves is not different from controls (34), in concordance with the bronchoscopic biopsy results of Howarth et al. in asthmatics (35), but in contrast to the studies of Ollerrenshaw et al. (32), using smaller airways from more severe asthmatics. As discussed above, eosinophils tend to accumulate near sensory nerve terminals during asthmatic inflammation (15).

Tachykinins or their receptors are increased in other chronic inflammatory states, such as inflammatory bowel disease (36) and arthritis (37). Increased levels of SP are found in the BAL and serum of asthmatics with further increases following allergen challenge (38–40). However, accurate determination of tachykinin concentration requires both HPLC and ELISA or RIA, so that studies not employing initial HPLC may have detected spurious tachykinin immunoreactivity. Thus Heaney and co-workers (41) were not able to detect SP in BAL fluid after HPLC, whereas NKA was detected in high concentration in both normal and mild asthmatic subjects, the level of NKA increasing further after allergen challenge in the asthmatics. The dermal response to SP increases with increasing severity of asthma (42), suggesting augmented receptor number or coupling, if indeed the effect is receptor mediated. We and others (6,43) have reported overexpression of NK-1 receptors in asthma, particularly in patients not receiving multiple therapies. Additionally, we have shown that expression levels of NK1Rs are modulated by proinflammatory stimuli such LPS and IL-β (44). In human peripheral lung explants, there appears to be marked plasticity in tachykinin receptor expression, i.e., fourfold increases in NK1 mRNA levels triggered by the mediators released by IgE receptor cross-linking (44). Passive overnight sensitization has been shown to increase contractile responsiveness to tachykinins in isolated human airways (45). This effect could be mediated by several mechanisms, one of which is enhanced NK-1R gene expression. Krishna and co-workers (46) have reported that ozone exposure reduces SP immunoreactivity in endobronchial biopsies in healthy humans. There was an inverse correlation between SP immunoreactivity and neutrophil influx and percent change in FEV$_1$ after ozone exposure, suggesting that SP could contribute to the bronchoconstriction and subsequent neutrophil infiltration into the airways. In a murine model of immune airway inflammation, Kaltreider and co-workers (47) have demonstrated upregulation of NK1Rs and increased secretion of SP in BAL fluid. Recruitment of inflammatory cells was significantly reduced by an NK1R antagonist.

Under normal conditions, the effects of released neuropeptides are usually probably short-lived because of the presence of specific endopeptidases, in particular, neutral endopeptidase (NEP). In asthmatic airways, the epithelium is often shed exposing sensory nerve endings, which may lead to increased direct or axon reflex release of tachykinin neuropeptides (48), and by removal of sources of degradative enzymes, epithelial damage may exaggerate tachykinin effects. Viruses can also decrease NEP activity (48).

Chronic infection may augment tachykinin receptor expression secondary to altered cytokine expression. Thus, following on from the pioneering work of McDonald and colleagues (49) using *Mycoplasma*-infected rats, where NK1-R receptor expression is increased leading to increased plasma extravasation following sensory nerve stimulation, Kraft and colleagues have recently reported increased expression of NK1-R in bronchial biopsies taken from a subset of individuals with serological PCR evidence of chronic *Mycoplasma* infection (50).

IV. Neurotrophic Cytokines

A variety of neurotrophic cytokines have been found that could induce the changes discussed above (Table 1). Several key observations suggest that leukemia inhibitory factor (LIF) is an important neurotrophic cytokine. First, injury or exposure of neural tissue (cultured rat dorsal root ganglia and sympathetic ganglia) to proinflammatory cytokines such as IL-1β (51) both increases the synthesis and release of LIF and coordinately increases mRNA and protein for substance P and NK-1 receptors. The observation that antibodies to LIF block the effect of IL-1 on tachykinin receptor expression suggests that LIF may also be an important intermediary, responsible for transducing the effects

Table 1 Cytokines with
Neurotrophic Effects

Leukemia inhibitory factor (LIF)
Ciliary neurotrophic factor (CNTF)
Nerve growth factor (NGF)
Brain-derived nerve factor (BDNF)
TGF beta 1
IL-6
IL-11
Fibroblast growth factor 2
Cardiotrophin 1
Oncostatin M

of other cytokines and mediators. Second, LIF-deficient mice show a diminished capacity to synthesize neuropeptides following nerve injury (52). Third, LIF induces neuropeptide synthesis and release in neurons (sympathetic) that do not normally produce neuropeptides (53). These findings emphasize the plasticity of peripheral autonomic neurons and raise the possibility that LIF may augment neuropeptide production in nonneuronal cell types that are known to potentially produce tachykinins. LIF is a 38–67-kDa variably glycosylated product (54) that has a diverse array of biological effects ranging from the differentiation of myeloid leukemic cells into macrophage lineage (55) to effects on bone metabolism (56), inflammation (57), neural development (58), embryogenesis (59), and the maintenance of implantation (60), but is best known as a cytokine at the forefront of the interaction between the immune and nervous systems (61). Most recently, LIF has been shown to be preferentially produced by TH2 cells (62). LIF, a product of chromosome 22, exists in soluble and matrix-bound forms and has been grouped within the IL-6 family of cytokines, which also includes IL-11, ciliary neurotrophic factor (CNTF), oncostatin-M (OSM), and, more recently, cardiotrophin-1 (CT-1) (63–65). This classification has been based on structural homology and common utilization of the gp130 signal transducer. Because of these features, the biological activities of this cytokine family overlap; e.g., all induce type 2 acute-phase proteins in hepatic cells. However, the family can be divided into three subgroups based on receptor patterns (66–68). First, LIF, OSM, and CT-1 each use receptors consisting of a heterodimeric complex of gp130 with the LIF receptor α-chain (LIFRα, sometimes known, confusingly, as LIFRβ!). Second, CNTF binds to a ligand-specific subunit (CNTFRα), which associates with a heterodimer of LIFRα and gp130. In contrast, functional IL-6 and IL-11 receptors are formed by an association of ligand-bound α-chains with gp130 homodimers with no involvement of LIFRα. IL-6 R and LIFR knockouts are lethal because of critical importance of the GP130 receptor in many biological processes and the importance of the LIFR for neuronal development (63). There is increasing evidence that the resulting signaling cascade initiated by ligand binding differs between cytokines. For example, although the JAK/STAT (STAT3 and STAT1) proteins are activated equally, STAT5 is much more prominently activated by LIF and OSM compared with IL-6 and thus there are both qualitative and quantitative differences between biological activities that are cell type dependent (66). Recent data have identified a new family of proteins induced rapidly in response to members of the IL-6 family, including LIF, named SOCS1-3 (or JAB or SSI-1), which act in a classic negative feedback loop to regulate cytokine signal transduction (67).

In keeping with its biological activity, LIF gene expression and protein have been localized to a variety of sites (51,69). Outside the uterus, however, LIF mRNA and protein are not readily detected in the basal state but are readily detected after endotoxin or at sites of inflammation (70). Within pulmonary tissue, until our studies, LIF had only been studied in cultured lung fibroblasts (71) where both IL-1 and MBP synergistically acted with TGFβ to increase LIF fourfold more than MBP or IL-1 alone. Whether LIF has IgE induction properties similar to IL-6 (72)—one of the few cytokines to nonisotypically induce IgE (IL-6 antibodies inhibit IgE production)—is unknown. LIF and related cytokines may play both direct and indirect roles in remodeling/proliferation. We have demonstrated immunoreactivity to LIF to airway epithelial cells, endothelial cells, submucosal glands, alveolar macrophages, and nerve bundles within human airways (73) (Fig. 3). Additionally, LIF is released from peripheral lung explants as well as from multiple isolated pulmonary cell types following inflammatory stimuli such as IL-1β. IL-6 itself releases LIF (74). Isolated eosinophils from atopic but not nonatopic subjects

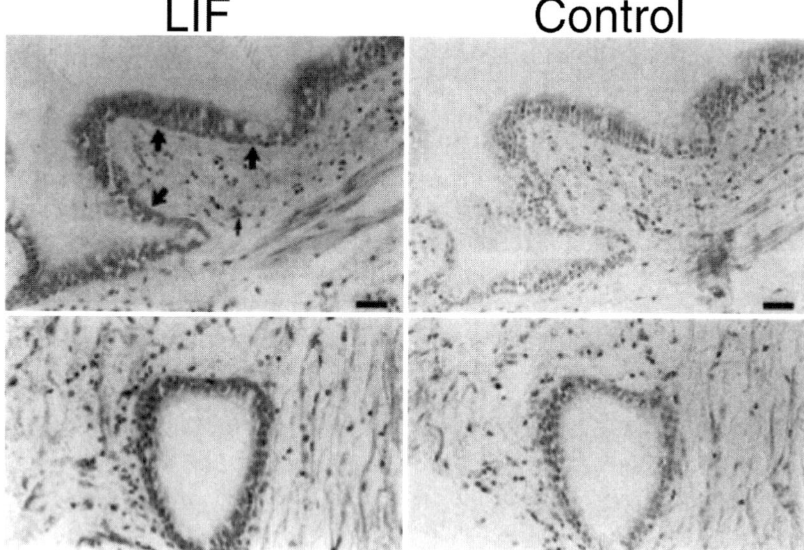

Figure 3 Localization of leukemia inhibitory factor (LIF) immunoreactivity in human airways to sites adjacent to the sensory neuron shown in Figure 2. LIF is a neurotrophic cytokine known to increase expression of neuropeptides in sensory neurons.

synthesize and release abundant amounts of LIF and serum LIF levels are increased in mild atopic asthma whereas serum levels are undetectable in normals. Subsequently, LIF was shown to enhance eosinophil chemotaxis to SP (75,76). LIF induces NK-1R gene expression, augmentation of airway smooth muscle contraction to NKA and capsaicin, and enhanced SP release from airway explants (73,76). In uterine endometrium, LIF has been shown to induce the secretion of fibronectin by trophoblasts (60). We speculate LIF may also induce fibronectin production in the airway. In airways epithelial and mesenchymal cells produce fibronectin, an important signal protein involved in the proliferation, migration, and attachment of cells at sites of injury and inflammation (77). LIF is also produced by mast cells (78). This ability, and proximity to nerves (24) and epithelial cells (79), may also be important in the proliferative response following mucosal damage. IL-6 has been shown to directly stimulate hyperplasia and hypertrophy of cultured airway smooth muscle cells (80) and is essential for PDGF-induced proliferation of human vascular smooth muscle cells and lung fibroblasts (81).

In addition to LIF and the IL-6 family, other candidate cytokines capable of modifying neuropeptide gene expression include the various nerve growth factors listed in Table 1. Thus, in culture, sensory neurons can be stimulated by nerve growth factor (NGF) released from lymphocytes to markedly increase gene transcription of PPT, the precursor for SP/NKA (82). NGF levels are increased in the serum of allergic asthma and levels correlate with asthma severity (83), although it is uncertain whether this is related to neurotrophic effects of NGF or other effects such as prolonged eosinophil survival (84).

V. Experimental Animal Models

In a variety of animal in vivo and in vitro models, there is abundant evidence for a major role for tachykinins in amplifying airway inflammation and/or airway hyperresponsiveness and parenchymal lung injury. Particularly germane are studies in pathogen-free versus chronically *M. pulmonis*–infected rats. ''Neurogenic inflammation'' is markedly upregulated by mycoplasma infection, secondary to increased expression of NK-1Rs, not only in the postcapillary venule, the usual site of permeability change, but in the capillaries as well (49). Depletion of tachykinins prevents the development of experimental allergic airways hyperresponsiveness (85), as well as cold-dry-air-induced bronchoconstriction in guinea pigs (86). Importantly, *dual* inhibition of NK-1 and NK-2 receptors is necessary to inhibit the development of airways hyperresponsiveness in *primates* in response to allergen challenge (87), reinforcing the need to use caution in interpreting experiments using single antagonists, given the ability of SP/NKA to activate all tachykinin receptors. In guinea pigs, the AHR induced by IL-5 (thought to be a critical cytokine in the induction of asthma) is solely mediated by activation of NK-2Rs following eosinophil infiltration and activation induced by IL-5 (88). In contrast, however, transgenic mice overexpressing NGF show enhanced airway neural growth, but not enhanced airways responsiveness (89).

Recent studies using an in vivo animal model of restricted epithelial damage and subsequent restitution have demonstrated that immediately post injury, the epithelial cells at the edge of the damaged area dedifferentiate, flatten, and rapidly migrate to provide a covering layer over the denuded basement membrane. In as little as 24 hr the new epithelial layer is tightly sealed, reinnervated, and the cells exhibit enhanced mitotic activity. The appearance of tachykinin-containing nerves appears coincident with the time of maximum cell proliferation and suggests that reinnervation and release of tachykinins may be contributing to the mitotic activity of these cells (90). Similarly, if the animals are neonataly capsaicinized to deplete the tachykinin content of the sensory nerves, the proliferation of epithelial cells is markedly inhibited in the first 72 hr after epithelial damage (91).

Our attempts, to date to induce or inhibit remodeling by manipulation of the tachykininergic system have been unsuccessful both in vivo in a guinea pig model and using airway explants. Thus constant in vivo infusion of SP via a pump did not induce airway remodeling in normal guinea pigs (92). Similarly, prior neuropeptide depletion with capsaicin pretreatment did not prevent the induction of smooth muscle growth in guinea pigs caused by chronic allergen challenge in vivo (93–95). Finally, guinea pig airway explants cultured over 7-days with SP and NEP inhibitors $\pm$ LIF did not show enhanced smooth muscle replication or cell hypertrophy (unpublished data).

Model 2: Neuropeptides as critical activators of airway inflammation and remodeling.

Recent research using a NK-1R knockout mouse model has provided strong evidence in support of the long-standing notion of a critical role for tachykinin neuropeptides in airway inflammation (96). Immune complexes that induce pulmonary capillary leakage and infiltration of inflammatory cells into the lungs in normal mice had no effect in NK1R knockout mice. Similarly, using NK1R+ or − knockouts, neutrophil influx induced by IL-1B in a similar model was also shown to be dependent on intact NK1Rs (97). As discussed above, the demonstration of effects of SP on dendritic cells, thought to be key initiating cells in immune reactions, is consistent with the results of the knock-out experiments (50).

VI. Conclusions

Although an attractive possibility, no conclusive evidence exists in support of a role for neural elements, particularly sensory neuropeptides, in the development of in vivo airway remodeling in asthma. However, there may be a sub-group of patients in whom the neural network is particularly important, via the interactions discussed above whereby neuropeptides augment inflammation and repair.

References

1. Bai TR, Roberts CR, Pare PD. Airway remodelling. In: Barnes PJ, Rodger IW, Thomson NC, eds. Asthma: Basic Mechanisms and Clinical Management. London: Academic Press, 1998:476–486.
2. Barnes PJ, Baraniuk JN, Belvisi MG. Neuropeptides in the respiratory tract. Part I. Am Rev Respir Dis 1991; 144:1187–1198.
3. Pascual DW, Beagley KW, Kiyono H, McGhee JR. Substance P promotes Peyer's patch and splenic B cell differentiation. Adv Exp Med Biol 1995; 371A: 55–59.
4. Helke CJ, Krause JE, Mantyh PW, Couture R, Bannon MJ. Diversity in mammalian tachykinin peptidergic neurons: multiple peptides, receptors, and regulatory mechanisms. FASEB J 1990; 4:1606–1615.
5. Roland J, Soranzo L, Launay JM, Vargaftig B. [Demonstration of the immunoreactivity of polynuclear eosinophils for bombesin and substance P. A new concept of the neuro-immune axis]. Bull Acad Natl Med 1996; 180:697–706; discussion 706–698. In French.
6. Bai TR, Zhou D, Weir T, Walker B, Hegele R, Hayashi S, McKay K, Bondy GP, Fong T. Substance P (NK1)- and neurokinin A (NK2)-receptor gene expression in inflammatory airway diseases. Am J Physiol 1995; 269:L309–317.
7. Colten HR, Krause JE. Pulmonary inflammation—a balancing act. N Engl J Med 1997; 336:1094–1096.
8. Mousli M, Bueb JL, Bronner C, Rouot B, Landry Y. G protein activation: a receptor-independent mode of action for cationic amphiphilic neuropeptides and venom peptides [see comments]. Trends Pharmacol Sci 1990; 11:358–362.
9. Myers A, Undem BJ. Tachykinin mediated stimulation of bronchial parasympathetic ganglian neurons. Am Rev Respir Dis 1992; 145:A261.
10. Bowden JJ, Gibbins IL. Relative density of substance P immunoreactive (SP-

IR) nerve fibres in the tracheal epithelium of a range of species. FASEB J 1992; 6:A1965.

11. Holzer P. Local effector functions of capsaicin-sensitive sensory nerve endings: involvement of tachykinins, calcitonin gene-related peptide and other neuropeptides. Neuroscience 1988; 24:739–768.

12. Coyle AJ, Perretti F, Manzini S, Irvin CG. Cationic protein-induced sensory nerve activation: role of substance P in airway hyperresponsiveness and plasma protein extravasation. J Clin Invest 1994; 94:2301–2306.

13. Coyle AJ, Uchida D, Ackerman SJ, Mitzner W, Irvin CG. Role of cationic proteins in the airway. Hyperresponsiveness due to airway inflammation. Am J Respir Crit Care Med 1994; 150:S63–71.

14. Coyle AJ, Ackerman SJ, Burch R, Proud D, Irvin CG. Human eosinophil-granule major basic protein and synthetic polycations induce airway hyperresponsiveness in vivo dependent on bradykinin generation. J Clin Invest 1995; 95:1735–1740.

15. Costello RW, Schofield BH, Kephart GM, Gleich GJ, Jacoby DB, Fryer AD. Localization of eosinophils to airway nerves and effect on neuronal M2 muscarinic receptor function. Am J Physiol 1997; 273:L93–103.

16. Okamoto Y, Shirotori K, Kudo K, Ishikawa K, Ito E, Togawa K, Saito I. Cytokine expression after the topical administration of substance P to human nasal mucosa. The role of substance P in nasal allergy. J Immunol 1993; 151:4391–4398.

17. Philip G, Sanico AM, Togias A. Inflammatory cellular influx follows capsaicin nasal challenge. Am J Respir Crit Care Med 1996; 153:1222–1229.

18. Germonpre PR, Lambrecht BN, Gepetti PP, Joos GF, Pauwels RA. Functional effect of neurokinin receptor blockade on dendritic cell induced T cell proliferation. Am J Respir Crit Care Med 1998; 157:A489.

19. Wiedermann FJ, Kahler CM, Reinisch N, Wiedermann CJ. Induction of normal human eosinophil migration in vitro by substance P. Acta Haematol 1993; 89:213–215.

20. Eglezos A, Andrews PV, Boyd RL, Helme RD. Tachykinin-mediated modulation of the primary antibody response in rats: evidence for mediation by an NK-2 receptor. J Neuroimmunol 1991; 32:11–18.

21. Blennerhassett MG, Janiszewski J, Bienenstock J. Sympathetic nerve contact alters membrane resistance of cells of the RBL-2H3 mucosal mast cell line. Am J Respir Cell Mol Biol 1992; 6:504–509.

22. Heaney LG, Cross LJ, Stanford CF, Ennis M. Substance P induces histamine release from human pulmonary mast cells. Clin Exp Allergy 1995; 25:179–186.

23. Kessler JA, Freidin MM, Kalberg C, Chandross KJ. Cytokines regulate substance P expression in sympathetic neurons. Regul Peptides 1993; 46:70–75.

24. Marshall JS, Waserman S. Mast cells and the nerves—potential interactions in the context of chronic disease. Clin Exp Allergy 1995; 25:102–110.

25. Solway J, Leff AR. Sensory neuropeptides and airway function. J Appl Physiol 1991; 71:2077–2087.

26. Bai TR, Zhou D. Substance P (SP) induces proliferation of human lung fibroblasts. Am J Respir Crit Care Med 1995; 151:A370.

27. Harrison NK, Dawes KE, Kwon OJ, Barnes PJ, Laurent GJ, Chung KF. Effects of neuropeptides on human lung fibroblast proliferation and chemotaxis. Am J Physiol 1995; 268:L278–283.

28. Nilsson J, von Euler AM, Dalsgaard CJ. Stimulation of connective tissue cell growth by substance P and substance K. Nature 1985; 315:61–63.

29. Parenti A, Amerini S, Ledda F, Maggi CA, Ziche M. The tachykinin NK1 receptor mediates the migration-promoting effect of substance P on human skin fibroblasts in culture. Naunyn-Schmiedebergs Arch Pharmacol 1996; 353:475–481.

30. Ellis JL, Undem BJ. Role of peptidoleukotrienes in capsaicin-sensitive sensory fibre-mediated responses in guinea-pig airways. J Physiol 1991; 436:469–484.

31. O'Connell F, Springall DR, Moradoghli-Haftvani A, Krausz T, Price D, Fuller RW, Polak JM, Pride NB. Abnormal intraepithelial airway nerves in persistent unexplained cough? Am J Respir Crit Care Med 1995; 152:2068–2075.

32. Ollerenshaw SL, Jarvis D, Sullivan CE, Woolcock AJ. Substance P immunoreactive nerves in airways from asthmatics and nonasthmatics. Eur Respir J 1991; 4:673–682.

33. Pilmane M, Luts A, Sundler F. Changes in neuroendocrine elements in bronchial mucosa in chronic lung disease in adults. Thorax 1995; 50:551–554.

34. Lilly CM, Bai TR, Shore SA, Hall AE, Drazen JM. Neuropeptide content of lungs from asthmatic and nonasthmatic patients. Am J Respir Crit Care Med 1995; 151:548–553.

35. Howarth PH, Djukanovic R, Wilson JW, Holgate ST, Springall DR, Polak JM. Mucosal nerves in endobronchial biopsies in asthma and non-asthma. Int Arch Allergy Appl Immunol 1991; 94:330–333.

36. Mantyh PW. Substance P and the inflammatory and immune response. Ann NY Acad Sci 1991; 632:263–271.

37. Levine JD, Dardick SJ, Roizen MF, Helms C, Basbaum AI. Contribution of sensory afferents and sympathetic efferents to joint injury in experimental arthritis. J Neurosci 1986; 6:3423–3429.

38. Cardell LO, Uddman R, Edvinsson L. Low plasma concentrations of VIP and elevated levels of other neuropeptides during exacerbations of asthma. Eur Respir J 1994; 7:2169–2173.

39. Tomaki M, Ichinose M, Miura M, Hirayama Y, Yamauchi H, Nakajima N, Shirato K. Elevated substance P content in induced sputum from patients with asthma and patients with chronic bronchitis. Am J Respir Crit Care Med 1995; 151:613–617.

40. Nieber K, Baumgarten CR, Rathsack R, Furkert J, Oehme P, Kunkel G. Substance P and beta-endorphin-like immunoreactivity in lavage fluids of subjects with and without allergic asthma. J Allergy Clin Immunol 1992; 90:646–652.

41. Heaney LG, Cross LJ, McGarvey LP, Buchanan KD, Ennis M, Shaw C. Neuroki-
     nin A is the predominant tachykinin in human bronchoalveolar lavage fluid in
     normal and asthmatic subjects. Thorax 1998; 53:357–362.

42. Nakai S, Iikura Y, Akimoto K, Shiraki K. Substance P-induced cutaneous and
     bronchial reactions in children with bronchial asthma. Ann Allergy 1991; 66:
     155–161.

43. Adcock IM, Peters M, Gelder C, Shirasaki H, Brown CR, Barnes PJ. Increased
     tachykinin receptor gene expression in asthmatic lung and its modulation by ste-
     roids. J Mol Endocrinol 1993; 11:1–7.

44. Knight DA, Zhou D, Weir T, Bai TR. Determination of predominant cell types
     expressing tachykinin receptors in human lung. Am J Respir Crit Care Med 1996;
     153:A161.

45. Ben-Jebria A, Marthan R, Rossetti M, Savineau JP. Effect of passive sensitiza-
     tion on the mechanical activity of human isolated bronchial smooth muscle in-
     duced by substance P, neurokinin A and VIP. Br J Pharmacol 1993; 109:131–136.

46. Krishna MT, Springall D, Meng QH, Withers N, Macleod D, Biscione G, Frew
     A, Polak J, Holgate S. Effects of ozone on epithelium and sensory nerves in the
     bronchial mucosa of healthy humans. Am J Respir Cri Care Med 1997; 156:
     943–950.

47. Kaltreider HB, Ichikawa S, Byrd PK, Ingram DA, Kishiyama JL, Sreedharan,
     SP, Warnock ML, Beck JM, Goetzl EJ. Upregulation of neuropeptides and neu-
     ropeptide receptors in a murine model of immune inflammation in lung paren-
     chyma. Am J Respir Cell Mol Biol 1997; 16:133–144.

48. Nadel JA. Neutral endopeptidase modulates neurogenic inflammation. Eur Re-
     spir J 1991; 4:745–754.

49. Baluk P, Bowden JJ, Lefevre PM, McDonald DM. Upregulation of substance P
     receptors in angiogenesis associated with chronic airway inflammation in rats.
     Am J Physiol 1997; 273:L565–571.

50. Chu HW, Kraft M, Krause JE, Cortright DN, Martin RJ. Neurokinin-1 (NK-
     1) and substance P (SP) expression in asthmatic airways–downregulation with
     clarithromycin. Am J Respir Crit Care Med 1998; 157:A24.

51. Ludlam WH, Chandross KJ, Kessler JA. LIF- and IL-1 beta-mediated increases
     in substance P receptor mRNA in axotomized, explanted or dissociated sympa-
     thetic ganglia. Brain Res 1995; 685:12–20.

52. Ohkawara Y, Yamauchi K, Tanno Y, Tamura G, Ohtani H, Nagura H, Ohkuda
     K, Takishima T. Human lung mast cells and pulmonary macrophages produce
     tumor necrosis factor-alpha in sensitized lung tissue after IgE receptor triggering.
     Am J Respir Cell Mol Biol 1992; 7:385–392.

53. Ludlam WH, Zang Z, McCarson KE, Krause JE, Spray DC, Kessler JA. mRNAs
     encoding muscarinic and substance P receptors in cultured sympathetic neurons
     are differentially regulated by Lif or CNTF. Dev Biol 1994; 164:528–539.

54. Gearing DP. The leukemia inhibitory factor and its receptor. Adv Immunol 1993;
     53:31–58.

55. Tomida M, Yamamoto-Yamaguchi Y, Hozumi M. Purification of a factor inducing differentiation of mouse myeloid leukemic M1 cells from conditioned medium of mouse fibroblast L929 cells. J Biol Chem 1984; 259:10978–10982.

56. Ishimi Y, Abe E, Jin CH, Miyaura C, Hong MH, Oshida M, Kurosawa H, Yamaguchi Y, Tomida M, Hozumi M, et al. Leukemia inhibitory factor/differentiation-stimulating factor (LIF/D-factor): regulation of its production and possible roles in bone metabolism. J Cell Physiol 1992; 152:71–78.

57. Noda M, Vogel RL, Hasson DM, Rodan GA. Leukemia inhibitory factor suppresses proliferation, alkaline phosphatase activity, and type I collagen messenger ribonucleic acid level and enhances osteopontin mRNA level in murine osteoblast-like (MC3T3E1) cells. Endocrinology 1990; 127:185–190.

58. Murphy M, Reid K, Hilton DJ, Bartlett PF. Generation of sensory neurons is stimulated by leukemia inhibitory factor. Proc Natl Acad Sci USA 1991; 88: 3498–3501.

59. Fry RC. The effect of leukaemia inhibitory factor (LIF) on embryogenesis. Reprod Fertil Dev 1992; 4:449–458.

60. Strickland S, Richards WG. Invasion of the trophoblasts. Cell 1992; 71:355–357.

61. Patterson PH. Leukemia inhibitory factor, a cytokine at the interface between neurobiology and immunology [comment]. Proc Natl Acad Sci USA 1994; 91: 7833–7835.

62. Piccinni MP, Beloni L, Livi C, Maggi E, Scarselli G, Romagnani S. Defective production of both leukemia inhibitory factor and type 2 T-helper cytokines by decidual T cells in unexplained recurrent abortions. Nature Med 1998; 4:1020–1024.

63. Taga T, Kishimoto T. Gp130 and the interleukin-6 family of cytokines. Annu Rev Immunol 1997; 15:797–819.

64. Kishimoto T, Akira S, Narazaki M, Taga T. Interleukin-6 family of cytokines and gp130. Blood 1995; 86:1243–1254.

65. Hirota H, Yoshida K, Kishimoto T, Taga T. Continuous activation of gp130, a signal-transducing receptor component for interleukin 6-related cytokines, causes myocardial hypertrophy in mice. Proc Natl Acad Sci USA 1995; 92: 4862–4866.

66. Kuropatwinski KK, De Imus C, Gearing D, Baumann H, Mosley B. Influence of subunit combinations on signaling by receptors for oncostatin M, leukemia inhibitory factor, and interleukin-6. J Biol Chem 1997; 272:15135–15144.

67. Starr R, Novak U, Willson TA, Inglese M, Murphy V, Alexander WS, Metcalf D, Nicola NA, Hilton DJ, Ernst M. Distinct roles for leukemia inhibitory factor receptor alpha-chain and gp130 in cell type-specific signal transduction. J Biol Chem 1997; 272:19982–19986.

68. Starr R, Willson TA, Viney EM, Murray LJ, Rayner JR, Jenkins BJ, Gonda TJ, Alexander WS, Metcalf D, Nicola NA, Hilton DJ. A family of cytokine-inducible inhibitors of signalling. Nature 1997; 387:917–921.

69. Arici A, Engin O, Attar E, Olive DL. Modulation of leukemia inhibitory factor gene expression and protein biosynthesis in human endometrium. J Clin Endocrinol Metab 1995; 80:1908–1915.

70. Rennick RE, Loesch A, Burnstock G. Endothelin, vasopressin, and substance P like immunoreactivity in cultured and intact epithelium from rabbit trachea. Thorax 1992; 47:1044–1049.

71. Elias JA, Zheng T, Whiting NL, Marcovici A, Trow TK. Cytokine-cytokine synergy and protein kinase C in the regulation of lung fibroblast leukemia inhibitory factor. Am J Physiol 1994; 266:L426–435.

72. Gosset P, Tsicopoulos A, Wallaert B, Joseph M, Capron A, Tonnel AB. Tumor necrosis factor alpha and interleukin-6 production by human mononuclear phagocytes from allergic asthmatics after IgE-dependent stimulation. Am Rev Respir Dis 1992; 146:768–774.

73. Knight D, McKay K, Wiggs B, Schellenberg RR, Bai T. Localization of leukaemia inhibitory factor to airway epithelium and its amplification of contractile responses to tachykinins. Br J Pharmacol 1997; 120:883–891.

74. Knight DA, Lydell CP, Zhou D, Weir TD, Schellenberg RR, Bai TR. Leukemia inhibitory factor (LIF) in human lung: distribution and regulation of LIF release. Am J Respir Cell Mol Biol 1999; 20(4):884–891.

75. Zheng X, Knight DA, Zhou D, Weir TD, Peacock C, Schellenberg RR, Bai TR. Leukemia inhibitory factor (LIF) is synthesized and released by human eosinophils and modulates activation state and chemotaxis. J Allergy Clin Immunol 1999; 104(1):136–144.

76. Zheng X, Zhou D, Bai TR. Enhanced LIF production from human eosinophils in atopic subjects. Am J Respir Crit Care Med 1999; 159:A92.

77. Rickard KA, Taylor J, Rennard SI, Spurzem JR. Migration of bovine bronchial epithelial cells to extracellular matrix components. Am J Respir Cell Mol Biol 1993; 8:63–68.

78. Marshall JS, Gauldie J, Nielsen L, Bienenstock J. Leukemia inhibitory factor production by rat mast cells. Eur J Immunol 1993; 23:2116–2120.

79. Lamb D, Lumsden A. Intra-epithelial mast cells in human airway epithelium: evidence for smoking-induced changes in their frequency. Thorax 1982; 37:334–342.

80. De S, Zelazny ET, Souhrada JF, Souhrada M. IL-1 beta and IL-6 induce hyperplasia and hypertrophy of cultured guinea pig airway smooth muscle cells. J Appl Physiol 1995; 78:1555–1563.

81. Roth M, Nauck M, Tamm M, Perruchoud AP, Ziesche R, Block LH. Intracellular interleukin 6 mediates platelet-derived growth factor-induced proliferation of nontransformed cells. Proc Nat Acad Sci USA 1995; 92:1312–1316.

82. Lindsay RM, Harmar AJ. Nerve growth factor regulates expression of neuropeptide genes in adult sensory neurons. Nature 1989; 337:362–364.

83. Bonini S, Lambiase A, Bonini S, Angelucci F, Magrini L, Manni L, Aloe L. Circulating nerve growth factor levels are increased in humans with

allergic diseases and asthma. Proc Natl Acad Sci USA 1996; 93:10955–10960.

84. Hamada A, Watanabe N, Ohtomo H, Matsuda H. Nerve growth factor enhances survival and cytotoxic activity of human eosinophils. Br J Haematol 1996; 93: 299–302.

85. Matsuse T, Thomson RJ, Chen XR, Salari H, Schellenberg RR. Capsaicin inhibits airway hyperresponsiveness but not lipoxygenase activity or eosinophilia after repeated aerosolized antigen in guinea pigs. Am Rev Respir Dis 1991; 144:368–372.

86. Solway J, Kao BM, Jordan JE, Gitter B, Rodger IW, Howbert JJ, Alger LE, Necheles J, Leff AR, Garland A. Tachykinin receptor antagonists inhibit hyperpnea-induced bronchoconstriction in guinea pigs. J Clin Invest 1993; 92:315–323.

87. Turner CR, Andresen CJ, Patterson DK, Keir RF, Obach S, Lee P, Watson JW. Dual antagonism of NK1 and NK2 receptors by CP-99994 and SR-48968 prevents AHR in primates. Am J Respir Crit Care Med 1996; 153:A160.

88. Kraneveld AD, Nijkamp FP, Van Oosterhout AJ. Role for neurokinin-2 receptor in interleukin-5-induced airway hyperresponsiveness but not eosinophilia in guinea pigs. Am J Respir Crit Care Med 1997; 156:367–374.

89. Hoyle GW, Graham RM, Finkelstein JB, Nguyen KP, Gozal D, Friedman M. Hyperinnervation of the airways in transgenic mice overexpressing nerve growth factor. Am J Respir Cell Mol Biol 1998; 18:149–157.

90. Erjefalt JS, Erjefalt I, Sundler F, Persson CG. In vivo restitution of airway epithelium. Cell Tissue Res 1995; 281:305–316.

91. Kim JS, McKinnis VS, Adams K, White SR. Proliferation and repair of guinea pig tracheal epithelium after neuropeptide depletion and injury in vivo. Am J Physiol 1997; 273:L1235–1241.

92. Wang Z, Pare PD, Bai TR. Effect of chronic infusion of substance P (SP) on in vivo airway responsiveness in guinea pigs. FASEB J 1993; 7:A505.

93. Wang ZL, Walker BA, Weir TD, Yarema MC, Roberts CR, Okazawa M, Pare PD, Bai TR. Effect of chronic antigen and beta 2 agonist exposure on airway remodeling in guinea pigs. Am J Respir Cri Care Med 1995; 152:2097–2104.

94. Lau E, Mckay KO, Pare PD, Bai TR. Prior neuropeptide depletion does not prevent airway smooth muscle proliferation induced by antigen exposure in vivo. Am J Repir Crit Care Med 1995; 151:A47.

95. Bai TR, Wang Z-L, Walker BM, Pare PD. Chronic allergic inflammation induces replication of airway smooth muscle cells in vivo in guinea pigs. Chest 1995; 107:93S.

96. Bozic CR, Lu B, Hopken UE, Gerard C, Gerard NP. Neurogenic amplification of immune complex inflammation. Science 1996; 273:1722–1725.

97. Ahluwalia AA, Defelipe C, Obrien J, Hunt SP, Perretti M. Impaired II-1-beta-induced neutrophil accumulation in tachykinin Nk1 receptor knockout mice. Br J Pharmacol 1998; 124:1013–1015.

10

The Influence of Pharmacological Therapy on Airway Remodeling in Asthma

PETER H. HOWARTH

Southampton General Hospital
Southampton, England

I. Introduction

While attention has focused largely on airway inflammation and the effects of treatment on the allergic inflammatory process over the last decade, it is only more recently that questions have been asked about the impact of therapy on the structural airway changes in asthma. Many changes are encompassed within the term "airway remodeling," both structural and functional. The functional changes may relate to a temporary alteration in behavior of an airway component, due to modulation by inflammatory processes, or may be a functional abnormality that arises because of a derangement of the morphological architecture of the airways. The former consequences should resolve with treatment that modifies the relevant inflammatory cascade, whereas the later may either be resistant to such therapy or have a different dose-response relationship to regulation than the initial inflammatory process. Before detailing the information available about the effects of differing asthma therapies on the airway remodeling process, it is pertinent to consider the remodeling changes within the airways that could be monitored and the physiological consequences, measurement of which may provide indirect information concerning drug intervention in asthma.

The range of structural airway changes include enhanced epithelial fragility, which is reflected by greater epithelial disruption in endobronchial biopsy samples and an increase in epithelial activation marker expression, an expansion of the myofibroblast phenotype within the airway mucosa, increased collagen deposition within the lamina propria beneath the true basement membrane, an increase in the extracellular matrix glycoprotein tenascin, a proliferation of mucus glands and goblet cells within the airways, an expansion of the airway vasculature, a possible neural plasticity, and both hyperplasia and hypertrophy of airway smooth muscle. A number of these structural airway changes, in particular those relating to the collagen deposition, the vasculature, and the smooth muscle, lead to airway wall thickening. This morphological change was highlighted as long ago as 1922 when Huber and Koessler reported, following detailed measurements of airway wall dimensions, that in bronchi of external diameter greater than 2 mm the thickness of the subepithelial layer, the thickness of the muscle layer, and the total wall thickness were all found to be increased in patients dying from asthma, as compared to a group of nonasthmatics dying from other causes (1). Subsequent studies have confirmed these findings and identified that this increase in wall area involves all airway groups: large cartilaginous airways both ≤10 mm and ≥10 mm internal perimeter and membranous airways of ≤2 mm and ≥2 mm internal perimeter (2). Comparable changes have also been described in resected and postmortem lung specimens from subjects with nonfatal asthma (3,4). Thus these changes appear relevant to the disease in general and not just fatal asthma. In milder asthma, however, the airway wall thickening is predominantly in the small (<2 mm internal perimeter) cartilaginous and membranous airways (3).

The contribution of individual components of the airway wall to the total increase in wall area has been analyzed. A number of studies have reported that the area of airway smooth muscle is substantially increased in both large and small airways (5–8). This is characterized predominantly by hyperplasia in the large airways and hypertrophy in the small airways (9). In fatal asthma, a greater proportion of the airway wall is occupied by mucus glands and other airway wall components (5,8,10). The epithelium, submucosa, vascular compartment, and adventitia have all been reported to be overrepresented in asthma and contribute, in part, to the total increase in airway wall size (2,4).

Part of the thickening within the lamina propria can be attributed to the enhanced deposition of collagen, which is evident both in postmortem examinations of airways and in endobronchial biopsy samples from patients with mild asthma (1,10–13). This thickened and denser deposition of collagen is predominantly composed of type III and type V collagen (14) and has been linked to the proliferation and activation of myofibroblasts within the airways (15). Evaluation of postmortem and resected lung tissue samples identifies that this enhanced collagen deposition is throughout the airways, involving both small and large airways (3).

These structural airway changes have relevance to the abnormal airway physiology in asthma, in that airway wall thickening has been linked both to the development of bronchial hyperresponsiveness (16) and to the persistent airflow obstruction that is incompletely reversible and is described in asthma (17–19), particularly in those whose disease is of longer duration (20,21). Thus information regarding the impact of therapy on airway remodeling in asthma may be derived not only from assessment of effects on the airway structural components, as evaluated directly through airway sampling at bronchoscopy, but also indirectly, through measurement of its effects on physiological measures, such as airflow obstruction, rate of decline in lung function, and bronchial hyperresponsiveness.

II. Rate of Decline in Lung Function and Airflow Obstruction

Asthmatics, as a group, experience an accelerated decline in spirometric lung function with time as compared to a nonasthmatic population (22–24). For example, one study from Australia identified a rate of decline in FEV_1, of 50 mL/year in asthmatics as compared to 35 mL/year in the control group (23). A more recent community-based survey over 15 years, the Copenhagen Heart Study, reported values of 38 mL/year and 22 mL/year, respectively (24). In both of these studies there was an additional effect with smoking, in that asthmatics who smoked had an even greater accelerated fall in lung function with time than the asthmatic nonsmokers.

With an exaggerated loss of lung function in asthma it would be anticipated that asthmatics would have lower lung function than age-, gender-, height-, and weight-matched controls. This is so even for patients with perceived mild disease and asthma is recognized as an obstructive airways disease. This obstruction is not always fully reversible with therapy (20,21,25).

The impact of treatment on this airflow obstruction can be assessed both in terms of reversibility and in terms of maintaining improved lung function and preventing an exaggerated decline in lung function with time. Understandably bronchodilator drugs such as short-acting β-agonists, long-acting β-agonists, and theophyllines all improve lung function in the short term but their effects are limited to the duration of action of the drug within the airway. Cessation of therapy leads to a rapid decline in lung function indicative that these protective effects are due to functional antagonism of bronchoconstriction and not related to any fundamental effect on airway structure. The same would also appear to apply to the leukotriene receptor antagonists although there are, as yet, inadequate long-term intervention studies to fully evaluate this with this class of drug therapy. The anti-inflammatory drugs, chromones and corticosteroids, do not have a rapid bronchodilator effect but lead to a progressive improvement in lung function over weeks to months (26–28). This has been attributed to their anti-inflammatory actions and indeed for corticosteroids this has been well established, with endobronchial biopsy and lavage studies demonstrating a reduction in airway eosinophils, mast cells, and T lymphocytes (29–37). The mechanism of action of chromones is less well established. There are few published reports of direct investigations into their airway anti-inflammatory potential in ''wild'' clinical asthma. A couple of studies with nedocromil sodium (4–8 mg q.i.d), one placebo-controlled, have found no effect on cell numbers in biopsies (38,39) although another with sodium cromoglycate (20 mg q.i.d) has reported a reduction in mucous eosinophils in bronchoalveolar lavage samples after a 3-month treatment period (40). A reduction in cell activation rather than cell recruitment may be more relevant to the effect of chromones. With corticosteroids, such as fluticasone, budesonide, and beclomethasone, and with chromones, such as sodium cromoglycate and nedocromil, not only is there improvement in baseline lung function with treatment but also a reduction in the amplitude of the diurnal variation in measures such as peak flow with continued use.

These changes in lung function, however, can all be explained by the airway anti-inflammatory effects of therapy and do not provide information as to whether intervention with these agents modifies the remodeling process within the airways. This is better evaluated in long-term studies. Surprisingly there are very few studies addressing the long-term impact of therapy on rate of decline of lung function. This is due to the clear benefit of intervention in asthma with anti-inflammatory therapies, such as inhaled corticosteroids, in reducing symptoms, improving lung function, and preventing exacerbations. It could thus be considered unethical to establish a long-term study in asthma in which there was an untreated control population. Thus the limited information available has come either from early studies comparing corticosteroids with β-agonists, from noncontrolled comparisons of groups on different treatments, or from follow-up of patients within one treatment group.

A publication by Dompeling and colleagues in patients with airflow obstruction, not all of whom had asthma, reported the impact of beclomethasone 800 µg b.d., as compared to placebo, over a 2-year period (42). Prior to initiating inhaled corticosteroid therapy this population's FEV_1 had been declining at 160 mL/year. During the first 6 months of therapy there was an improvement in lung function, with FEV_1 increasing by 460 mL. However, in the subsequent follow-up, lung function declined despite the steroid therapy at 100 mL/year. This study is compounded by the inclusion of smoking-related airflow obstruction, as subsequent studies have identified that after an initial plateau, inhaled corticosteroids do not modify the rate of decline in lung function in smoking-related COPD (42). The suggestion from the Dompeling study was, however, that the protective effect of corticosteroids in preventing loss of lung function was more marked in the asthmatics although not statistically significant.

A further study by Haahtela and colleagues, in patients with mild asthma, initially reported a comparison of budesonide 600 µg b.d. and terbutaline 375 µg b.d. over a 2-year period, which confirmed the clinical benefit of corticosteroid therapy in improving symptoms, lung function, and bronchial reactivity (26). Over the 2-year period at this dose of inhaled steroid, there does not appear to have been any decline in lung function in these subjects, although data are only available as mean values for the group and only from those who remained in the study over the period of observation. However, an extension of this study, for a further year, reported that subsequent treatment of the terbutaline-treated patients with budesonide 600 µg b.d. failed to improve either lung function or bronchial reactivity to the level that had been achieved when this treatment was given as first-line therapy to the other group (43). This can be interpreted as indicating that delay in initiating anti-inflammatory therapy leads to structural airway changes with loss of reversibility and, by implication, that the early use of steroid therapy in the other group must have prevented this.

Consistent with this is a retrospective analysis by Agertoft and Pedersen of children who, following their diagnosis, were treated for asthma with either corticosteroids or with other therapies, including chromones, theophyllines, and regular β-agonists (44). The non-steroid-treated children who were subsequently transferred to inhaled corticosteroid therapy had a reduced annual improvement in percent predicted FEV_1 as they grew, in comparison with the primary steroid treatment group, suggesting that early intervention with corticosteroid therapy had prevented loss of lung function. A further retrospective analysis from Finland of adults with asthma also found that duration of asthma prior to initiating corticosteroid therapy was an important determinant of maximal improvement in lung function (Fig. 1), with the greatest benefit being identified with therapy introduced early in the disease (45). All these reports indicate that early treatment with inhaled corticosteroid therapy may prevent the development of airway events, presumed to be those associated with structural remodeling, that lead to irreversibility in lung function but do not reverse these changes once they have arisen. Such a conclusion is supported by a recently published prospective study of 101 asthmatics by Grol et al. that reported change in lung function in a cohort of patients who were reviewed when aged 5–14 years, 22–32 years, and finally 32–42 years (46). Those asthmatics who received inhaled corticosteroids for their asthma had a significantly smaller annual decline in lung function (FEV_1) from visit 2 to visit 3, when this change was adjusted for their FEV_1 at visit 2. Thus this study, in conjunction with the other findings already detailed, provides indirect evidence to suggest that maintenance inhaled steroid therapy in asthma provides protec-

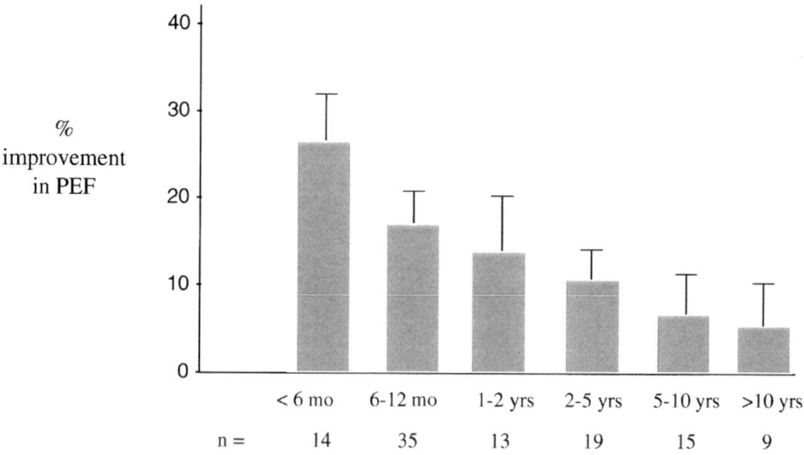

Figure 1 Percent improvement in peak expiratory flow (PEF) after treatment with inhaled corticosteroid therapy in steroid-naive asthmatics depending upon the duration of their asthma before the initiation of this therapy. (From Ref. 45.)

tion against the development of structural remodeling. The presence in the literature, however, of conflicting reports of decline in lung function in asthma despite steroid therapy (21,25,47) might suggest that this protective effect is only partial or that it may require a higher dose than that which is standardly employed to see a consistent effect in all patients.

III. Bronchial Hyperresponsiveness

An exaggerated airway narrowing to a diverse range of potential constrictor stimuli occurs in asthma and this phenomenon is termed bronchial hyperresponsiveness. While a number of mechanisms, including epithelial disruption (33), may contribute to this enhanced responsiveness, it has been proposed that structural airway changes, in particular those associated with airway wall thickening, are a substantial determinant of this physiological abnormality (16). Initially it was considered that the increase in airway smooth muscle in asthma would lead to an increased shortening in response to a set stimulus, particularly if the increase in adventitial area led to uncoupling of the smooth muscle from the opposing and limiting effects of the parenchymal elastic recoil (48). Subsequently, computer modeling emphasized the importance of the airway wall thickening in the exaggerated constrictor stimulus (16). For the same degree of smooth muscle constriction as in a normal airway, a thickened airway wall in asthma would cause considerably greater encroachment on the internal lumen and thereby lead to enhanced airway constriction with stimuli. The application of this model to measurements obtained from postmortem specimens predicted not only this greater effect on airways resistance in asthma, with modest smooth muscle shortening, but that such a response could occur even when the thickened airway wall had little if any impact on baseline airways resistance (49). Thus the magnitude of airway wall thickening that is observed in the airways of subjects, even with apparently mild asthma, is likely to significantly contribute to bronchial hyperresponsiveness. In a subsequent extension to this model it was concluded that the increase in submucosal thickening, adventitial thickening, and the increase in smooth muscle mass were all important contributors but that the smooth muscle component was likely to have a much greater impact in the smaller conducting airways, which have smooth muscle that completely encircles the airway lumen, than in the more central airways (50). Consistent with this belief, that bronchial hyperresponsiveness, at least in part, provides a surrogate physiological marker for airway wall remodeling, is the reported positive correlation between the annual decline in FEV_1 in asthma and airway responsiveness to inhaled histamine (23,51).

A. Bronchodilators

Any drug that relaxes airway smooth muscle per se will functionally antagonize constrictor stimuli and will thus modify bronchial responsiveness during the period of pharmacological activity. Thus both short- and long-acting β-agonists as well as theophyllines will modify PC_{20} values under such circumstances (52–56). This change does not, however, reflect an alteration in airway remodeling as no long-lasting effect is evident in clinical asthma on discontinuation of therapy (53–55). Although salmeterol has been shown to inhibit the proliferation of smooth muscle cells grown in culture, through a cyclic AMP-dependent mechanism (57), and inhibition of repeated airway narrowing in vivo might be anticipated to modify smooth muscle hypertrophy, there does not appear to be any fundamental effect on airway reactivity with either long-acting β-agonists or theophyllines when used as sole long-term therapy in asthma (53–55).

B. Receptor Antagonists

Both H_1-receptor antagonists and, more recently, antagonists of leukotrienes (LTs) at the $cystLT_1$ receptor have been assessed in asthma, with the leukotriene receptor antagonists (LTRAs) being licensed for use as both sole and add-on treatment for asthma because of their beneficial effects in improving lung function, decreasing symptoms, and reducing the requirement for rescue bronchodilator medication. H_1 antihistamines modify the airway response to histamine but, unless they also coexhibit other receptor antagonism, do not modify the airway response to a non-histamine-mediated bronchoconstrictor stimulus (58,59). Thus H_1 antihistamines have no effect on bronchial reactivity in perennial clinical asthma.

Similarly there is little evidence for a concerted effect of LTRAs on bronchial reactivity in placebo-controlled studies in naturally occurring disease. There is only one report of an improvement, a 1.87-fold shift in the threshold dose of methacholine inducing bronchoconstriction over a 4-week period with oral pranlukast (225 mg b.i.d.) (60). Despite the conduct of a methacholine dose-response curve the PC_{20} was not provided in this publication and this change in sensitivity was apparent without any improvement in baseline lung function (FEV_1). It may be that a more consistent and greater effect would be seen with more prolonged therapy. As studies in vitro have identified that LTD_4 can induce smooth muscle hyperplasia in the presence of epidermal growth factor or platelet-derived growth factor, it is possible that inhibition of leukotriene activity within the airways might lead to a reduction in the smooth muscle remodeling and improve bronchial reactivity (61). Until, however, there are consistent and repeatable reports of LTRAs modifying airway reactivity in asthma, the balance of probabilities suggest that $cystLT_1$ receptor antagonists do not modify airway reactivity and are thus unlikely at the standard clinical dose to modify airway remodeling.

C. Chromones

As chromones are considered anti-inflammatory in their mode of action they might thus be anticipated to modify airway reactivity with prolonged use. Although a number of uncontrolled studies report improvement in bronchial responsiveness with treatment (62–64), there is limited evidence from placebo-controlled studies that either sodium cromoglycate or nedocromil fundamentally modifies airway hyperreactivity (65,66). The reports that chromones reduce the airway response to stimuli such as sulfur dioxide (67), hypertonic saline (68), and ''fog'' (69) could be explained by the inhibitory pharmacological effect of chromones on afferent ''c'' fiber activity (70). Such a neurogenic effect to explain the protection under these circumstances, rather than a fundamental one on the bronchial hyperresponsiveness, is the failure to find any effect on direct-acting smooth muscle stimuli, such as methacholine, with regular use (71–77). These studies thus indirectly suggest that it is unlikely that chromones would have a long-term effect in modifying airway remodeling once it has arisen. This class of drug does, however, protect against laboratory allergen-challenge-induced increments in airway reactivity (78) and there are reports, albeit not always consistent, of chromones protecting against seasonal increases in bronchial responsiveness in pollen-sensitive subjects when used on a regular prophylactic basis (79). These shorter-term stimuli are likely to induce airway reactivity changes linked to airway wall edema and inflammatory cell influx rather than due to structural changes. Direct evidence is thus needed to clarify whether chromones either prevent or modify such structural events.

D. Corticosteroids

Early studies investigating the benefits of oral steroids reported only small effects in improving airway reactivity measures with not all studies reporting a reduction in bronchial hyperresponsiveness. This is in contrast to studies with inhaled corticosteroids, which when used for periods longer than 2 weeks led to improvements in measures of histamine and methacholine reactivity (26,29,71–73,77). One study comparing the effects of inhaled budesonide (120 µg/day) and oral prednisolone (12.5 mg/day), in a crossover study design in asthma, found that although both treatments improved lung function, only the inhaled corticosteroid improved airway reactivity (80). This suggests the importance of the topical activity in the improvement of bronchial hyperresponsiveness.

Studies in both children and adults (26,27,81) have identified that with prolonged therapy there can be a progressive improvement in bronchial hyperresponsiveness that does not plateau until after 9–18 months of treatment (Fig. 2). This progressive improvement, in contrast to lung function measures, which improve over 2–4 weeks, would be consistent with a gradual reduction in the airway remodeling. This improvement in reactivity is associated, in mild asthma, with a limitation in the maximum airway narrowing achievable with bronchoconstrictor stimuli such as methacholine, indicative of a fundamental change in airway behavior.

Although several potential mechanisms exist for the improvement in bronchial reactivity with inhaled corticosteroids, it is probable that while the rapid improvement seen in bronchial reactivity over the first month may relate

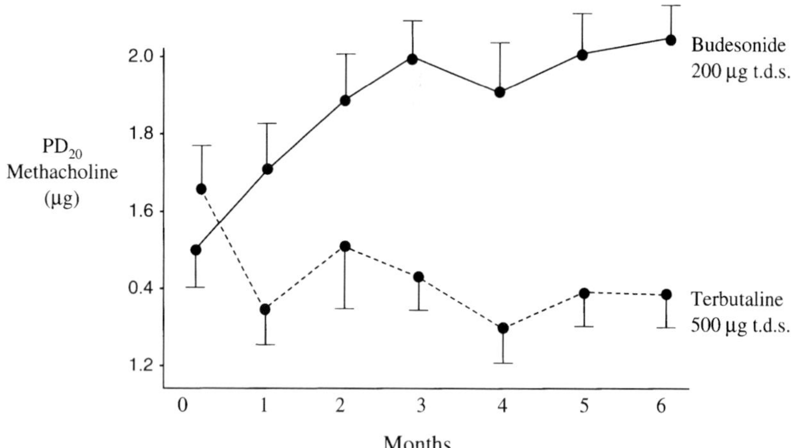

Figure 2 Change in PC_{20} methacholine with budesonide 200 µg t.d.s. and terbutaline 500 µg t.d.s. over a 6-month treatment period in children with asthma. (From Ref. 27.)

to a reduction in inflammation and a decrease in epithelial activation, the longer-term gradual improvement is likely to relate to resolution of airway remodeling. Consistent with this, it has been identified that asthma rapidly regresses within 1 week of stopping treatment, after short-duration inhaled steroid therapy (6 weeks) but there is long-lasting improvement (greater than 3 months) after continuous treatment for 1 year (43,82,83).

IV. Endobronchial Biopsy and Lavage Studies

The final arbiter as to whether treatment modifies the airway wall remodeling process comes from direct assessment of airway events before and after the initiation of treatment. Endobronchial biopsies sample large airways and provide information about airway ultrastructure, cell activation, and airway morphology, while bronchoalveolar lavage samples distal airways and allows measurements of growth factors and lumenal markers relevant to the remodeling process (84). Within the biopsies it is possible to assess epithelial morphology and activation, sub-basement membrane collagen thickness, collagen phenotype expression, and vessel numbers. It is not possible to get an index of smooth muscle bulk or airway wall thickness. As large airway events have been found in resected lung and postmortem tissue examination to reflect small airway events, it is presumed that the effect of treatment as assessed in these biopsies from large airways reflects change throughout the airways. This would be reasonable provided treatment is evenly distributed throughout the airways and for inhaled therapy that the local concentration of drug is the same, which is probably not the case.

A. Epithelial Morphology and Activation

Corticosteroid treatment in asthma has been reported to improve epithelial morphology in asthma, returning the disrupted appearance evident on endobronchial biopsies toward an intact, normal-appearing epithelium (85,86). The first study reporting this was an uncontrolled study by Lundgren and colleagues, who examined biopsies obtained before and up to 10 years after starting inhaled corticosteroid therapy. A subsequent careful transmission electron micrographic analysis of biopsies from non-steroid-treated asthmatics transferred to inhaled budesonide also reported an improvement in morphology with 16 weeks' treatment. Initially the epithelium had lost both cilliated and goblet cells and was reported to be comprised predominantly of undifferentiated cells containing microvilli. After 16 weeks' inhaled corticosteroid therapy, in addition to a resolution in the inflammatory cell number in the epithelium, the epithelium predominantly consisted of cilliated cells with considerable improvement in the structure. The epithelium was still, however, abnormal with evidence of intracellular edema and the presence of epithelial cells in transitional phases of cellular differentiation.

The epithelium is recognized as an active cell population potentially contributing significantly to cell recruitment and retention within the airways through cytokine and chemokine release and also contributing to matrix remodeling events through the release of growth factors such as endothelin, TGF-β, and FGF. The epithelial expression of endothelin is reduced in steroid-treated and -responsive asthmatics (87) and in contrast to non-steroid-treated asthmatics, who have raised endothelin levels in bronchoalveolar lavage (BAL); such steroid-treated patients as a group do not have BAL endothelin levels different from those in healthy nonasthmatics (88). There is, however, considerable interindividual variation with considerable overlap in the BAL endothelin levels between the groups. In addition, in more severe steroid-treated but still symptomatic subjects there is abnormal epithelial endothelin immunoreactivity, suggesting in these subjects that there are still persistent epithelial abnormalities despite treatment (89). It is uncertain under such circumstances whether the failure to restore epithelial activation to normality is a reflection of the inability of such treatment to fully modify the response due to an altered gene sensitivity to regulation in such patients or whether there is an overwhelming presence of factors maintaining epithelial disruption in this severe form of disease.

B. Extracellular Matrix and Basement Membrane

The extracellular matrix (ECM) is composed of macromolecules, such as polysaccharide glycosaminoglycans, proteoglycans, and fibrous proteins. The latter can be divided into two functional types, those that are functional in nature, e.g., collagen and elastin, and those that are adhesive and involved in cell interactions, e.g., fibronectin and laminin. Abnormalities of these components have been described in asthma, with an increase in collagen (12–14), a decrease in elastin fibers (90), enhanced fibronectin expression (14), and increased laminin β_2 along the basement membrane (91). There is also increased expression of tenascin, a glycoprotein that is reexpressed within the airway epithelial basement membrane in asthma (92). This increased expression is considered to be a reflection of the increased epithelial turnover and is thus a marker of the damage and repair cycle in asthma. Tenascin immunoreactivity is increased within the airways in pollen-sensitive asthmatics during seasonal exposure. This enhanced expression has been shown to be decreased by the prophylactic use of inhaled budesonide (400 μg b.d) in comparison to placebo (92). One uncontrolled study has also reported a reduction in tenascin expression with regular salbutamol therapy (39).

Beneath the true basement membrane, which is composed of type IV collagen, is the enhanced airway deposition of collagen, predominantly composed of types III and V collagen (14). As this collagen layer is clearly visible in endobronchial biopsy samples it has been the most assessed component of airway remodeling (Table 1). The first reported studies that compared collagen thickness before and after inhaled corticosteroids reported no influence of treatment on this abnormality, even with up to 10 years' treatment, despite significant improvements in symptoms and bronchial reactivity as well as a reduction in airway mucosal inflammation (29,30,85). The possibility that this process could be reversible, however, was indicated in a follow-up of patients with toluene diisocyanate (TDI)-induced occupational asthma (93). Removal of these individuals from their work environment and high-dose steroid therapy were associated with a significant decrease in the thickness of the sub-basement membrane collagen thickness. Subsequent studies in mild asthma

Table 1 Influence of Treatment on Collagen Thickness in Bronchial Biopsies in Asthma

		Collagen thickness (μm)	
Source	Treatment/duration	Pre	Post
Lundgren et al., 1988 (85)	Variable 10 years	7.0	5.8
Jeffery et al., 1992 (30)	Bud 200 μg b.i.d. 4/12	11.0	10.8
	Terb 500 μg q.d.s. 4/52	11.5	9.9
Trigg et al.,[a] 1994 (31)	BDP 500 μg b.i.d. 4/12	29.7	19.9[b]
	Placebo 4/12	23.1	20.8
Olivieri et al., 1997 (94)	FP 250 μg b.i.d. 6/52	14.0	10.7[b]
	Placebo 6/52	10.8	10.1
Hoshino et al., 1998 (95)	BDP 400 μg b.i.d. 6/12	8.31	6.07[b]
	Placebo 6/12	8.09	8.62

[a] Type III collagen thickness.
[b] Corticosteroid significant effect.
Bud = budesonide; Terb = terbutaline; BDP = beclomethasone diproprionate; FP = fluticasone propionate.

have reported that inhaled steroids modify the thickness of the collagen layer, with low-dose fluticasone (250 μg b.i.d) for 6 weeks (94) and beclomethasone 400 μg b.i.d for 6 months (95) both being reported to decrease the sub-basement collagen deposition (Fig. 3). A significant reduction in collagen type III thickness has also been reported with 4 months' treatment with beclomethasone in a placebo-controlled study design (31). The link between this marker of airway wall remodeling and bronchial hyperresponsiveness has been suggested by the reported inverse correlation between bronchial hyperresponsiveness measures in asthma and the thickness of type III collagen (96). The same study reported similar correlations with the thickness of the type V collagen and the basement membrane tenascin.

Thus, although not the major airway change contributing to bronchial hyperresponsiveness, the presence of collagen is a marker of remodeling events within the airways evident in bronchial biopsies and its modulation is likely to be a marker of more widespread effects of treatment on remodeling with corticosteroids. This link is further supported by the clinical study of Sont et al. in which corticosteroid treatment for asthma was adjusted depending on the level of bronchial hyperresponsiveness and found, in comparison to a group in whom treatment adjustments were not made on the basis of this measure, that after 2 years, those in whom attempts had been made to normal-

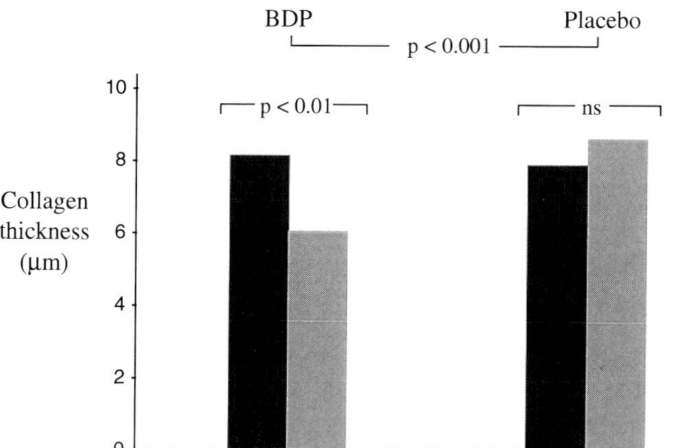

Figure 3 Change in collagen thickness in endobronchial biopsy samples in a randomized, placebo-controlled trial of beclomethasone diproprionate 400 μg b.d. ($n = 12$) in 24 asthmatics with treatment for a 6-month period. Biopsies were taken before and at completion of the study. (From Ref. 95.)

ize bronchial reactivity had better lung function, less exacerbations, and had a significant reduction in the thickness of their sub-basement membrane collagen in endobronchial biopsy samples (96). There is thus accumulating evidence that corticosteroids can modify the remodeling process in asthma. Further information is required as to the extent and dose-response relationship of this. At present none of the other asthma therapies has been clearly found to modify collagen deposition and by implication the other remodeling processes within the airways.

V. Conclusions

Considerable evidence points toward the structural airway changes in asthma as being important in the progression and persistence of the disease. To date much attention has focused on the effect of treatment on airway inflammation and treatments for asthma are currently classified into those that are predominantly bronchodilator in their effects, such as β-agonists, theophylline, and leukotriene receptor antagonists, or those that are predominantly anti-inflammatory, such as chromones or corticosteroids. This subdivision is largely based on whether there is a rapid improvement in lung function with administration and whether the treatment is primarily directed toward relaxing airway smooth muscle rather than inhibiting the underlying cell recruitment and activation. Drugs that modify cell recruitment, such as eosinophil recruitment, are considered to be disease modifying whereas those that primarily bronchodilate are not. Such a consideration, however, overlooks the impact of therapy on structural airway events and the presumption is made that structural events are a consequence of inflammation and that if inflammation is modified, the structural changes will also be modified. Although inflammation can certainly be linked to the development of structural changes, it is far from certain that this is a sine qua non and it is important that the impact of therapy on these events should be considered separately from effects on inflammation. This is because there are many uncertainties. It is not known whether the mechanisms of airway remodeling differ from those of inflammation, whether the time course of resolution of structural changes differs from resolution of inflammation, what the dose-response relationships are for resolution of these events, and whether the timing of intervention is critical, such that treatment may prevent airway remodeling but not resolve changes that have already arisen. These considerations remain to be resolved, as does the question how does one best measure/monitor airway remodeling in asthma? Is there one marker of remodeling or do many have to be measured as several differing structural components are involved in the remodeling process?

The evidence to date from both indirect and direct evaluations, however, reveals that corticosteroids appear to be the only pharmacological treatment that may fundamentally alter the development and progression of the remodeling process and are best administered by the inhaled route in this respect. There are still, however, many questions relating to the extent and range of these effects, and the potential that combination therapy may have a more extensive effect remains to be evaluated.

References

1. Huber HL, Koessler KK. The pathology of bronchial asthma. Arch Intern Med 1922; 30:689–760.
2. James AL, Pare PD, Hogg JC. The mechanics of airway narrowing in asthma. Am Rev Respir Dis 1989; 139:242–246.
3. Carroll N, Elliot J, Morton A, James A. The structure of large and small airways in nonfatal and fatal asthma. Am Rev Respir Dis 1993; 147:405–410.
4. Kuwano K, Bosken CH, Pare PD, Bai TR, Wiggs BR, Hogg JC. Small airways dimensions in asthma and in chronic obstructive pulmonary disease. Am Rev Respir Dis 1993; 148:1220–1225.
5. Dunnill MS, Massarella GR, Anderson JA. A comparison of the quantitative anatomy of the bronchi in normal subjects, in status asthmaticus, in chronic bronchitis, and in emphysema. Thorax 1969; 24:176–179.
6. Heard BE, Hossain S. Hyperplasia of bronchial smooth muscle in asthma. J Pathol 1972; 110:319–331.
7. Hossain S. Quantitative measurements of bronchial muscle in men with asthma. Am Rev Respir Dis 1973; 107:99–109.
8. Takizawa T, Thurlbeck WM. Muscle and mucous gland size in the major bronchi of patients with chronic bronchitis, asthma, and asthmatic bronchitis. Am Rev Respir Dis 1971; 104:331–336.
9. Ebina M, Takahashbi T, Chiba T, Motomiya M. Cellular hypertrophy and hyperplasia if airway smooth muscles underlying bronchial asthma: a 3-D morphometric study. Am Rev Respir Dis 1993; 148:720–726.
10. Glynn AA, Michaels L. Bronchial biopsy in chronic bronchitis and asthma. Thorax 1960; 15:142–153.
11. Dunnill MS. The pathology of asthma, with special reference to changes in the bronchial mucosa. J Clin Pathol 1960; 13:27–33.
12. Beasley R, Roche WR, Roberts JA, Holgate ST. Cellular events in the bronchi in mild asthma and after bronchial provocation. Am Rev Respir Dis 1989; 139: 806–817.

13. Jeffery PK, Wardlaw AJ, Nelson FC, Collins JV, Kay AB. Bronchial biopsies in asthma: an ultrastructural, quantitative study and correlation with hyperreactivity. Am Rev Respir Dis 1989; 140:1745–1753.

14. Roche WR, Beasley R, Williams JH, Holgate ST. Subepithelial fibrosis in the bronchi of asthmatics. Lancet 1989; 1:520–524.

15. Brewster CEP, Howarth PH, Djukanovic R, Wilson J, Holgate ST, Roche WR. Myfibroblasts and subepithelial fibrosis in bronchial asthma. Am J Respir Cell Mol Biol 1990; 3:507–511.

16. Wiggs BR, Moreno R, Hogg JC, Hilliam C, Pare PD. A model of the mechanics of airway narrowing. J Appl Physiol 1990; 69:849–860.

17. Minshall EM, Leung DYM, Martin RJ, Song YL, Cameron L, Ernst P, Hamid Q. Eosinophil-associated TGF-B1 mRNA expression and airways fibrosis in bronchial asthma. Am J Respir Cell Mol Biol 1997; 17:326–333.

18. Chetta A, Foresi A, Del Donno M, Bertorelli G, Pesci A, Olivieri D. Airways remodelling is distinctive feature of asthma and is related to severity of disease. Chest 1997; 111:852–857.

19. Hoshino M, Nakamura Y, Sim J, Shimojo J, Isogai S. Bronchial subepithelial fibrosis and expression of matrix metalloproteinase-9 in asthmatic airway inflammation. J Allergy Clin Immunol 1998; 102(5):783–788.

20. Brown JP, Grenville WH, Finucane KE. Asthma and irreversible airflow obstruction. Thorax 1984; 39:131–136.

21. Connolly CK, Chan NS, Prescott RJ. The relationship between age and duration of asthma and the presence of persistent obstruction in asthma. Postgrad Med J 1988; 64(752):422–425.

22. Schacter EN, Doyle CA, Beck GJ. A prospective study of asthma in a rural community. Chest 1984; 85:623–630.

23. Peat JK, Woolcock AJ, Cullen K. Rate of decline in lung function in subjects with asthma. Eur J Respir Dis 1987; 70:171–179.

24. Lange P, Parner J, Vestbo J, Schnohr P, Jensen G. A 15-year follow-up study of ventilatory function in adults with asthma. N Engl J Med 1998; 339:1194–1200.

25. Backman KS, Greenberger PA, Patterson R. Airways obstruction in patients with long-term asthma consistent with "irreversible asthma." Chest 1997; 112:1234–1240.

26. Haahtela T, Jarvinen M, Kava T, et al. Comparison of a beta 2-agonist, terbutaline, with an inhaled corticosteroid, budesonide, in newly detected asthma. N Engl J Med 1991; 325:388–392.

27. Kerrebijn KF, VAN Essen-Zandvliet EEM, Neijens JJ. Effect of long-term treatment with inhaled corticosteroids and beta-agonists on the bronchial responsiveness in children with asthma. J Allergy Clin Immunol 1987; 79:653–659.

28. de Jong JW, Postma DS, de Monchy JGR, Koeter GH. A review of nedocromil sodium in asthma therapy. Eur Respir Rev 1993; 3:511–519.

29. Djukanovic R, Wilson JW, Britten KM, Wilson SJ, Walls AF, Roche WR, How-

arth PH, Holgate ST. Effect of an inhaled corticosteroid on airway inflammation and symptoms in asthma. Am Rev Respir Dis 1992; 145:669–674.

30. Jeffery PK, Godfrey RW, Adelroth E, Nelson F, Rogers A, Johansson S-A. Effects of treatment on airway inflammation and thickening of basement membrane reticular collagen in asthma: a quantitative light and electron microscopic study. Am Rev Respir Dis 1992; 145:890–899.

31. Trigg CJ, Manolitsas ND, Wang J, Calderon M, McAulay A, Jorden SE, Herman MJ, Jhalli N, Duddle JM, Hamilton S, Devalia JL, Davies RJ. Placebo-controlled immunopathologic study of four months on inhaled corticosteroids in asthma. Am J Respir Crit Care Med 1994; 150:17–22.

32. Booth H, Richmond I, Ward C, Gardiner PV, Harkawat R, Walters EH. Effect of high dose inhaled fluticasone propionate on airway inflammation in asthma. Am J Respir Crit Care Med 1995; 152:45–52.

33. Bentley AM, Hamid Q, Robinson DS, et al. Prednisolone treatment in asthma. Reduction in the numbers of eosinophils, T cells, tryptase-only positive mast cells, and modulation of IL-4, IL-5, and interferon-gamma cytokine gene expression within the bronchial mucosa. Am J Respir Crit Care Med 1996; 153:551–556.

34. Hoshino M, Nakamura Y. Anti-inflammatory effects of inhaled beclomethasone diproprionate in nonatopic asthmatics. Eur Respir J 1996; 9(4):696–702.

35. Burke CM, Sreenan S, Pathmakanthan S, Patterson J, Schmekel B, Poulter LW. Relative effects of inhaled corticosteroids on immunopathology and physiology in asthma: a controlled study. Thorax 1996; 51:993–999.

36. Djukanovic R, Homeyard S, Gratziou C, et al. The effect of treatment with oral corticosteroids on asthma symptoms and airway inflammation. Am J Respir Crit Care Med 1997; 155:826–832.

37. Laitinen A, Altraja A, Kampe M, Linden M, Virtanen I, Laitinen LA. Tenascin is increased in airway basement membrane of asthmatics and decreased by an inhaled steroid. Am J Respir Crit Care Med 1997; 156:951–958.

38. Manolitsas ND, Wang J, Devalia JL, Trigg CJ, McAulay AE, Davies RJ. Regular albuterol, nedocromil sodium, and bronchial inflammation in asthma. Am J Respir Crit Care Med 1995; 151:1925–1930.

39. Altraja A, Laitinen A, Meriste S, Marran S, Martson T, Sillastu H, Laitinen LA. Effect of regular nedocromil sodium or albuterol on bronchial inflammation in asthma. J Allergy Clin Immunol 1996; 98:S58–66.

40. Diaz P, Galleguillos FR, Gonzalez MC, Pantin CFA, Kay AB. Bronchoalveolar lavage in asthma: the effect of disodium cromoglycate (cromolyn) on leukocyte counts, immunoglobulins and complement. J Allergy Clin Immunol 1984; 74:41–48.

41. Dompeling E, Van Schay KCP, Van Grunsven PM, Van Herwaarden CLA, Akkermans R, Molema J, Folgering H, Van Weel C. Slowing the deterioration of asthma and chronic obstructive pulmonary disease during bronchodilator therapy by adding inhaled corticosteroids. Ann Intern Med 1993; 118:770–778.

42. Pauwels RA, Lofdahl CG, Laitinen LA, Schouten JP, Postma DS, Prode NB, Ohlsson SV. Long-term treatment with inhaled budesonide disease who continue smoking. N Engl J Med 1999; 340(35):1948–1953.

43. Haahtela T, Jarvinen M, Kava T, Kiviranta K, Koskinen S, Lehtonen K, Nikander K, Persson T, Selroos O, Sovijarvi A, Stenius-Aarniala B, Scahn T, Tammivaara R, Laitinen LA. Effects of reducing or discontinuing inhaled budesonide in patients with mild asthma. N Engl J Med 1994; 331:700–705.

44. Agertoft L and Pedersen S. Effects of long-term treatment with inhaled corticosteroid or growth and pulmonary function in asthmatic children. Respir Med 1994; 88:373–381.

45. Selroos O, Pietinalho A, Lofroos AB, Riska H. Effect of early vs late intervention with inhaled corticosteroids in asthma. Chest 1995; 108:1228–1234.

46. Grol MH, Gerritsen J, Vonk JM, et al. Risk factors for growth and decline of lung function in asthmatic individuals up to age 42 years. A 30-year follow-up study. Am J Respir Crit Care Med 1999; 160:1830–1837.

47. Ulrik CS, Lange P. Decline of lung function in adults with bronchial asthma. Am J Respir Crit Care Med 1994; 150:629–634.

48. Moreno RH, Hogg JC, Pare PD. Mechanics of airway narrowing. Am Rev Respir Dis 1986; 133:1171–1180.

49. Wiggs DB, Bosken C, Pare PD, James A, Hogg JC. A model of airway narrowing in asthma and in chronic obstructive pulmonary disease. Am Rev Respir Dis 1992; 145:1251–1258.

50. Lambert RK, Wiggs BR, Kuwano K, Hogg JC, Pare PD. Functional significance of increased airway smooth muscle in asthma and COPD. J Appl Physiol 1993; 74:2771–2881.

51. Redline S, Tager IB, Segal MR, Gold D, Speizer FE, Weiss ST. The relationship between longitudinal change in pulmonary function and nonspecific airway responsiveness in children and young adults. Am Rev Respir Dis 1989; 140(1): 179–184.

52. Gungora HC, Wisniewski AF, Tattersfield AE. A single-dose comparison of inhaled albuterol and two formulations of salmeterol on airway reactivity in asthmatic subjects. Am Rev Respir Dis 1991; 144:626–629.

53. Wilding P, Clark M, Coon JT, Lewis S, Rushton L, Bennett J, Oborne J, Cooper S, Tattersfield AE. Effect of long-term treatment with salmeterol on asthma control: a double-blind, randomised cross-over study. Br Med J 1997; 314:1441–1446.

54. Rosenthal RP, Busse WW, Kemp JP, Baker JW, Kalberg C, Emmett A, Rickard KA. Effect of long term salmeterol therapy compared with as needed albuterol use on airway hyperresponsiveness. Chest 1999; 116:595–662.

55. Roberts JA, Bradding P, Britten KM, Walls AF, Wilson S, Gratziou C, Holgate ST, Howarth P. The long-acting β_2-agonist salmeterol xinafoate: effects on airway inflammation in asthma. Eur Respir J 1999; 14:275–282.

56. McWilliams BC, Menendez R, Kelly HW, Howick J. Effects of theophylline on

inhaled methacholine and histamine in asthmatic children. Am Rev Respir Dis 1984; 130:193–197.

57. Tomlinson PR, Wilson JW, Stewart AG. Salbutamol inhibits the proliferation of human airway smooth muscle cells grown in culture: relationship to elevated cAMP levels. Biochem Pharmacol 1995; 49:1809–1819.

58. Woenne R, Kattan M, Orange RP, Levison H. Bronchial hyperreactivity to histamine and methacholine in asthmatic children after inhalation of SCH1000 and chlorpheniramine malcate. J Allergy Clin Immunol 1978; 62:119–123.

59. Rafferty P, Holgate ST. Terfenadine (seldure) is a potent and selective histamine H_1-receptor antagonist in asthmatic airways. Am Rev Respir Dis 1987; 135:181–184.

60. Nakamura Y, Hoshino M, Sim JJ, Ishii K, Hosaka K, Sakamoto T. Effect of the leukotriene receptor antagonist pranlukast on cellular infiltration in the bronchial mucosa of patients with asthma. Thorax 1998; 53:835–841.

61. Panettieri RA, Tan EML, Ciocca V, Luffman MA, Leonard TB, Hay DWP. Effects of LTD_4 on human airway smooth muscle cell proliferation, matrix expression and contraction in vitroL differential sensitivity to cysteinyl leukotriene receptor antagonists. Am J Respir Cell Mol Biol 1998; 19:453–461.

62. Orefice U, Struzzo P, Dorigo R, Peraoner A. A long term treatment with sodium cromoglycate, nedocromil sodium and beclomthasone diproprionate reduces bronchial responsiveness in asthmatic subjects. Respiration 1992; 59:97–101.

63. Wasserman SI, Furukawa CT, Henochowicz SI, Marcoux JP, Prenner BM, Findlay SR, Gross GN, Hudson Level D, Myers DJ, Steinberg P. Asthma symptoms and airway hyperresponsiveness are lower during treatment with nedocromil sodium than during treatment with regular inhaled albuterol. J Allergy Clin Immunol 1995; 95:541–547.

64. Groot CA, Lammers SW, Molema J, Festen J, Herwaarden CL. Effect of inhaled beclomethasone and nedocromil sodium on bronchial responsiveness to histamine and distilled water. Eur Respir J 1992; 5:1075–1082.

65. Bel EH, Timmers MC, Hermans J, Dijkman JH, Sterk PJ. The long term effects of nedocromil sodium and beclomethasone diproprionate on bronchial responsiveness to methacholine in nonatopic asthmatic subjects. Am Rev Respir Dis 1990; 141:21–28.

66. Fiocchi A, Riva E, Sanini I, Bernardo L, Sala M, Mirri GP. Effect of nedocromil sodium on bronchial hyperreactivity in children with nonatopic asthma. Ann Allergy Asthma Immunol 1997; 79:503–506.

67. Dixon CMS, Fuller RW, Barnes PJ. Effect on nedocromil sodium on sulphur dioxide induced bronchoconstriction. Thorax 1987; 42:462–465.

68. Rodwell LT, Anderson SD, Du Toit J, Seale JP. Nedocromil sodium inhibits the airway response to hyperosmolar challenge in patients with asthma. Am Rev Respir Dis 1992; 146:1149–1155.

69. Robushi M, Vaghi A, Simone P, Bianco S. Presentation of fog induced bronchospasm by nedocromil sodium. Clin Allergy 1987; 17:69–74.

70. Myers AC, Riccio MM, Undem BJ. Effect of nedocromil sodium on neurogenic mechanisms in vitro. J Allergy Clin Immunol 1996; 98:S107–S111.
71. Baki A, Karaguzel G. Short term effects of budesonide, nedocromil sodium and salmeterol on bronchial hyperresponsiveness in childhood asthma. Acta Paediatr Jpn 1998; 40:247–251.
72. Svendsen UG, Frolund L, Madsen F, Nielsen NH, Holstein-rathton NH, Weeke B. A comparison of the effects of sodium cromoglycate and beclomethasone diproprionate on pulmonary function and bronchial hyperreactivity in subjects with asthma. J Allergy Clin Immunol 1987; 80:68–74.
73. Molema J, Van Herwaarden CL, Folgering HT. Effects of long term treatment with inhaled cromoglycate and budesonide on bronchial hyperresponsiveness in patients with allergic asthma. Eur Respir J 1989; 2:308–316.
74. Griffin MP, MacDonald N. McFadden ER. Short and long term effects of cromolyn sodium on the airway reactivity of asthmatics. J Allergy Clin Immunol 1983; 71:331–338.
75. Patel KR. Sodium cromoglycate in histamine and methacholine reactivity in asthma. Clin Allergy 1984; 14:143–145.
76. Laitinen LA, Venlo K, Poppins H. A controlled study of the effect of treatment with cromolyn sodium pressurised aerosol on bronchial reactivity in patients with asthma. Ann Allergy 1986; 56:270–273.
77. Sont JK, Bel EH, Dijkman JH, Sterk PJ. The long term effect of nedocromil sodium on the maximal degree of airway narrowing to methacholine in atopic asthmatic subjects. Clin Exp Allergy 1992; 22:534–560.
78. Cockcroft DW, Murdock KY. Comparative effects of inhaled salbutamol, sodium cromoglycate and beclomethasone diproprionate on allergen-induced early asthmatic responses, late asthmatic responses and increased bronchial responsiveness to histamine. J Allergy Clin Immunol 1987; 79:734–740.
79. Lowhagen O, Rak I. Modification of bronchial hyperreactivity after treatment with sodium cromoglycate during pollen season. J Allergy Clin Immunol 1985; 75:460–467.
80. Jenkins CR, Woolcock AJ. Effect of prednisolone and beclomethasone diproprionate on airway responsiveness in asthma: a comparative study. Thorax 1988; 43:378–384.
81. Woolcock AJ, Yan K, Salome Carol Martin. Effect of therapy on bronchial hyperresponsiveness in the long term management of asthma. Clin Allergy 1988; 18:165–176.
82. Vathenen AS, Knox AJ, Wisniewski A, Tattersfield AE. Time course of change in bronchial reactivity with an inhaled corticosteroid in asthma. Am Rev Respir Dis 1991; 143:1317–1321.
83. Juniper EF, Kline PA, Vanzieleghem MA, Ramsdale EH, O'Byrne PM, Hargreave FE. Effect of long term treatment with an inhaled corticosteroid (budesonide) on airway hyperresponsiveness and clinical asthma in nonsteroid-dependent asthmatics. Am Rev Respir Dis 1990; 142:832–836.

84. Howarth PH. What is the nature of asthma and where are the therapeutic targets? Respir Med 1997; 91(Suppl):2–8.

85. Lundgren R, Soderberg M, Horstedt P, Sterling R. Morphological studies of bronchial mucosal biopsies from asthmatics before and after ten years of treatment with inhaled steroids. Eur Respir J 1988; 1:883–889.

86. Laitinen LA, Laitinen A, Heino M, Haahtela T. Eosinophilic airway inflammation during exacerbation of asthma and its treatment with inhaled corticosteroid. Am Rev Respir Dis 1991; 143:423–427.

87. Redington AE, Springall DR, Meng Q-H, Tuck A, Holgate ST, Polak JM, Howarth PH. Immunoreactive endothelin in bronchial biopsy specimens: Increased expression in asthma and modulation by corticosteroid therapy. J Allergy Clin Immunol 1997; 100:544–552.

88. Redington AE, Springall DR, Ghatei MA, Madden J, Bloom SR, Frew AJ, Polak JM, Holgate ST, Howarth PH. Airway endothelin levels in asthma: influence of endobronchial allergen challenge and maintenance corticosteroid therapy. Eur Respir J 1997; 10:1026–1032.

89. Springall DR, Howarth PH, Counihan H, Djukanovic R, Holgate ST, Polak JM. Endothelin immunoreactivity of airway epithelium in asthmatic patients. Lancet 1993; 337:697–701.

90. Bousquet J, Lacoste JY, Chanez P, Vic P, Godard P, Michel FB. Bronchial elastic fibers in normal subjects and asthmatic patients. Am J Respir Crit Care Med 1996; 153:1648–1654.

91. Altraja A, Laitinen A, Virtanen I, Kampe M, Simonsson BG, Karlson S-E, Hakansson L, Verge P, Sillastu H, Laitinen LA. Expression of laminins in the airways in various types of asthmatic patients: a maphometric study. Am J Respir Cell Mol Biol 1996; 15:482–488.

92. Laitinen A, Altraja A, Kampe M, Linden M, Virtanen I, Laitinen LA. Tenascin is increased in airway basement membrane of asthmatics and decreased by inhaled steroid. Am J Respir Crit Care Med 1997; 156:951–958.

93. Saetta M, Maestrelli P, Turato G, Mapp CE, Milani G, Pivirotto LM, Fabbri LM, di Stefano A. Airway wall remodelling after cessation of exposure to isocyanates in sensitised asthmatic subjects. Am J Respir Crit Care Med 1995; 151: 489–494.

94. Olivieri D, Chetta A, Del Donno M, Bertorelli G, Casalini A, Pesci A, Testi R, Foresi A. Effect of short-term treatment with low-dose inhaled fluticasone propionate on airway inflammation and remodelling in mild asthma: a placebo controlled study. Am J Respir Crit Care Med 1997; 155:1864–1871.

95. Hoshino M, Nakamura Y, Sim JJ, et al. Inhaled corticosteroid reduced lamina reticularis of the basement membrane by modulation of insulin-like growth factor (IGF)-I expression in bronchial asthma. Clin Exp Allergy 1998; 28(5):568–577.

96. Sont JK, Willems LN, Bel EH, Van Krieken JH, Vandenbroncke JP, Sterk PJ. Clinical control and histopathologic outcome of asthma when using airway hyperresponsiveness as an additional guide to long term treatment. The AMPUL study group. Am J Respir Crit Care Med 1999; 159:1043–1057.

11

The Human Eosinophil and Its Role in Airway Remodeling

PER VENGE

University of Uppsala
Uppsala, Sweden

I. Introduction

The eosinophil granulocyte is produced in the bone marrow with a production rate of 10^{10} and 10^{11} eosinophils per day. Most eosinophils enter the tissues and stay there for several days to weeks and the eosinophil should probably be regarded as a tissue cell (1). Production of eosinophils is regulated by growth factors such as the interleukins 3 (IL-3) and 5 (IL-5) and the granulocyte-macrophage-colony stimulating factor (GM-CSF). The same cytokines are also important activators of mature eosinophils and probably regulate their attraction to and accumulation in tissues. The view of the biological role of the human eosinophil has dramatically changed in the last decades and focused on the cell being a proinflammatory cell with potent cytotoxic capabilities. Findings during recent years have suggested that the eosinophil also may be active in tissue repair processes, as activated eosinophils are commonly found in fibrotic diseases. It is, however, still an open question whether the activities of the eosinophil are responsible for the basal membrane thickening in the bronchi that is so typically observed in patients with bronchial asthma. This chapter will briefly review some important aspects of the biochemistry and function of the human eosinophil and discuss the evidence and possible role of this cell in tissue remodeling

II. Biochemistry and Function of the Human Eosinophil

The eosinophil is primarily a secretory cell (2). The biological activities exerted by the eosinophil are related to the biological activities of the products produced by and released from the cell. The preformed mediators are stored in the granules of the eosinophil. The four major proteins of eosinophil granules are eosinophil cationic protein (ECP), eosinophil peroxidase (EPO), eosinophil protein x/eosinophil–derived neurotoxin (EPX/EDN), and major basic protein (MBP). One characteristic of the four proteins is their extremely high cationic charge, which makes them very sticky. The granules also contain a number of other protein molecules of which the family of cytokines is of considerable interest. Some of these cytokines are IL-2, IL-6, IL-8, TGF-α, TGF-β1, and GM-CSF. In addition, the human eosinophil contains in its granules certain enzymes with collagenolytic activities, i.e., MMP-3, also called stromelysin, and MMP-9, also called 92-kDa collagenase IV (3), and also other enzymatic activities such as an arylsulfatase B, histaminase, and phospholipase activities (1).

Upon stimulation the eosinophil forms a number of nonpreformed mediators such as prostaglandins, leukotrienes, platelet-activating factor, and the reactive oxygen species (ROS) $O2^-$, H_2O_2, OH, and NO. The human eosinophil is a potent producer of ROS and the lipid mediators and in this regard fully comparable to other potent cells such as the neutrophil and the mast cell.

Another molecule produced in large amounts by the eosinophil is the Charcot-Leyden crystal (CLC) protein, which presumably is a plasma membrane protein. The CLC protein is shed from the eosinophils and forms extracellular needle-like crystals in tissues of heavy eosinophil infiltration. The CLC protein is a lysophospholipase and has interesting biological activities (4), which may be of importance to the role of the eosinophil in allergic inflammation.

Attraction of eosinophils to tissues and accumulation of eosinophils in tissues is a complex process. One early step is the adhesion of eosinophils to the endothelial cells through the interaction between specific receptor molecules on the respective cell. In allergic inflammation these molecules involve the expression of VCAM-1 and ICAM-1 on endothelial cells and VLA-4 and CD11b/CD18 on the eosinophil (5,6). Another important step is the priming of circulating eosinophils. This includes the increased expression of adhesion molecules on the cell surface and the enhanced responsiveness to chemotactic signals (7). In allergic inflammation IL-5 seems to be an important priming factor. The production and generation of chemotactic signals at the site of allergic inflammation is probably a necessary step in the subsequent attraction and guidance of eosinophils to move from the vascular compartment into the tissues. Numerous molecules with chemotactic properties for eosinophils have been identified and include molecules such as PAF, C5a, LTB$_4$, RANTES (8), IL-4 (9), IL-5, IL-8 (10), eotaxin (11), and MIP-1α (6,12,13). In the asthmatic lung IL-5, IL-8, and RANTES seemed to be of the greatest importance with IL-5 being a cofactor to the two chemotactic principles (10). Others have, however, shown that PAF, C5a, and eotaxin are very potent in stimulating transepithelial migration (14,15). Thus, the relative role of these different chemotactic molecules is not clear and their role may vary depending on the conditions. Thus, one set of molecules may be operative during the allergic inflammation and another set during the attraction of eosinophils to a fibrotic process. Still another mechanism that may be important in the accumulation of eosinophils is prevention of the normal turnover of eosinophils, i.e., enhancement of the survival of the eosinophils in the tissues. Such mechanisms have been proposed and involve generation of the growth factors IL-3, IL-5, and GM-CSF, since these growth factors prevent the apoptotic alterations of the eosinophils (16,17). The effects of these survival enhancing factors may, however, be counteracted by other cytokines such as TGF-β1 (18). The knowledge of the processes governing the attraction and accumulation of eosinophils in tissues is of the greatest importance in our attempts to regulate the activities of these cells.

A. Some Properties of the Major Granule Proteins

ECP is a heterogeneous protein with molecular weight varying from 16 to 22 kDa (2). The heterogeneity is partly due to differences in glycosylation of the molecule. At least six distinct variants have been recognized in preparations of ECP originating from pools of cells from several hundred blood donors (Trulson et al. submitted). ECP is a weak ribonuclease and a potent cytotoxic molecule with the capacity to kill mammalian as well as nonmammalian cells such as parasites and bacteria. The cytotoxic activity of ECP is attributed to one particular variant, which is uniquely identified by one monoclonal antibody produced against ECP, i.e., Mab 652. The mechanism of cytotoxicity is due to the capacity of ECP to make pores in cell membranes. ECP also has a number of noncytotoxic activities one of which includes the alteration of glycosaminoglycan production and storage by human fibroblasts (19) (see below). An activity of particular interest to the present discussion is the effects of ECP on fibrinolysis, since ECP was shown to enhance fibrinolysis by the enhancement of plasminogen activator activation of plasminogen (20). The possible consequence of this property will be discussed further below.

EPX and EDN are two names of the same protein. EPX/EDN is a one-chain basic protein with a molecular size of 18 kDa, and as opposed to ECP, only one variant has been described. EPX/EDN and ECP share a large degree of amino acid sequence homology, but EPX/EDN is a far more potent ribonuclease than ECP, but much less cytotoxic.

EPO is a two-chain basic protein with a total molecular weight of 67 kDa. Together with halides or SCN^- and H_2O_2, EPO constitutes a potent cytotoxic mechanism, which among other things kills parasites. The peroxidase activity of EPO is involved in the inactivation of some lipid mediators, notably the leukotrienes.

Major basic protein (MBP) forms the typical crystalloid structures in the human eosinophil granules. MBP is a single-chain basic protein with a molecular weight of 13.9 kDa. The major biological functions of MBP are related to the cytotoxic activities of the molecule and involve the killing and damage of a variety of parasites and mammalian cells. MBP also has some noncytotoxic biological activities on various cells. One such effect is the interaction with Il-1α and TGF-β1 in the stimulation of fibroblast production of various cytokines (21).

III. The Interaction Between Eosinophils and Fibroblasts In Vivo

A. Clinical Studies

Endomyocardial fibrosis is a sign of hypereosinophilia, whether the cause of eosinophilia is unknown as in the hypereosinophilic syndrome (HES) or whether it is caused by parasite infestation (22). In these cases it is assumed that the development of fibrosis is the direct consequence of the presence of huge numbers of eosinophils in the endomyocardium. In pulmonary fibrosis the eosinophil is present in high numbers in the bronchoalveolar lavage fluid (BAL) (23) and the levels of ECP in the fluid are raised dramatically (24), in some patients more than 1000-fold the normal levels. Correlations between the raised levels and the severity of the disease as measured by various lung function tests were also shown. Also in patients with systemic sclerosis (25,26) and cystic fibrosis (27) high levels of ECP and other eosinophil secretory proteins were found in serum, sputum, and BAL as signs of increased eosinophil involvement in the disease processes. Thus, it seems as if the eosinophil is an obligatory participant in the processes of fibrosis in humans. Studies on patients with asthma, either seasonal, chronic, or occupational, attempted to address this question further, and indeed increased subepithelial deposition in the reticular basement membrane of the matrix proteins tenascin, laminin, and collagen was demonstrated (28–30) in asthmatic patients in whom increased mucosal numbers of eosinophils also were seen. The extent of the deposition varied between the patient groups and the expression of tenascin was reduced by inhaled glucocorticosteroids. However, no direct correlations were found between the number of EG2-positive eosinophils and the expression of the matrix proteins, although the mucosal expression of MMP-9 and TIMP-1 (tissue inhibitor of metalloproteinases) showed such a correlation.

B. Animal Studies

In studies on wound healing it was shown that TGF-α and TGF-β1 were sequentially expressed in the tissues and that a cellular source of these two cytokines were the infiltrating eosinophils (31,32). It was concluded that the eosinophils may help in the regulation of critical processes of wound healing. Induction of fibrosis by means of bleomycin is probably mediated by an oxygen radical mediated process (33) and invariably causes excessive lung eosinophilia. In a recent report it was shown that in this process, both lung eosinophilia and pulmonary fibrosis were completely inhibited by treatment of the animals with antibodies against IL-5, clearly suggesting a causative role of the eosinophil in the development of fibrosis in this model (34,35).

IV. The Interaction Between Eosinophils and Fibroblasts In Vitro

The first demonstrations of an effect of eosinophils on fibroblast behavior in vitro were published no more than about 10 or 15 years ago. One such publication investigated the effects of guinea pig eosinophil material on fibroblast replication and found that both extracts and released material from the eosinophils stimulated this process (36).

This investigation was extended to human eosinophils grown in the presence of GM-CSF and IL-3 and IL-5 and showed an increase in the soluble and cell-associated fibroblast glycosaminoglycan production as well as an increase in collagen production (37). These findings largely supported those of others showing increased replication of fibroblasts by eosinophil-derived conditioned medium (38). The conclusions of these studies were that eosinophils might be active contributors to fibrotic diseases, but that the actual molecular mechanisms behind the effects on fibroblasts remained unknown. Recent studies have shown that several mechanisms may be operative. One such mechanism is related to the activities of the granule proteins ECP (19) and MBP (21). Another to the production by the eosinophils of TGF-α (39) and TGF-β (40). A third mechanism may be the production by the eosinophils of reactive oxygen species, as it is well established that fibroblasts respond with an increased proliferation to the exposure to ROS (41).

In the early studies on ECP it was found that ECP stimulated proteoglycan and hyaluronan synthesis by human fibroblasts (42). In subsequent studies ECP was shown to inhibit proteoglycan degradation in fibroblasts, which led to the accumulation of proteoglycans within the fibroblast (19). The specificity of ECP was indicated by the lack of effects of other highly charged peptides such as protamine and poly-L-lysine and by the fact that antibodies to ECP inhibited the effect. In more recent studies these data were confirmed, but extended in the sense that it was shown that different variants of ECP had different and seemingly opposing effects. Thus, one variant did induce accumulation of proteoglycans, whereas another variant actually increased the extracellular secretion of proteoglycans (Malmström et al., to be published). Whether these different variants with seemingly opposing effects on fibroblasts are posttranslational modifications of ECP or actually are different gene products is at present not known, but raises the interesting possibility that the production of different molecular species predisposes to different end results. In one case the result is a purposeful fibrotic process and in the other case the result may be excessive fibrosis and disease.

Another interesting property of ECP in this context is, as mentioned above, its capacity to enhance the urokinase-mediated conversion of plasminogen to plasmin (20). This enhancement was due to a stoichiometric 1:1 molecular interaction between ECP and plasminogen and resulted in a three- to fivefold increased generation of plasmin. Conversion of proMMP-3 and proMMP-9 to their enzymatically active counterparts may both be mediated by plasmin. Therefore, ECP has the potential to greatly accelerate this process, which may lead to the increased generation of collagenolytic activity in the airways and contribute to airway remodeling.

MBP was shown to regulate the IL-1- and TGF-β1-induced production of IL-6-type cytokines by fibroblasts, but did not affect fibroblast proliferation or collagen synthesis. The effects of MBP were synergistic with IL-1 and TGF-β1, since MBP had no effects on its own (21). These findings add to the knowledge that eosinophils and fibroblasts interact at several levels, as it was shown previously that fibroblasts also produce cytokines, in particular GM-CSF, that enhance the survival and activation of eosinophils (43,44).

V. The Role of Eosinophils in Airway Remodeling: Conclusion and Hypothesis

From the above it seems likely that the eosinophil is an active participant in wound healing processes and in the development of fibrosis. The mechanisms by which this is brought about are mediated through the secretion of granule proteins such as ECP, MBP, and the metalloproteinases MMP-3 and MMP-9, and also by the production and secretion of various cytokines of which the transforming growth factors seem to be some of the key molecules. In addition, the production of reactive oxygen species by the eosinophil may be important. Whether these mechanisms are also operative in the basal membrane thickening seen in the bronchi of asthmatic patients is uncertain. Some support, however, has been derived from clinical observations showing increased expression of TGF-β1 in lung eosinophils in asthmatics (45,46). Also, the fact that an increased number of eosinophils and basal membrane thickening are the two unique and early findings in children subsequently developing asthma may support this notion (Roche et al., reported at the European Respiratory Society, 1998), although no direct relationships between signs of remodeling in the asthmatic lung, i.e., tenascin and laminin deposition in the basal membrane, and submucosal infiltration of eosinophils could be found.

In Figure 1 a hypothesis as to the role of the eosinophil in airways remodeling is shown. In this hypothesis the key molecules and interactions are 1) the induction of fibroblast proliferation by TGFs; 2) the alteration by ECP variants of fibroblast synthesis and breakdown of proteoglycans, hyaluronan, and collagen; 3) the production and secretion of collagenolytic activities; and 4) the enhancement by ECP of the plasmin-mediated conversion of the pro-forms of MMP-3 and MMP-9. It is understood in this model that the eosinophil may not be the sole source of TGFs, MMPs, and ROS, but that neutrophils and macrophages and possibly several other cells may be important contributors also, although in asthma, eosinophils may be the major source.

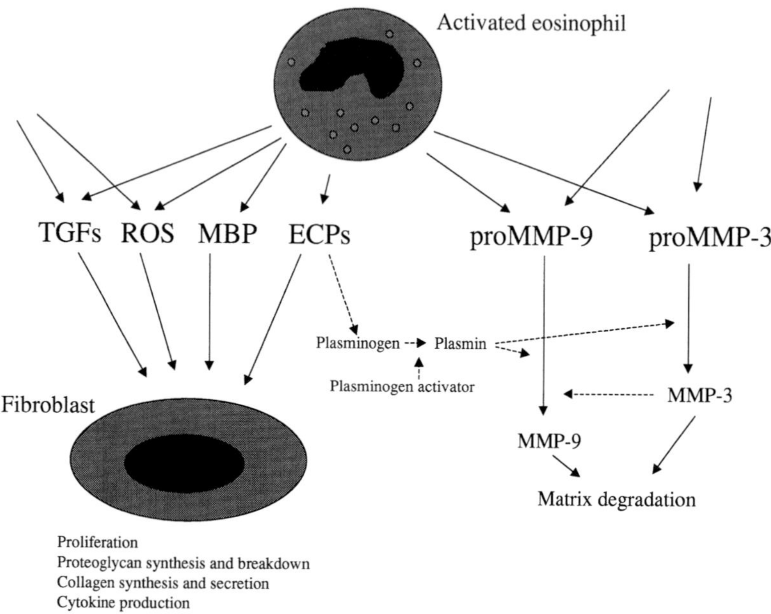

Figure 1 The role of the eosinophil in tissue remodeling: a hypothesis. The eosinophil may affect fibroblast activities in several ways, leading to fibroblast replication and altered synthesis and handling of matrix proteins and cytokines. The secretion of ECP from the eosinophils may enhance the rate of plasmin-dependent conversion of the proforms of the metalloproteinases proMMP-3 and proMMP-9 to their active collagenolytic counterparts.

VI. Targets for Future Therapy

From the model depicted in Figure 1 it may also be deduced that one strategy of pharmacological intervention to prevent fibroblast activation and tissue remodeling should be directed toward the eosinophil and its products. In asthma it is assumed that cytokines such as IL-5 are key activators of the eosinophil and the prevention of this activation pathway should be successful. This is probably the pathway that is downregulated by corticosteroids and one of the reasons for the success of these drugs in controlling asthmatic inflammation. The involvement of IL-5 in generating fibrosis is indeed also suggested by the animal studies on bleomycin-induced fibrosis as discussed above (35), but the therapeutic success with corticosteroids in fibrotic diseases in humans is, in spite of this, very limited. This could have two explanations. One is that the patients are treated too late and when the process has become irreversible. Early intervention in asthma has been shown beneficial and may prevent irreversible airways changes (47). Another possibility is that other pathways are operative in humans. A major question, therefore, is whether the molecular mechanisms involved in the attraction and activation of eosinophils in fibrotic diseases are the same as those involved in the asthmatic inflammation. From studies on cystic fibrosis this does not seem to be the case, as in these patients the attraction and activation of eosinophils was related to a different cytokine panel from that seen in asthma (48). Thus, it is obvious that eosinophils can be attracted and activated by several different mechanisms of which some may not be as sensitive to corticosteroids as the Th2-mediated pathways. One strategy for future drug development should therefore, as mentioned above, be directed toward the search for specific principles that control the eosinophils.

Acknowledgments

Unpublished work cited in this review was supported by the Swedish Medical Research Council and Vårdalstiftelsen.

References

1. Venge P. Eosinophils. In: Barnes PJ, Rodger IW, Thomson NC, eds. Asthma. Basic Mechanisms and Clinical Management, 3rd ed. San Diego: Academic Press, 1998:141–158.
2. Venge P, Byström J. Eosinophil cationic protein (ECP). Int J Biochem Cell Biol 1998; 30:433–437.
3. Ståhle-Bäckdahl M, Sudbeck BD, Eisen AZ, Welgus HG, Parks WC. Expression of 92-kDa type IV collagenase mRNA by eosinophils associated with basal cell carcinoma. J Invest Dermatol 1992; 99(4):497–503.
4. Gomolin HI, Yamaguchi Y, Paulpillai AV, Dvorak LA, Ackerman SJ, Tenen DG. Human eosinophil Charcot-Leyden crystal protein: cloning and characterization of a lysophospholipase gene promoter. Blood 1993; 82(6):1868–1874.
5. Bevilacqua MP. Endothelial-leukocyte adhesion molecules. Annu Rev Immunol 1993; 11:767–804.
6. Walsh GM. Human eosinophils: their accumulation, activation and fate. Br J Haematol 1997; 97:701–709.
7. Håkansson L, Heinrich C, Rak S, Venge P. Priming of eosinophil adhesion in patients with birch pollen allergy during pollen season: effect of immunotherapy. J Allergy Clin Immunol 1997; 99:551–562.

8.   Alam R, Stafford S, Forsythe P, Harrison R, Faubion D, Lett-Brown MA, et al. RANTES is a chemotactic and activating factor for human eosinophils. J Immunol 1993; 150(8):3442–3447.

9.   Dubois GR, Bruijnzeel Koomen CA, Bruijnzeel PL. IL-4 induces chemotaxis of blood eosinophils from atopic dermatitis patients, but not from normal individuals. J Invest Dermatol 1994; 102:843–846.

10. Venge J, Lampinen M, Håkansson L, Rak S, Venge P. Identification of IL-5 and RANTES as the major eosinophil chemoattractants in the asthmatic lung. J Allergy Clin Immunol 1996; 97:1110–1115.

11. Lilly CM, Nakamura H, Kesselman H, Nagler-Anderson C, Asano K, Garcia-Zepeda EA, et al. Expression of eotaxin by human lung epithelial cells—induction by cytokines and inhibition by glucocorticoids. J Clin Invest 1997; 99:1767–1773.

12. Alam R, York J, Boyars M, Stafford S, Grant JA, Lee J, et al. Increased MCP-1, RANTES, and MIP-1α in bronchoalveolar lavage fluid of allergic asthmatic patients. Am J Respir Crit Care Med 1996; 153:1398–1404.

13. Ponath PD, Qin SX, Ringler DJ, Clark-Lewis I, Wang J, Kassam N, et al. Cloning of the human eosinophil chemoattractant, eotaxin—expression, receptor binding, and functional properties suggest a mechanism for the selective recruitment of eosinophils. J Clin Invest 1996; 97:604–612.

14. Okada S, Kita H, George TJ, Gleich GJ, Leiferman KM. Transmigration of eosinophils through basement membrane components in vitro: synergistic effects of platelet-activating factor and eosinophil-active cytokines. Am J Respir Cell Mol Biol 1997; 16:455–463.

15. Liu LX, Zuurbier AE, Mul FP, Verhoeven AJ, Lutter R, Knol EF, et al. Triple role of platelet-activating factor in eosinophil migration across monolayers of lung epithelial cells: eosinophil chemoattractant and priming agent and epithelial cell activator. J Immunol 1998; 161:3064–3070.

16. Simon HU, Yousefi S, Schranz C, Schapowal A, Bachert C, Blaser K. Direct demonstration of delayed eosinophil apoptosis as a mechanism causing tissue eosinophilia. J Immunol 1997; 158:3902–3908.

17. Walsh GM. Mechanisms of human eosinophil survival and apoptosis. Clin Exp Allergy 1997; 27:482–487.

18. Alam R, Forsythe P, Stafford S, Fukuda Y. Transforming growth factor β abrogates the effects of hematopoietins on eosinophils and induces their apoptosis. J Exp Med 1994; 179:1041–1045.

19. Hernäs J, Särnstrand B, Lindroth P, Peterson CGP, Venge P, Malmström A. Eosinophil cationic protein alters proteoglycan metabolism in human lung fibroblast cultures. Eur J Cell Biol 1992; 59:352–363.

20. Dahl R, Venge P. Enhancement of urokinase-induced plasminogen activation by the cationic protein of human granulocytes. Thromb Res 1979; 14(4/5):599–608.

21. Rochester CL, Ackerman SJ, Zheng T, Elias JA. Eosinophil-fibroblast interac-

tions—granule major basic protein interacts with IL-1 and transforming growth factor-β in the stimulation of lung fibroblast IL-6-type cytokine production. J Immunol 1996; 156:4449–4456.

22. Spry CJF. Eosinophils. A Comprehensive Review and Guide to the Scientific and Medical Literature. Oxford: Oxford University Press, 1988.

23. Davis WB, Fells GA, Sun X-H, Gadek JE, Venet A, Crystal RG. Eosinophil-mediated injury to lung parenchymal cells and interstitial matrix A possible role for eosinophils in chronic inflammatory disorders of the lower respiratory tract. J Clin Invest 1984; 74:269–278.

24. Hällgren R, Bjermer L, Lundgren R, Venge P. The eosinophil component of the alveolitis in idiopathic pulmonary fibrosis. Signs of eosinophil activation in the lung are related to impaired lung function. Am Rev Respir Dis 1989; 139:373–377.

25. Gustafsson R, Fredens K, Nettelbladt O, Hällgren R. Eosinophil activation in systemic sclerosis. Arthritis Rheum 1991; 34(4):414–422.

26. Cox D, Earle L, Jimenez SA, Leiferman KM, Gleich GJ, Varga J. Elevated levels of eosinophil major basic protein in the sera of patients with systemic sclerosis. Arthritis Rheum 1995; 38:939–945.

27. Koller DY, Gotz M, Eichler I, Urbanek R. Eosinophilic activation in cystic fibrosis. Thorax 1994; 49:496–499.

28. Altraja A, Laitinen A, Virtanen I, Kämpe M, Simonsson BG, Karlsson SE, et al. Expression of laminins in the airways in various types of asthmatic patients: a morphometric study. Am J Respir Cell Mol Biol 1996; 15:482–488.

29. Laitinen A, Altraja A, KΣmpe M, Linden M, Virtanen I, Laitinen LA. Tenascin is increased in airway basement membrane of asthmatics and decreased by an inhaled steroid. Am J Respir Crit Care Med 1997; 156:951–958.

30. Hoshino M, Nakamura Y, Sim J, Shimojo J, Isogai S. Bronchial subepithelial fibrosis and expression of matrix metalloproteinase-9 in asthmatic airway inflammation. J Allergy Clin Immunol 1998; 102:783–788.

31. Todd R, Donoff BR, Chiang T, Chou MY, Elovic A, Gallagher GT, et al. The eosinophil as a cellular source of transforming growth factor alpha in healing cutaneous wounds. Am J Pathol 1991; 138(6):1307–1313.

32. Wong DTW, Donoff RB, Yang J, Song B-Z, Matossian K, Nagura N, et al. Sequential expression of transforming growth factors α and β₁ by eosinophils during cutaneous wound healing in the hamster. Am J Pathol 1993; 143(1):130–142.

33. Chandler DB, Fulmer JD. The effect of deferoxamine on bleomycin-induced lung fibrosis in the hamster. Am Rev Respir Dis 1985; 131:596–598.

34. Gharaee-Kermani M, McGarry B, Lukacs N, Huffnagle G, Egan RW, Phan SH. The role of IL-5 in bleomycin-induced pulmonary fibrosis. J Leukocyte Biol 1998; 64:657–666.

35. Gharaee-Kermani M, Phan SH. The role of eosinophils in pulmonary fibrosis (Review). Int J Mol Med 1998; 1:43–53.

36. Pincus SH, Ramesh KS, Wyler DJ. Eosinophils stimulate fibroblast DNA synthesis. Blood 1987; 70(2):572–574.

37. Birkland TP, Cheavens MD, Pincus SH. Human eosinophils stimulate DNA synthesis and matrix production in dermal fibroblasts. Arch Dermatol Res 1994; 286:312–318.

38. Shock A, Rabe KF, Dent G, Chambers RC, Gray AJ, Chung KF, et al. Eosinophils adhere to and stimulate replication of lung fibroblasts "in vitro." Clin Exp Immunol 1991; 86:185–190.

39. Walz TM, Nishikawa BK, Malm C, Wasteson Å. Production of transforming growth factor alpha by normal human blood eosinophils. Leukemia 1993; 7(10): 1531–1537.

40. Wong DT, Weller PF, Galli SJ, Elovic A, Rand TH, Gallagher GT, et al. Human eosinophils express transforming growth factor alpha. J Exp Med 1990; 172: 673–681.

41. Murrell GA, Francis MJ, Bromley L. Modulation of fibroblast proliferation by oxygen free radicals. Biochem J 1990; 265:659–665.

42. Särnstrand B, Westergren-Thorsson G, Hernäs J, Peterson CGB, Venge P, Malmström A. Eosinophil cationic protein and transforming growth factor-A stimulates synthesis of hyaluronan and proteoglycan in human fibroblast cultures. 5th International Colloquium on Pulmonary Fibrosis, 1988, abstract.

43. Owen WF, Rothenberg ME, Silberstein DS, Gasson JC, Stevens RL, Austen KF, et al. Regulation of human eosinophil viability, density, and function by granulocyte/macrophage colony-stimulating factor in the presence of 3T3 fibroblasts. J Exp Med 1987; 166:129–141.

44. Takafuji S, Shoji S, Ito K, Yamamoto K, Nakagawa T. Eosinophil degranulation in the presence of lung fibroblasts. Int Arch Allergy Immunol 1998; 117:52–54.

45. Ohno I, Nitta Y, Yamauchi K, Hoshi H, Honma M, Woolley K, et al. Transforming growth factor b1 (TGFb1) gene expression by eosinophils in asthmatic airway inflammation. Am J Respir Cell Mol Biol 1996; 15:404–409.

46. Minshall EM, Leung DY, Martin RJ, Song YL, Cameron L, Ernst P, et al. Eosinophil-associated TGF-b1 mRNA expression and airways fibrosis in bronchial asthma. Am J Respir Cell Mol Biol 1997; 17:326–333.

47. Haahtela T, Järvinen M, Kava T, Kiviranta K, Koskinen S, Lehtonen K, et al. Comparison of a B2-agonist, terbutaline, with an inhaled corticosteroid, budesonide, in newly detected asthma. N Engl J Med 1991; 325(6):388–392.

48. Koller DY, Nething I, Otto J, Urbanek R, Eichler I. Cytokine concentrations in sputum from patients with cystic fibrosis and their relation to eosinophil activity. Am J Respir Crit Care Med 1997; 155:1050–1054.

12

Role of Macrophages in Airway Remodeling in Asthma
Future Therapeutic Target

ANTONIO MAURIZIO VIGNOLA,
LIBORIA SIENA,
ROSALIA GAGLIARDO, and
GIOVANNI BONSIGNORE

Institute of Lung Pathophysiology
Italian National Research Council (CNR)
Palermo, Italy

PHILIPPE GODARD and
JEAN BOUSQUET

Montpellier University and
Service des Maladies Respiratoires–
  INSERM U454
Hôpital Arnaud de Villeneuve
Montpellier, France

PASCAL CHANEZ and
GISELE MAUTINO

Service des Maladies Respiratoires–
  INSERM U454
Hôpital Arnaud de Villeneuve
Montpellier, France

I. Introduction

Lung macrophages are the pulmonary representatives of the mononuclear phagocyte system, which consists of a migratory, specialized family of cells derived from hematopoietic precursors that circulate in blood as monocytes and are widely distributed as macrophages in tissues and body fluids.

Based upon their localization, function, and morphology, macrophages in the lung are categorized as alveolar macrophages (AM), interstitial macrophages, monocytes, dendritic cells, Langerhans cells, and pleural macrophages (1). Macrophages are mobile and thus can move to regions where they are needed.

Lung macrophages play a central role in maintaining lung structure and function through their different capacities. Macrophages have a central role in host defense against infection and in inflammatory processes. The endocytic and phagocytic machinery of macrophages is particularly potent and their secretory potential is large and diverse. Because of these multiple functions, macrophages also possess the capacity to injure normal structures, leading to tissue repair and remodeling.

II. Function of Macrophages in Health and Disease

Normal lung macrophages possess different functional capacity: mobility, phagocytosis, antigen presentation, and release of a wide variety of mediators, cytokines, and growth factors. These functional capabilities allow the macrophages to have a major role in helping to maintain normal lung structure and function.

In inflammation, macrophages are very abundant and have much wider functions in biology and pathology (2). They have the fundamental role in specific immunity through a relationship within lymphocytes (3) and possess wide metabolic properties (4). Tissue macrophages present a very large number of functions that are dependent on their microenvironment, state of activation, and differentiation and make them very versatile (5). Many of these function are turned off or operate at low level in the resting state but are upregulated when the cells are activated.

Activated macrophages have the potential to secrete a wide variety of products, many of which are involved in tissue inflammation, injury, and remodeling (Fig. 1). The spectrum of biological activities induced is phenomenal for a single cell (2,6,7). Furthermore, the versatility of the macrophage is such

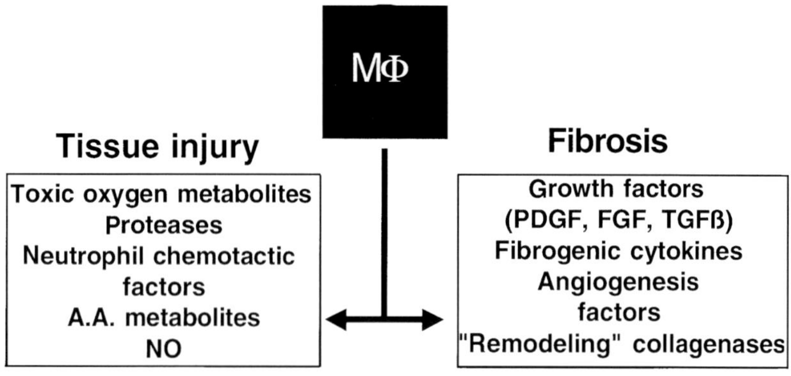

Figure 1 Mediators released by macrophages in tissue injury and repair.

that secretions of this product can be regulated (increased or decreased) by interactions between the cells and its environment, other cells, extracellular matrix (ECM) components such as fibronectin and serum (complement), as well as exogenous agents. Thus, macrophages may become "deactivated" favoring resolution of the inflammatory response.

III. Macrophages in Airway Inflammation in Asthma

Mononuclear phagocytes are likely to be involved in the pathogenesis of asthma (8) as macrophages are among the cells present in the airways inflammatory infiltrate (9–12), particularly in nonatopic asthma (12). Macrophages are present even in mild asthmatics (13) and in patients with newly diagnoses asthma (14). However, the increase in the numbers of macrophages in the airways was first described in a group of young smokers (15) and is far greater in chronic bronchitis than in asthma or control subjects, particularly in bronchioles and surrounding alveoli (16,17).

Alveolar macrophages (AM) recovered by bronchoalveolar lavage (BAL) have been extensively studied in asthma and most studies have revealed their increased activation (18–24) and shown a significant correlation between their activation and the severity of asthma (25,26). Using Percoll density fractionation, it was shown that AM of asthmatics are hypodense compared to those of normal subjects (27). Endobronchial challenge with allergen has induced the activation of AM (28–31) and they are also activated during the late-phase reaction following allergen challenge (32). Cytokines that usually downregulate AM, such as IL-4, are less effective in asthmatic patients than in control subjects (23,24).

Macrophages may be also involved in generation of the airways obstruction and regulation of the airways inflammation through release enzymes (19), eicosanoids (33), PAF (34), oxygen free radicals and cytokines (22,23), and mucus secretagogues (35) that are likely to be deleterious for the bronchi. Macrophages can also modulate the immune response (36,37).

IV. Role of Macrophages in Airway Remodeling in Asthma

The pathogenesis of airway remodeling can be considered a multistep process, in which an important role is played by the following factors.

1. The persistence of activated inflammatory cells within the bronchial mucosa

2. The release of cytokines and growth factors able to modulate the proliferation and activation of mesenchymal cells (fibroblasts and myofibroblasts)
3. The altered homeostasis of the extracellular matrix components

In each of these biological steps, airway macrophages are able to play an important role, contributing to the pathogeneis of many of the structural alterations of the bronchial architecture characterizing bronchial asthma.

A. Persistence of Macrophages in the Airways of Asthmatics

The survival of inflammatory cells in airway tissues depends on survival factors. Apoptosis, a dynamic process involved in the control of the "tissue load" of cells at inflamed sites, tends to limit inflammatory tissue injury and to promote resolution rather than progression of inflammation (38,39). Since the initiation of apoptosis serves to terminate the inflammatory process by reducing the number of inflammatory cells within the bronchial mucosa, the persistence of inflammation may be due to abnormalities in the regulation of cell apoptosis leading to a chronic and self-perpetuating inflammatory cell survival and accumulation. Thus, once at the site of airways inflammation, their survival as activated cells is increased (40) as a consequence of reduced apoptosis (41,42). We studied the survival of tissue macrophages in asthmatic and chronic bronchitis subjects, and found that the absolute number of apoptotic macrophages was significantly lower in asthma than in chronic bronchitis, and inversely correlated with the severity of asthma (43). These data suggest that the chronic accumulation of macrophages in asthma is due to an increased recruitment of these cells in the airways (11) as well as by an inhibition of their programmed cell death.

B. Release of Fibrogenic Growth Factors

Macrophages may also be involved in regulation of the airway remodeling through the secretion of growth-promoting factors for fibroblasts, cytokines, as well as growth factor, such as platelet-derived growth factor (PDGF), basic fibroblast growth factor (b-FGF), transforming growth factor-β (TGF-β) (44), and insulin growth factor (IGF) (45,46), which can play an important role in fibrosis (47).

Airway macrophages appear to play a crucial role in the pathogenesis of fibrotic lung processes (48,49) since the suppression of monocyte-macrophage infiltration in healing wounds blocks the evolution of fibrotic lesions (50).

In interstitial lung diseases, airway macrophages directly participate to the remodeling of the airways by releasing cytokines, plasminogen activator, and a fibrinolytic inhibitor MIP-1α (51–53), hepatocyte growth factor (54), and PDGF-β chain (55–58). In bleomycin-induced pulmonary fibrosis TGF-β is directly involved (59). In patients with fibrotic lung diseases, increased TGF-β production colocalized with areas of increased fibrotic ECM protein deposition has been demonstrated in biopsies (60).

Similarly to interstitial lung disease, in asthma, airway macrophages can participate in tissue repair and remodeling by releasing a wide range of fibrogenic mediators. We found a greater TGF-β release by AM in asthmatics and chronic bronchitics than in controls (61). TGF-β is increased after allergen challenge in the BAL fluid (62). TGF-β is considered to be a major fibrogenic cytokine (47,63), and its overexpression in asthma was correlated to some markers of airway remodeling, such as the thickness of the reticular layer of the basement membrane and the number of fibroblasts (64). In addition to TGF-β, airway macrophages can express other profibrotic growth factors in asthma, such as PDGF-β (65), and endothelin. Platelet-derived growth factor can be produced by most inflammatory cell types of the airways inflammation, and appears to be involved in tissue repair via the induction of the migration and proliferation of connective tissue cells, including smooth muscle (66,67). In asthma, transcripts for PDGF (68) have been found in eosinophils infiltrating the airways. However, PDGF immunoreactivity does not seems to be greater in the airways of asthmatics than in those of normal subjects (69,70). The lack of an increased production of PDGF in asthma may explain, at least in part, why airway remodeling in this disease is a slow process, and does not evolve rapidly toward severe fibrosis, as observed in fibrotic lung diseases (71) or even COPD in which PDGF immunoreactivity is increased (69).

Airway macrophages can also produce endothelin, another growth factor involved in tissue repair and remodeling. Endothelin can modulate the activation and proliferation of fibroblasts, myofibroblasts (72), and airway smooth muscle thereby contributing to the increased muscle mass and to bronchial obstruction observed in asthma (73). Endothelin immunoreactivity is overexpressed in bronchial biopsies of asthmatic patients (74), and its concentrations in BAL fluid are higher in asthmatic than in normal subjects (75,76), and after bronchial allergen challenge (62). In asthma, AM not only release endothelin in greater amounts than in controls (24), but they also respond to endothelin stimulation by releasing increased levels of fibronectin and TNF-α, two mediators involved in tissue repair and remodeling (24,77). TNF-α can, in turn, stimulate endothelin secretion from cultured airway smooth muscle cells, accelerating the proliferation of mesenchymal cells and the expression of GM-CSF mRNA in the human fetal lung fibroblast (78).

In asthma, it is likely that airway macrophages participate in a dynamic cellular network in which autocrine and paracrine stimulations lead to an over-production of fibrogenic growth factors responsible for tissue damage, repair, and remodeling (Fig. 2).

C. Homeostasis of the ECM

Connective tissue cells produce and secrete an array of macromolecules forming a complex network filling the extracellular space of the submucosa called the ECM (79). Extracellular matrix is a complex and dynamic meshwork. The macromolecules that constitute the ECM consist of fibrous proteins (collagen, elastin) and structural or adhesive proteins (fibronectin and laminin) embedded in a hydrated polysaccharide gel containing several glycosaminoglycans including hyaluronic acid (HA). The glucosaminoglycans, proteoglycans, and structural proteins trap water molecules to form a highly hydrated gel-like ''ground substance'' in which the insoluble fibrous proteins are embedded, giving the matrix strength, rigidity, and resilience. The ECM is a dynamic structure and an equilibrium between synthesis (80) and degradation of ECM

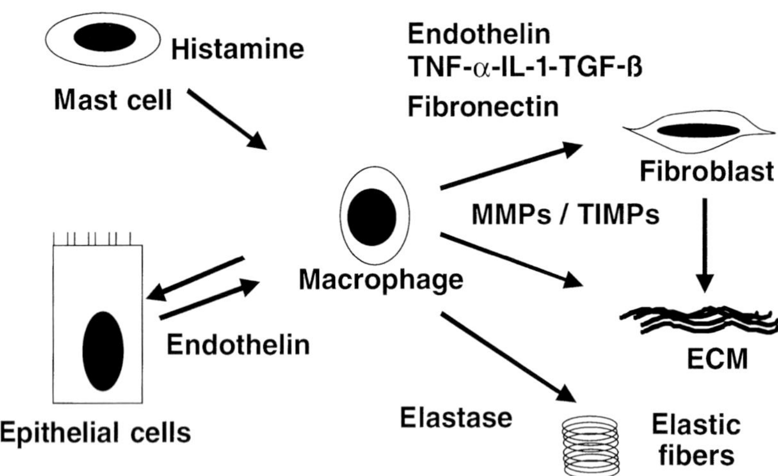

Figure 2   Role of macrophages in the cellular network underlying airway inflammation and remodeling in asthma.

components is required for the maintenance of its homeostasis. Matrix metalloproteinases (MMPs) are major proteolytic enzymes that are involved in extracellular matrix (ECM) turnover, due to their ability to cleave all the proteins constituting ECM (81). MMP-9 is the major metalloprotease found in the airways and its major inhibitor is tissue inhibitor metalloprotease-1 (TIMP-1).

Airway macrophages participate in the homeostasis and turnover of ECM by releasing several ECM components, such as fibronectin. In asthma, the spontaneous release of fibronectin by AM is increased in comparison to controls (61) and appears to be modulated by endothelin and histamine (24,82).

The turnover of ECM is regulated, at least in part, by MMP-9 and TIMP-1. In a recent study we found that in sputum of asthmatic and chronic bronchitis subjects the levels of TIMP-1 are significantly increased as compared with those of control subjects (83), and that the molar ratio between MMP-9 and TIMP-1 is significantly lower than in control subjects, suggesting the existence of a protease-antiprotease imbalance in these diseases. High levels of TIMP-1 can lead to an increased deposition of ECM components and may increase myofibroblast proliferation acting through its cell-growth-promoting activity (84). These data, together with the absence of activated MMP-9 probably associated with the excess of TIMP-1, suggest a trend toward fibrosis in both asthma and chronic bronchitis. Hence, the high levels of TIMP-1 may potentially contribute to the pathogenesis of the increased thickness of the basement membrane in asthma (85) and of the ECM deposition in the airway wall in chronic bronchitis (86). In asthma we also found an inverse correlation between MMP-9/TIMP-1 molar ratio and airway obstruction. Although eosinophils, neutrophils, and epithelial cells can release MMPs and TIMPs, airway macrophages appear to be important cells. MMP-9 was found to be increased in supernatants from AM recovered from untreated asthmatics, in comparison to control healthy subjects, patients suffering from chronic bronchitis, and asthmatic patients treated with inhaled corticosteroids (87). Moreover, TIMP-1 was also found to be increased in AM from asthmatics and the MMP-9 to TIMP-1 molar ratio was lower in untreated asthmatics (88). The presence of an excess of TIMP-1 over MMP-9 in asthma may protect the bronchi against metalloproteinase-degrading activity, but it may also interfere with tissue repair and also contribute to fibrosis by its inhibition of MMP-9 or other MMP in vivo. The increased levels of TIMP-1 found in asthma and chronic bronchitis can be the result of the effects of several mediators released during the development of airway inflammation in these diseases, among which TGF-β may be of great importance (63).

Airway macrophages can directly control the turnover of ECM by producing other proteases and protease inhibitors (81,89) including elastase (90). Human macrophage metalloelastase (HME) is a recent addition to the matrix metalloproteinase (MMP) family that was initially found to be expressed in AM of cigarette smokers. The elastolytic activity of lung macrophages has also been shown to be modulated by inflammatory mediators and, to a lesser extent, by phagocytosis (90,91). The ability of AM to exert an elastolytic activity may play an important role in airway remodeling in asthma but no data are available yet. Finally, it has been shown that macrophages can influence the expression of metalloproteases generated by other cell types, such as the interstitial collagenase (MMP-13; collagenase-3) gene from fibroblastic cells within silicotic lung granulomas. This activity is dependent on the combined effects of TNF-α and 12-lipoxygenase-derived arachidonic acid metabolites, and involved the induction of nuclear activator protein-1 activity (92).

D. Angiogenesis

Several recent pieces of evidence lend support to the hypothesis that asthma is characterized by an increased mucosal angiogenesis. An increase in vessel area has been demonstrated in asthma (93,94), and it may play an important role in the pathogenesis of a thickened airway wall (95) in this disease. Although a direct role of AM in angiogenesis in asthma has not yet been demonstrated, these cells have the potential to release various endothelial growth factors involved in tissue angiogenesis, such as vascular endothelial growth factor (VEGF) (96), bFGF, platelet-derived endothelial cell growth factor (PD-ECGF), HGF, prostaglandins, TGF-α, and PDGF. In primary pulmonary hypertension the vascular remodeling is characterized by inflammatory infiltrates, endothelial cell proliferation, and a high expression of 5-lipoxygenase and five lypoxygenase activating protein (FLAP) in AM which are more frequently found in clusters in the vicinity of remodeled blood vessels, suggesting that these cells have the potential to play an important role in vascular remodeling (97). This hypothesis is also supported by the evidence that in acute and chronic hyperoxia-induced lung injury AM can produce high levels of TNF-α, contributing to alveolar-capillary membrane remodeling, including microvessel wall thickening and interstitial fibrosis (98). It is therefore likely that macrophages have the potential to participate in most processes in healing from acute and chronic inflammation through angiogenesis (99,100), proliferation of endothelial and mesenchymal cells, and the regulation of ECM synthesis and degradation possibly leading to fibrosis (101).

V. Pharmacological Control of Airway Remodeling

The effects of anti-inflammatory drugs on the process of airways remodeling are little studied (102), but there is an increasing need to understand whether and to what extent the use of anti-inflammatory drugs can reduce or reverse the structural changes of the airway mucosa due to tissue remodeling. Compelling evidence has been obtained showing that AM can directly influence the evolution of airway remodeling in asthma, contributing either directly or through the stimulation of other cells to the production of huge amounts of substances capable of altering the original architecture of the airways. It is therefore conceivable to consider AM of asthmatic subjects as an important target for the development of effective therapeutically strategies for the control of airway remodeling in asthma.

References

1. van-Furth R. Production and migration of monocytes and kinetics of macrophages. In: van-Furth R, ed. Mononuclear Phagocytes. Dordrecht, NL: Kluwer Academic Publishers, 1992:3–12.
2. Johnston R Jr. Current concepts: immunology. Monocytes and macrophages. N Engl J Med 1988; 318:747–752.
3. Unanue ER, Cerottini JC. Antigen presentation. FASEB J 1989; 3:2496–2502.
4. Sibille Y, Reynolds HY. Macrophages and polymorphonuclear neutrophils in lung defense and injury. Am Rev Respir Dis 1990; 141:471–501.
5. Stein M, Keshav S. The versatility of macrophages. Clin Exp Allergy 1992; 22:19–27.
6. Nathan CF. Secretory products of macrophages. J Clin Invest 1987; 79:319–326.
7. Werb Z, Underwood J, Rappolee D. The role of macrophage-derived growth factors in tissue repair. In: van-Furth R, ed. Mononuclear Phagocytes. Dordrecht: Kluwer Academic Press, 1992:404–409.
8. Bousquet J, Chanez P, Arnoux B, Vignola AM, Damon M, Michel FB, Godard Ph. Monocytes and macrophages and asthma. Immunopharmacol Allergic Dis 1996; 8:263–286.
9. Poulter LW, Power C, Burke C. The relationship between bronchial immunopathology and hyperresponsiveness in asthma. Eur Respir J 1990; 3:792–799.
10. Bradley BL, Azzawi M, Jacobson M, Assoufi B, Collins JV, Irani AM, Schwartz LB, Durham SR, Jeffery PK. Eosinophils, T-lymphocytes, mast cells, neutrophils, and macrophages in bronchial biopsy specimens from atopic subjects with asthma: comparison with biopsy specimens from atopic subjects

without asthma and normal control subjects and relationship to bronchial hyper-responsiveness. J Allergy Clin Immunol 1991; 88:661–674.

11. Poston RN, Chanez P, Lacoste JY, Litchfield T, Lee TH, Bousquet J. Immuno-histochemical characterization of the cellular infiltration in asthmatic bronchi. Am Rev Respir Dis 1992; 145:918–921.

12. Bentley AM, Menz G, Storz C, Robinson DS, Bradley, Jeffery PK, Durham SR, Kay AB. Identification of T lymphocytes, macrophages, and activated eosinophils in the bronchial mucosa in intrinsic asthma. Relationship to symptoms and bronchial responsiveness. Am Rev Respir Dis 1992; 146:500–506.

13. Vignola AM, Chanez P, Campbell AM, Souques F, Lebel B, Enander I, Bousquet J. Airway inflammation in mild intermittent and in persistent asthma. Am J Respir Crit Care Med 1998; 157:403–409.

14. Laitinen LA, Laitinen A, Haahtela T, Vilkka V, Spur BW, Lee TH. Leukotriene E4 and granulocytic infiltration into asthmatic airways. Lancet 1993; 341:989–990.

15. Niewoehner D, Kleinerman J, Rice D. Pathologic changes in the peripheral airways of young cigarette smokers. N Engl J Med 1974; 278:1355–1360.

16. Saetta M, Di-Stefano A, Maestrelli P, Ferraresso A, Drigo R, Potena A, Ciaccia A, Fabbri LM. Activated T-lymphocytes and macrophages in bronchial mucosa of subjects with chronic bronchitis. Am Rev Respir Dis 1993; 147:301–306.

17. O'Shaughnessy TC, Ansari TW, Barnes NC, Jeffery PK. Inflammation in bronchial biopsies of subjects with chronic bronchitis: inverse relationship of CD8+ T lymphocytes with FEV_1. Am J Respir Crit Care Med 1997; 155:852–857.

18. Godard P, Chaintreuil J, Damon M, Coupe M, Flandre O, Crastes-de-Paulet A, Michel FB. Functional assessment of alveolar macrophages: comparison of cells from asthmatics and normal subjects. J Allergy Clin Immunol 1982; 70:88–93.

19. Joseph M, Tonnel AB, Torpier G, Capron A, Arnoux B, Benveniste J. Involvement of immunoglobulin E in the secretory processes of alveolar macrophages from asthmatic patients. J Clin Invest 1983; 71:221–230.

20. Fuller RW, O'Malley G, Baker AJ, MacDermot J. Human alveolar macrophage activation: inhibition by forskolin but not beta-adrenoceptor stimulation or phosphodiesterase inhibition. Pulm Pharmacol 1988; 1:101–106.

21. Rankin JA. The contribution of alveolar macrophages to hyperreactive airway disease. J Allergy Clin Immunol 1989; 83:722–729.

22. Borish L, Mascali JJ, Dishuck J, Beam WR, Martin RJ, Rosenwasser LJ. Detection of alveolar macrophage-derived IL-1 beta in asthma. Inhibition with corticosteroids. J Immunol 1992; 149:3078–3082.

23. Chanez P, Vignola AM, Paul-Eugene N, Dugas B, Godard P, Michel FB, Bousquet J. Modulation by interleukin-4 of cytokine release from mononuclear phagocytes in asthma. J Allergy Clin Immunol 1994; 94:997–1005.

24. Chanez P, Vignola AM, Albat B, Springall DR, Polak JM, Godard P, Bousquet

J. Involvement of endothelin in mononuclear phagocyte inflammation in asthma. J Allergy Clin Immunol 1996; 98:412–420.

25. Cluzel M, Damon M, Chanez P, Bousquet J, Crastes-de-Paulet A, Michel FB, Godard P. Enhanced alveolar cell luminol-dependent chemiluminescence in asthma. J Allergy Clin Immunol 1987; 80:195–201.

26. Kelly C, Ward C, Stenton CS, Bird G, Hendrick DJ, Walters EH. Number and activity of inflammatory cells in bronchoalveolar lavage fluid in asthma and their relation to airway responsiveness. Thorax 1988; 43:684–692.

27. Chanez P, Bousquet J, Couret I, Cornillac L, Barneon G, Vic P, Michel FB, Godard P. Increased numbers of hypodense alveolar macrophages in patients with bronchial asthma. Am Rev Respir Dis 1991; 144:923–930.

28. Tonnel AB, Joseph M, Gosset P, Fournier E, Capron A. Stimulation of alveolar macrophages in asthmatic patients after local provocation test. Lancet 1983; 1: 1406–1408.

29. Metzger WJ, Zavala D, Richerson HB, Moseley P, Iwamota P, Monick M, Sjoerdsma K, Hunninghake GW. Local allergen challenge and bronchoalveolar lavage of allergic asthmatic lungs. Description of the model and local airway inflammation. Am Rev Respir Dis 1987; 135:433–440.

30. Calhoun WJ, Reed HE, Moest DR, Stevens CA. Enhanced superoxide production by alveolar macrophages and air-space cells, airway inflammation, and alveolar macrophage density changes after segmental antigen bronchoprovocation in allergic subjects. Am Rev Respir Dis 1992; 145:317–325.

31. Calhoun WJ, Jarjour NN, Gleich GJ, Stevens CA, Busse WW. Increased airway inflammation with segmental versus aerosol antigen challenge. Am Rev Respir Dis 1993; 147:1465–1471.

32. Gosset P, Tsicopoulos A, Wallaert B, Vannimenus C, Joseph M, Tonnel AB, Capron A. Increased secretion of tumor necrosis factor alpha and interleukin-6 by alveolar macrophages consecutive to the development of the late asthmatic reaction. J Allergy Clin Immunol 1991; 88:561–571.

33. Damon M, Chavis C, Daures JP, Crastes-de-Paulet A, Michel FB, Godard P. Increased generation of the arachidonic metabolites LTB4 and 5-HETE by human alveolar macrophages in patients with asthma: effect in vitro of nedocromil sodium. Eur Respir J 1989; 2:202–209.

34. Arnoux B, Jouvin-Marche E, Arnoux A, Chrétien J, Benveniste J. Release of paf-acether from human monocytes. Agents Action 1982; 12:713–716.

35. Sperber K, Chanez P, Bousquet J, Goswami S, Marom Z. Detection of a novel macrophage-derived mucus secretagogue (MMS-68) in bronchoalveolar lavage fluid of patients with asthma. J Allergy Clin Immunol 1995; 95:868–876.

36. Aubas P, Cosso B, Godard P, Michel FB, Clot J. Decreased suppressor cell activity of alveolar macrophages in bronchial asthma. Am Rev Respir Dis 1984; 130:875–878.

37. Poulter LW, Janossy G, Power C, Sreenan S, Burke C. Immunological/physiological relationships in asthma: potential regulation by lung macrophages. Immunol Today 1994; 15:258–261.

38. Haslett C, Savill JS, Whyte MK, Stern M, Dransfield I, Meagher LC. Granulocyte apoptosis and the control of inflammation. Philos Trans R Soc Lond B Biol Sci 1994; 345:327–333.

39. White E. Life, death, and the pursuit of apoptosis. Genes Dev 1996; 10:1–15.

40. Ohnishi T, Sur S, Collins DS, Fish JE, Gleich GJ, Peters SP. Eosinophil survival activity identified as interleukin-5 is associated with eosinophil recruitment and degranulation and lung injury twenty-four hours after segmental antigen lung challenge. J Allergy Clin Immunol 1993; 92:607–615.

41. Woolley KL, Gibson PG, Carty K, Wilson AJ, Twaddell SH, Woolley MJ. Eosinophil apoptosis and the resolution of airway inflammation in asthma. Am J Respir Crit Care Med 1996; 154:237–243.

42. Walsh G. Mechanisms of human eosinophil survival and apoptosis. Clin Exp Allergy 1997; 27:482–487.

43. Vignola AM, Chanez P, Chiappara G, Merendino AM, Reina C, Gagliardo R, Profita M, Bousquet J, Bonsignore J. Evaluation of apoptosis of eosinophils, macrophages and T-lymphocytes in mucosal biopsies of asthmatic and chronic bronchitis patients. J Allergy Clin Immunol 1999; 103:563–573.

44. Rennard SI, Hunninghake GW, Bitterman PB, Crystal RG. Production of fibronectin by the human alveolar macrophage: mechanism for the recruitment of fibroblasts to sites of tissue injury in interstitial lung diseases. Proc Natl Acad Sci USA 1981; 78:7147–7151.

45. Aston C, Jagirdar J, Lee TC, Hur T, Hintz RL, Rom WN. Enhanced insulin-like growth factor molecules in idiopathic pulmonary fibrosis. Am J Respir Crit Care Med 1995; 151:1597–1603.

46. Homma S, Nagaoka I, Abe H, Takahashi K, Seyama K, Nukiwa T, Kira S. Localization of platelet-derived growth factor and insulin-like growth factor I in the fibrotic lung. Am J Respir Crit Care Med 1995; 152:2084–2089.

47. Kovacs E, DiPietro L. Fibrogenic cytokines and connective tissue production. FASEB J 1994; 8:854–861.

48. Assoian RK, Fleurdelys BE, Stevenson HC, et al. Expression and secretion of type beta transforming growth factor by activated human macrophages. Proc Natl Acad Sci USA 1987; 84:6020–6024.

49. Shaw R, Kelly J. Macrophages/monocytes. In: Phan S, Thrall R, eds. Pulmonary Fibrosis. New York: Marcel Dekker, 1995:405–444.

50. Leibovich S, Ross R. The role of the macrophage in wound repair. Am J Pathol 1975; 78:71–100.

51. Chapman HA, Allen CL, Stone OL. Abnormalities in pathways of alveolar fibrin turnover among patients with interstitial lung disease. Am Rev Respir Dis 1986; 133:437–443.

52. Lyberg T, Nakstad B, Hetland O, Boye NP. Procoagulant (thromboplastin) activity in human bronchoalveolar lavage fluids is derived from alveolar macrophages. Eur Respir J 1990; 3:61–67.

53. Piguet PF, Ribaux C, Karpuz V, Grau GE, Kapanci Y. Expression and localiza-

tion of tumor necrosis factor-alpha and its mRNA in idiopathic pulmonary fibrosis. Am J Pathol 1993; 143:651–655.

54. Sakai T, Satoh K, Matsushima K, et al. Hepatocyte growth factor in bronchoalveolar lavage fluids and cells in. Am J Respir Cell Mol Biol 1997; 16:388–397.

55. Antoniades HN, Bravo MA, Avila RE, et al. Platelet-derived growth factor in idiopathic pulmonary fibrosis. J Clin Invest 1990; 86:1055–1064.

56. Marinelli WA, Polunovsky VA, Harmon KR, Bitterman PB. Role of platelet-derived growth factor in pulmonary fibrosis [comment]. Am J Respir Cell Mol Biol 1991; 5:503–504.

57. Vignaud JM, Allam M, Martinet N, Pech M, Plenat F, Martinet Y. Presence of platelet-derived growth factor in normal and fibrotic lung is specifically associated with interstitial macrophages, while both interstitial macrophages and alveolar epithelial cells express the c-sis proto-oncogene [see comments]. Am J Respir Cell Mol Biol 1991; 5:531–538.

58. Shaw RJ, Benedict SH, Clark RA, King T, Jr. Pathogenesis of pulmonary fibrosis in interstitial lung disease. Alveolar macrophage PDGF(B) gene activation and up-regulation by interferon gamma. Am Rev Respir Dis 1991; 143:167–173.

59. Khalil N, Bereznay O, Sporn M, Greenberg AH. Macrophage production of transforming growth factor beta and fibroblast collagen synthesis in chronic pulmonary inflammation. J Exp Med 1989; 170:727–737.

60. Broekelmann TJ, Limper AH, Colby TV, McDonald JA. Transforming growth factor beta 1 is present at sites of extracellular matrix gene expression in human pulmonary fibrosis. Proc Natl Acad Sci USA 1991; 88:6642–6646.

61. Vignola A, Chanez P, Chiappara G, et al. Release of transforming growth factor-β and fibronectin by alveolar macrophages in airway diseases. Clin Exp Immunol 1996; 106:114–119.

62. Redington AE, Madden J, Frew AJ, et al. Transforming growth factor-beta 1 in asthma. Measurement in bronchoalveolar lavage fluid. Am J Respir Crit Care Med 1997; 156:642–647.

63. Border W, Noble N. Transforming growth factor β in tissue fibrosis. N Engl J Med 1994; 331:1286–1292.

64. Vignola AM, Chanez P, Chiappara G, et al. Transforming growth factor-β expression in mucosal biopsies in asthma and chronic bronchitis. Am J Respir Crit Care Med 1997; 156:591–599.

65. Taylor IK, Sorooshian M, Wangoo A, et al. Platelet-derived growth factor-beta mRNA in human alveolar macrophages in vivo in asthma. Eur Respir J 1994; 7:1966–1972.

66. Ross R. Platelet-derived growth factor. Lancet 1989; 1:1179–1182.

67. Heldin CH. Structural and functional studies on platelet-derived growth factor. EMBO J 1992; 11:4251–4259.

68. Ohno K, Ammann P, Fasciati R, Maier P. Transforming growth factor beta 1

preferentially induces apoptotic cell death in rat hepatocytes cultured under pericentral-equivalent conditions. Toxicol Appl Pharmacol 1995; 132:227–236.

69. Chanez P, Vignola M, Steinger R, Vic P, Michel F, Bousquet J. Platelet-derived growth factor in asthma. Allergy 1995; 50:878–883.

70. Aubert JD, Hayashi S, Hards J, Bai TR, Pare PD, Hogg JC. Platelet-derived growth factor and its receptor in lungs from patients with asthma and chronic airflow obstruction. Am J Physiol 1994; 266:L655–663.

71. Lama M. Pulmonary fibrosis: Human and experimental disease. Connec Tissue Health Dis 1990; 1:123–188.

72. Takuwa N, Takuwa Y, Yanagisawa M, Yamashita K, Masaki T. A novel vasoactive peptide endothelin stimulates mitogenesis through inositol lipid turnover in Swiss 3T3 fibroblasts. J Biol Chem 1989; 264:7856–7861.

73. Luscher TF. Endothelin: systemic arterial and pulmonary effects of a new peptide with potent biologic properties. Am Rev Respir Dis 1992;146:S56–60.

74. Springall DR, Howarth PH, Counihan H, Djukanovic R, Holgate ST, Polak JM. Endothelin immunoreactivity of airway epithelium in asthmatic patients. Lancet 1991; 337:697–701.

75. Nomura A, Uchida Y, Kameyana M, Saotome M, Oki K, Hasegawa S. Endothelin and bronchial asthma [letter]. Lancet 1989; 2:747–748.

76. Kraft M, Beam WR, Wenzel SE, Zamora MR, O'Brien RF, Martin RJ. Blood and bronchoalveolar lavage endothelin-1 levels in nocturnal asthma. Am J Respir Crit Care Med 1994; 149:946–952.

77. Thrall RS, Vogel SN, Evans R, Shultz LD. Role of tumor necrosis factor-alpha in the spontaneous development of pulmonary fibrosis in viable motheaten mutant mice. Am J Pathol 1997; 151:1303–1310.

78. Xu J, Zhong NS. The interaction of tumour necrosis factor alpha and endothelin-1 in pathogenetic models of asthma. Clin Exp Allergy 1997; 27:568–573.

79. Alberts B, Bray D, Lewis J, Raff M, Roberts K, Watson J. Cell Adhesion, Cell Junctions, and the Extracellular Matrix. New York: Garland, 1989:792–834.

80. Mosher D, Sottile J, Wu C, McDonald J. Assembly of extracellular matrix. Curr Opin Cell Biol 1992; 4:810–818.

81. Matrisian LM. The matrix-degrading metalloproteinases. Bioessays 1992; 14:455–463.

82. Vignola AM, Chanez P, Paul-Lacoste P, Paul-Eugene N, Godard P, Bousquet J. Phenotypic and functional modulation of normal human alveolar macrophages by histamine. Am J Respir Cell Mol Biol 1994; 11:456–463.

83. Vignola AM, Riccobono L, Mirabella A, et al. Sputum MMP-9/TIMP-1 ratio correlates with airflow obstruction in asthma and chronic bronchitis. Am J Crit Care Med 1998; 158:1945–1950.

84. Hayakawa T. Tissue inhibitors of metalloproteinase and their cell growth-promoting activity. Cell Struct Funct 1994; 19:109–114.

85. Roche WR, Beasley R, Williams JH, Holgate ST. Subepithelial fibrosis in the bronchi of asthmatics. Lancet 1989; 1:520–524.

86. Thurlbeck WM. Pathology of chronic airflow obstruction. Chest 1990; 97:6S–10S.
87. Mautino G, Oliver N, Chanez P, Bousquet J, Capony F. Increased release of matrix metalloproteinase-9 in bronchoalveolar lavage fluid and by alveolar macrophages of asthmatics. Am J Respir Cell Mol Biol 1997; 17:583–591.
88. Mautino G, Henriquet C, Oliver N, Bousquet J, Capony F. Elevated levels of tissue inhibitor of metalloproteinase-1 in bronchoalveolar lavage of asthmatic patients. Lab Invest 1999; 79:39–47.
89. O'Connor CM, FitzGerald MX. Matrix metalloproteases and lung disease. Thorax 1994; 49:602–609.
90. Werb Z, Gordon S. Elastase secretion by stimulated macrophages: characterization and regulation. J Exp Med 1975; 142:361–377.
91. White R, Lin HS, Kuhn C. Elastase secretion by peritoneal exudative and alveolar macrophages. J Exp Med 1977; 146:802–808.
92. Mariani TJ, Sandefur S, Roby JD, Pierce RA. Collagenase-3 induction in rat lung fibroblasts requires the combined. Mol Biol Cell 1998; 9:1411–1424.
93. Kuwano K, Bosken CH, Pare PD, Bai TR, Wiggs BR, Hogg JC. Small airways dimensions in asthma and in chronic obstructive pulmonary disease. Am Rev Respir Dis 1993; 148:1220–1225.
94. Saetta M, Di-Stefano A, Rosina C, Thiene G, Fabbri LM. Quantitative structural analysis of peripheral airways and arteries in sudden fatal asthma. Am Rev Respir Dis 1991; 143:138–143.
95. James AL, Pare PD, Hogg JC. The mechanics of airway narrowing in asthma. Am Rev Respir Dis 1989; 139:242–246.
96. Brown DL, Kao WW, Greenhalgh DG. Apoptosis down-regulates inflammation under the advancing epithelial wound edge: delayed patterns in diabetes and improvement with topical growth factors. Surgery 1997; 121:372–380.
97. Wright L, Tuder RM, Wang J, Cool CD, Lepley RA, Voelkel NF. 5-Lipoxygenase and 5-lipoxygenase activating protein (FLAP) immunoreactivity in lungs from patients with primary pulmonary hypertension. Am J Respir Crit Care Med 1998; 157:219–229.
98. Horinouchi H, Wang CC, Shepherd KE, Jones R. TNF alpha gene and protein expression in alveolar macrophages in acute and chronic hyperoxia-induced lung injury. Am J Respir Cell Mol Biol 1996; 14:548–555.
99. Sunderkötter C, Steinbrink K, Goebeler M, Bhardawaj R, Sorg C. Macrophages and angiogenesis. J Leukocyte Biol 1994; 55:410–422.
100. Wahl LM, Shankavaram U, Zhang Y. Role of macrophages in vascular tissue remodelling. Transplant Immunol 1997; 5:173–176.
101. Shaw RJ. The role of lung macrophages at the interface between chronic inflammation and fibrosis. Respir Med 1991; 85:267–273.
102. Laitinen LA, Laitinen A. Remodeling of asthmatic airways by glucocorticosteroids. J Allergy Clin Immunol 1996; 97:153–158.

13

Airway Smooth Muscle as a Target for Novel Antiasthma Drugs Acting on Airway Wall Remodeling

ALASTAIR G. STEWART

University of Melbourne
Parkville, Victoria, Australia

I. Introduction

Airway wall thickening was first described in the 1920s and confirmed by several groups, most notably by Dunnill and colleagues (1). Recent studies have confirmed and extended these observations by demonstrating that both hypertrophy and hyperplasia contribute to the increase in volume of the airway wall occupied by airway smooth muscle (2). The notion that airway wall remodeling contributes significantly to airway hyperresponsiveness (AHR) in asthma and chronic obstructive pulmonary disease is largely based on the work of Hogg and colleagues, whose studies of postmortem material have shown that there is a severity-dependent increase in the overall dimensions of the airway. When modeled mathematically, the resulting airway wall thickening appears to be capable of accounting for much of the AHR in asthma (3).

AHR shows a major underlying component that is relatively resistant to drug treatment and a smaller component that is seasonal in its severity and is amenable to drug treatment. Interestingly, similar seasonal increases in airway responsiveness are reported to occur in atopic, nonasthmatic subjects without AHR outside the allergen season (4). In some patients, prolonged allergen avoidance may be sufficient to reduce the levels of AHR to those observed in healthy individuals (5). Collectively, these findings indicate that AHR and, by inference, airway wall remodeling are at least partly reversible. If airway wall remodeling is spontaneously reversible, it is highly likely that reversal can be influenced by appropriate drug treatment. However, if the smooth muscle component of AHR is to be a useful independent drug target, then reductions in AHR should impact on asthma severity. Longitudinal studies simultaneously measuring AHR and asthma symptoms during seasonal fluctuations in asthma severity indicate a strong association between these

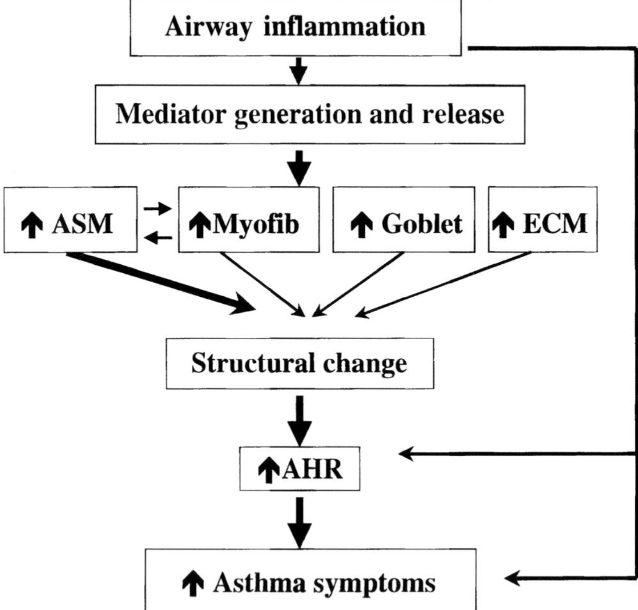

Figure 1 Relationship between airway inflammation, structural changes, and asthma symptoms. The dominant influence of increases in volume occupied by airway smooth muscle justifies it as a primary target for drugs acting on airway wall remodeling.

parameters (5). It seems reasonable to suggest that AHR is necessary (but not sufficient) for asthma symptoms and therefore its reduction will impact on clinical asthma.

A. Is Airway Smooth Muscle a Rational Therapeutic Target?

The relative importance of the changes in airway wall volume occupied by smooth muscle compared with other cellular compartments is a consideration in assessing whether smooth muscle per se is a rational target for new agents (Fig. 1). The other cellular compartments that contribute to the remodeling response include mucus cell metaplasia (6), subepithelial fibrosis (7), angiogenesis (8), and fibroblasts, which may be activated to a myofibroblast phenotype (9). Mathematical simulations showing that increases in smooth muscle volume have the largest impact of any of the changes in different cell types on airway narrowing in responses to smooth muscle shortening (10) provide the logic for the assertion that airway smooth muscle hyperplastic and hypertrophic growth are legitimate novel drug targets for antiasthma agents. The remainder of this chapter will examine what is known of the effects of existing agents on airway smooth muscle growth and will discuss strategies that could provide drug treatments for this key feature of asthma pathology that are complementary to current regimens.

II. Why Does Asthmatic Airway Smooth Muscle Grow Excessively?

It is commonly asserted that chronic inflammation in the airways is responsible for many, if not all, aspects of the remodeling process (11,12), but there is no definitive evidence for this mechanism from clinical studies. An important role for inflammation in remodeling is supported by the ability to mimic remodeling in animal models of chronic antigen-induced bronchoconstriction. Nevertheless, it is not yet possible to exclude a genetic basis for remodeling. Observations of strain differences between Fisher and Lewis rats in airway smooth muscle content that correlate with AHR are consistent with genetic factors having a role in determining airway wall thickness (13). Airway smooth muscle cultured from these two strains maintains a differential growth rate in vitro in response to PDGF suggesting that the differences are inherent to the airway smooth muscle (14).

A. Chemical Mediators

At the molecular level, the specific mediators contributing to remodeling have not been distinguished from the plethora of mediators that have the potential to elicit hyperplasia, hypertrophy (Table 1), and increased deposition of extracellular matrix. Many growth factors and stimuli have so far been described for airway smooth muscle and it is indeed reasonable to expect that there are many more yet to be described. In cardiovascular disease, angiotensin II plays a dominant role in the hypertrophic response, whereas basic fibroblast growth factor (bFGF) appears to be the dominant mediator of cell proliferation. It is not yet clear whether there are equivalent dominant factors in asthma and chronic obstructive pulmonary disease. The application of immunohistochemistry and in situ hybridization techniques to biopsy and explant culture material have revealed the presence of a large number of growth factors within inflammatory and structural cells in the epithelial and subepithelial regions that are poised to act on the underlying airway smooth muscle (15–17). The epithelium, which is subjected to repeated episodes of injury (18), shows a high level of expression of transforming growth factor-α (TGF-α) and epidermal growth factor (EGF). The cycle of injury and repair of the epithelial layer may entail a spillover of these growth factors onto the underlying airway smooth muscle (11). The immediate proximity of mast cells to the airway smooth muscle (19) is possibly of the greatest importance to smooth muscle proliferation, as mast cells are replete with a wide array of factors known to stimulate airway smooth muscle growth. These factors include histamine, bFGF, tryptase, and cytokines such as tumor necrosis factor-α (TNFα), which have complex growth effects depending on concentration, duration of exposure, and recruitment and involvement of other cell types such as T lymphocytes (20–22). It has recently become apparent that smooth muscle cells themselves have the capacity to make a number of direct and indirect growth-modulatory mediators including granulocyte-macrophage colony-stimulating factor (GM-CSF), interleukin-6, and transforming growth factor-β (TGF-β) (23). Thus, complex and variable patterns of growth factor expression contribute to growth of airway smooth muscle. Antagonism of any single one of these growth factors is unlikely to have a sufficiently significant impact on the process to arrest the remodeling response.

B. Physical Factors

Investigation of cell proliferation has been pursued more extensively than hypertrophy, even though the latter response is well evidenced and possibly more

Table 1 Factors That Influence Growth of Airway Smooth Muscle[a]

Proliferative	Antiproliferative	Hypertrophic	Antihypertrophic
Histamine	Prostaglandin E_2	Interleukin-1	?
Substance P	Epinephrine	Interleukin-6	
Neurokinin A	Hydrocortisone	Transforming growth factor-β	
Leukotriene D_4	VIP	Cyclical strain (stretch)	
Thromboxane A_2	Angiotensin II		
Endothelin-1	Dehydroepiandrosterone		
	2-Methoxyestradiol		
	Heparin		
	Interleukin-1		
Platelet-derived growth factor	Tumor necrosis factor-α		
Epidermal growth factor	Transforming growth factor-β		
Basic fibroblast growth factor			
Insulin-like growth factor			
Transforming growth factor-α			
Transforming growth factor-β	Isoprenaline		
Interleukin-1	Salbutamol		
Interleukin-6	Salmeterol		
Tumor necrosis factor-α	Dexamethasone		
	Beclomethasone dipropionate		
Thrombin	Fluticasone propionate		
Tryptase	Methylprednisolone		
β-Hexosaminidase	Rapamycin (PI3K)		
	ST638 (PTK)		
	Ro 318220 (PKC)		
	SB203580 (p38[HOG])		
	PD98059 (MEK1)		
	Wortmannin (PI3K)		
	H_2O_2		

[a] See text for discussion and references.

important in asthmatics (2). Transforming growth factor-β (TGF-β) (24) and interleukins-1 and -6 (25,26) increase smooth muscle size. Angiotensin II, which is an established causative factor in cardiac and vascular smooth muscle cell hypertrophy, also induces hypertrophy of human cultured airway smooth muscle through induction of TGF-β (27).

The impact of strain and stress upon growth of smooth muscle in the airway wall has not been extensively explored. Smith and co-workers have shown that increased strain generated by culture of airway smooth muscle on flexible silastic membranes results in an increase in cell size and cell number together with an increase in the expression of contractile proteins such as smooth-muscle-specific α-actin (28,29). It is unusual, but not without precedent [e.g., IL-1 (25)], that a single stimulus increases cell size and proliferation, and appears to promote the contractile phenotype of the airway smooth muscle. Time-course studies may indicate whether these responses are indeed simultaneous, sequential, or whether they are occurring in distinct cell populations. It has been suggested that strain will be increased in the asthmatic airway, but this is at variance with the well-established fibrotic component of the airway wall remodeling process, which may limit bronchodilatation in severe asthmatics with a component of fixed airway obstruction (30). Strain (the stretching of cells) would be opposed by fibrosis. Fibrosis may therefore provide feedback inhibition of the growth-promoting effects of strain. On the other hand, stress, the force generated per unit area, causes muscle shortening and therefore opposes the effects of strain. Contractile agents may also antagonize the effects of strain on muscle growth responses. Strain increases both fibroblast (31) and smooth muscle (32) production of collagen types that may indirectly enhance the proliferative response (33). Simulation of cyclical strain in cultured airway smooth muscle stimulates both DNA synthesis and hypertrophy (28), the latter response occurring only when cells reach confluence (29). Thus, the capacity of bronchoconstrictors to induce cell proliferation may be underestimated in cell culture studies, in which substrate attachment prevents the development of increased strain and there is no cyclical variation due to tidal breathing. The influence of interactions between strain, stress, and extracellular matrix deposition on airway smooth muscle proliferation requires further investigation.

In asthmatic patients, airway smooth muscle is subjected to greater stress than that of healthy individuals as a result of increased exposure of the airway smooth muscle to contractile stimuli. Equilibrium length and tension measurements have not provided evidence of hypercontractility of asthmatic smooth muscle, but there is increasing interest in the importance of velocity of shortening as a component of AHR in asthma (34). Increased velocity of shortening may enable significant obstruction to occur within the expiratory phase of the cycle and may explain the absence of a bronchodilator effect of a prior deep inspiration in asthmatic subjects (34–37).

C. Growth Responses of Cultured Airway Smooth Muscle

Contractile Mediators Regulating Growth Responses

In general, agents that are primarily stimulants of the contractile response have not proved to be powerful stimulants of airway smooth muscle proliferation. Thus, neither cysteinyl leukotrienes (CysLTs) nor endothelin-1 (ET-1) increases airway smooth muscle cell number in culture, despite appearing to produce a small increase in DNA synthesis (38). Both constrictors synergize with growth factors that activate receptor tyrosine kinases (39,40). Leukotriene D_4 (LTD$_4$) has been implicated in the proliferative response to endothelin-1 in rabbit airway smooth muscle through an indirect pathway involving thromboxane A_2 and enhanced secretion of an insulin-like growth factor binding protein (IGF-BP) protease, which releases IGF from inhibition (41,42). In human airway smooth muscle LTD$_4$ acts, by stimulation of CysLT1 receptors, as a comitogen with PDGF (40). Histamine stimulates proliferation of canine (43) and human cultured airway smooth muscle cells (44). Substance P and neurokinin A elicit growth of rabbit tracheal muscle (45), but not human airway muscle (Stewart, unpublished observations). TxA$_2$ mimetics have also been shown to stimulate DNA synthesis (38,46), possibly through the secondary production of LTs (46). The regulatory role for IGF-BP released from the cell surface is achieved through activation and release of matrix metalloproteinases (MMPs) (47). Thus, IGFs secreted by airway smooth muscle stimulate proliferation when their concentration exceeds the binding capacity of IGF binding protein (IGF-BP) (47).

Studies of contractile agents have used cultured airway smooth muscle cells likely to be in the synthetic rather than contractile phenotype (48). The influence of contractile agonists on growth of native smooth muscle remains to be established.

Peptide Growth Factors

Platelet-derived growth factor (PDGF) (43,49), epidermal growth factor (EGF), and basic fibroblast growth factor (bFGF) (38) are more active and more potent than bronchoconstrictors in eliciting airway smooth muscle proliferation. In addition, serine proteases including thrombin (38,50) and mast-cell-derived tryptase (51) are powerful growth stimuli. Cleavage-dependent generation of a nascent amino terminus that acts as a tethered ligand for the protease-activated receptors (PAR) raises the possibility that transient exposure to these proteases could lead to sustained growth responses. Lysosomal hydrolases derived from inflammatory cells such as β-hexosaminidase have also been identified as airway smooth muscle mitogens acting via stimulation of a mannose receptor (52).

Proinflammatory Cytokines

The growth-promoting actions of several cytokines have been evaluated. Interleukin-1β (IL-1β) elicits both proliferation and hypertrophy secondary to the release of PDGF (25,26). Tumor necrosis factor-α (TNFα) stimulates (20,53) or inhibits growth responses depending on the concentration and duration of incubation; short incubation periods at high concentrations result in inhibition of DNA synthesis (20).

D. Intracellular Signaling Mechanisms

Evidence from a variety of cell types including airway smooth muscle supports an important regulatory role for the ras/raf/MEK1/ERK pathway (54–56) as an essential upstream signaling cascade that ultimately leads to activation of the cyclin D1 promoter (57). Signal transduction of proliferation is complex and there may be redundancies in the pathways activated by mitogens. The proximal signals activated by growth factors include phospholipase C, elevation of intracellular calcium (Ca^{2+}_i), phosphoinositol-3-kinase (P13K), protein kinase C (PKC), and tyrosine kinases (PTK) (50,58,59). Elevation of Ca^{2+}_i does not appear to be required for the proliferative response (50,58). However, none of the growth factors yet investigated fails to activate ERKs, which are members of the MAPK family of kinases. MAP kinases, and ERKs in particular, are believed to play an obligatory role in the signaling cascade that enables cells to pass through the restriction point of the cell cycle, although the relative contributions of the many different MAPK isoforms remains unclear (60). In bovine tracheal muscle, persistent ERK activation appears to be required for DNA synthesis (54) and similar observations have been made for human airway smooth muscle (61). Inhibition of ERK by PD98059, which prevents activation of the upstream kinase MEK1, inhibits proliferation induced by thrombin in human airway smooth muscle (61), PDGF in bovine tracheal airway smooth muscle (55), and ET-1 in rat airway smooth muscle (62), and decreases levels of cyclin D1 (56,61). However, both the DNA synthesis and cyclin D1 increases in response to higher concentrations of bFGF are resistant to inhibition by PD98059, despite inhibition of ERK activity, suggesting the existence of an alternative pathway leading to elevation of cyclin D1 protein levels under certain conditions. For example, we have observed that the p38^{HOG} inhibitor SB203580 reduces DNA synthesis in response to both thrombin and bFGF (Ravenhall, Fernandes, and Stewart, unpublished observations). Cyclin D1 partners cyclin-dependent kinase 4 (cdk4), which phosphorylates the restriction protein retinoblastoma (pRb) (63). Upon phosphorylation, pRb dissociates from and disinhibits the transcription factor complex E2F allowing the synthesis of genes essential for DNA synthesis and further cell cycle progression. Regulation of the levels of cyclin-dependent kinase inhibitors (cdki), p21^{cip1}/p27^{Kip1}/P57^{kip2}, and the INK family represents an alternative means of regulating cell-cycle progression. In G1 phase of the cell cycle the relative amounts and association of cyclin/cdk complexes with the cdki's determines the phosphorylation of key targets such as pRb (64,65). The links between the early signaling events and pRb phosphorylation are not well understood and may differ from those described for transformed cell lines.

III. Synthetic Activities of Airway Smooth Muscle

A. Mediator Production

There is increasing evidence that airway smooth muscle cells produce mediators that contribute to or modulate the inflammatory response (23). Exposure of airway smooth muscle to cytokines such as IL-1β, TNFα, and IFN-γ generates increased levels of secretory phospholipase A$_2$ (66), which acts in concert with increased expression of inducible cycle-oxygenase (COX-2) in human airway smooth muscle in vitro to elevate the cellular release of PGE$_2$ and PGF$_{2\alpha}$ (66–69). The bronchodilator PGE$_2$ is the main prostanoid produced by airway smooth muscle. Thus, glucocorticoids, which repress COX-2 and secretory PLA$_2$, would inhibit bronchoprotective processes (67), such as airway smooth muscle relaxation and inhibition of proliferation (70). Since PGE$_2$ is an effective regulator of airway smooth muscle DNA synthesis with a greater capacity than β_2-agonists for elevation of cAMP, repression of cytokine-induced COX-2 by GCS may limit the beneficial effects of GCS by preventing the operation of this endogenous regulatory mechanism (71).

Airway smooth muscle not only responds to, but also produces, a number of cytokines, including TGE-β (72), RANTES (73), and GM-CSF (74).

Glucocorticoids inhibit the production of GM-CSF (74) and the chemokine RANTES (73), but not TGF-β (72) from human airway smooth muscle cells in culture. Of these cytokines, TGF-β is known to influence growth.

B. Extracellular Matrix

Cultured synthetic-state smooth muscle cells produce and are able to modify their extracellular matrix (ECM). Release of proteases, including matrix metalloproteinase (MMP) activity, alters the collagen network in the cell microenvironment and may be permissive for airway smooth muscle proliferation (42). Studies in vascular smooth muscle indicate that the synthetic state of airway smooth muscle may be promoted by fibronectin, thrombospondin, and type I collagen and reinforced by smooth muscle production of these ECM components. Conversely, basement membrane collagen type IV and heparin promote the contractile phenotype and inhibit proliferation (33). Growth factors such as thrombin, bFGF, and TGF-β may be sequestered in the ECM and mobilized when the ECM is degraded by inflammatory cell-derived enzymes, resulting in airway smooth muscle proliferation. The profibrotic cytokine TGF-β, which elicits complex growth patterns in many cell types including airway smooth muscle (24,72), also stimulates airway smooth muscle production of hyaluronan, which may lead to airway wall thickening due to water retention in the ECM (72).

IV. How Do Existing Antiasthma Drugs Influence Airway Smooth Muscle Proliferation?

Much of what is known about existing antiasthma drugs and airway smooth muscle growth responses has been inferred from studies of smooth muscle cells in culture, since there are no satisfactory methods for imaging of smooth muscle in situ. Furthermore, bronchial biopsies are too shallow to provide a full-thickness sample of the airway wall incorporating the full muscularis, and postmortem studies cannot accurately relate structural findings to drug therapy. Several animal models of airway smooth muscle hyperplasia and hypertrophy have been investigated. The Brown Norway model of chronic allergic bronchoconstriction is the best characterized for structural change, its relationship to AHR, and the causative factors (75). Similar increases in airway smooth muscle volume in chronically challenged guinea pigs and naturally sensitized cats have been reported (76). However, there has not yet been a systematic investigation of the influence of antiasthma drugs on airway wall structural change in these models. Interestingly, chronic exposure to aerosols of fenoterol appear to induce as much AHR and smooth muscle increase as chronic antigen challenge in the guinea pig, but it is not clear how the dose of fenoterol compared to those used clinically (77). Surprisingly, there appear to be no published studies of the effects of glucocorticoids on volumetric increases in airway smooth muscle animal models of chronic allergic bronchoconstriction. In the Brown Norway rat model of chronic antigen-induced bronchoconstriction, the late response, the increase in airway wall thickness, and AHR are all reduced by CysLT1 receptor antagonism (78). Such actions may explain the slow onset of inhibition of airway hyperresponsiveness during LT receptor antagonist therapy in human asthmatics (79), which is consistent with a role for LTs in AHR (80,81). Nevertheless, in the more chronic inflammation occurring in human asthma it seems likely that multiple growth factors contribute, perhaps synergistically, to the overall remodeling responses.

A. Antiasthma Drugs and Airway Smooth Muscle Proliferation

Endogenous adenylate cyclase stimulants including adrenaline acting on β_2-adrenoceptors (70,82,83), PGE_2 (38,84), and VIP (44) inhibit airway smooth muscle DNA synthesis and proliferation, but their effects on hypertrophic responses have not been described. The effect of adrenaline is a classic effect of β_2-adrenoceptor agonists and has also been described for the nonselective β-agonist isoprenaline (82), for the short-acting β_2-selective agonist salbutamol (70,85) and for the long-acting β_2-selective agonist salmeterol (85). The mechanisms of the antiproliferative effects differ from those of the relaxant actions, as regulation of Ca^{2+}_i does not appear to be important (38). The addition of β_2-agonist, and hence the elevation of cAMP, can occur late in the G1 phase of the cell cycle and still cause G1 arrest, indicating that regulation of passage through the restriction point may be the target (86). Thus, salbutamol reduces the levels of cyclin D1 (87,88) and the phosphorylation of pRb without affecting cyclic D1 mRNA levels by a mechanism that appears to involve activation of proteasome degradation of cyclin D1 (88), which has recently been shown to play a role in regulation of cyclin D1 levels (89).

   Glucocorticoids inhibit proliferation of cultured airway smooth muscle from human (90), rabbit (82), and bovine (85) airways. The mechanism appears to involve suppression of cyclin D1 mRNA levels with a consequent reduction in cyclin D1 protein and retinoblastoma phosphorylation (61). Although both β_2-adrenoceptor agonists and glucocorticoids reduce cyclin D1 protein levels (61,87,88), neither consistently influences ERK activity in human cultured airway smooth muscle (61). There are substantial differences in the sensitivity of DNA synthesis induced by different mitogens to the inhibitory effects of glucocorticoids, with thrombin being the most sensitive and bFGF and EGF the least sensitive, which is similar to the profile of activity of salbutamol (Fig. 2).

Heparin inhibits DNA synthesis induced by FCS, but not by PDGF (91,92), indicating that it acts on a proximal and mitogen-specific signaling mechanism, probably upstream of the common ERK pathway, and not by preventing modulation of airway smooth muscle from the contractile to the synthetic phenotype (93). Some endogenous antimitogens such as TGF-β have small direct stimulatory effects on DNA synthesis, but with prolonged incubation (48 hr) inhibit responses to other mitogens (24,72). A similar profile of activity was observed with tumor necrosis factor- α(TNFα) (20). The temporal dependence of the actions of these cytokines may relate to different actions on distinct cell subpopulations, since TGF-β also induces hypertrophy (72).

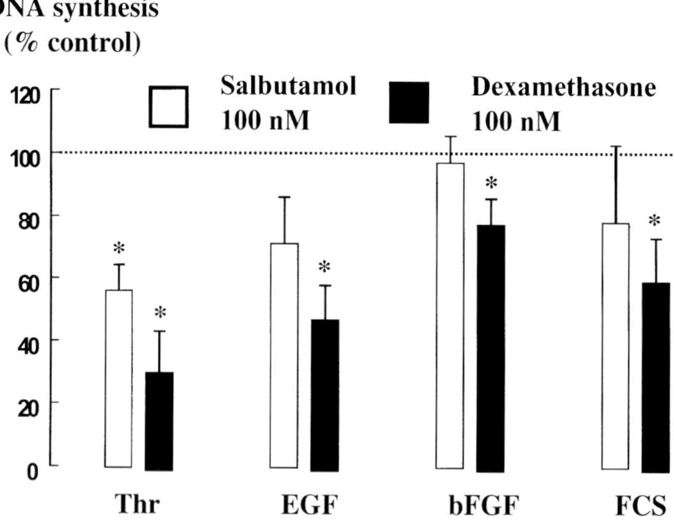

Figure 2   Comparison of the effects of salbutamol and dexamethasone on DNA synthesis induced by maximally effective concentrations of thrombin (Thr 0.3 units/mL), epidermal growth factor (EGF, 300 pM), basic fibroblast growth factor (bFGF, 300 pM), and fetal calf serum (FCS, 10% v/v). *$p < 0.05$.

The phosphodiesterase inhibitors (PDEI) have not been subjected to extensive investigation. We showed that the nonselective PDEI isobutylmethylxanthine (IBMX) directly inhibited airway smooth muscle DNA synthesis and enhanced the inhibitory effects of salbutamol (70), consistent with the role of cAMP in the effects of β_2-agonists (38). More recently, we have investigated the effects of PDEI in combination with β_2-adrenoceptor agonists under conditions in which the latter agents had reduced maximum responses to strong mitogenic stimulation produced by higher concentrations of FCS (94). IBMX increased the magnitude of the maximum inhibitory effect to a level equivalent to that achieved with either PGE_2 or 1 mM 8-bromo-cAMP, suggesting that the level of cAMP generated by β_2-adrenoceptor stimulation is not optimal for regulation of airway smooth muscle DNA synthesis. Combinations of β_2-adrenoceptor agonists and subtype-selective PDEIs may therefore constitute a superior combination for control of the airway smooth muscle remodeling in asthma.

Combinations of isoprenaline and methylprednisolone have synergistic inhibitory actions (82) as could be expected by their actions on distinct components of the mitogen signaling pathways. While both classes of antiasthma agents reduce cyclin D1 protein levels, glucocorticoids reduce mRNA levels, whereas β_2-agonists enhance degradation of cyclin D1 protein levels. However, the maximum effects of these agents are not increased by their combination. Furthermore, the maximum inhibitory effects achieved with β_2-adrenoceptor agonists and glucocorticoids are mitogen-dependent and are modest with powerful growth factors such as bFGF and EGF (Fig. 2).

V. Potential Drug Targets

The diversity of receptors for growth factors and the existence of physical stimuli for growth such as strain indicate that fundamental and common components of growth pathways need to be targeted to achieve adequate control of the process (Table 2). Thus, the use of agents with high levels of specificity is not likely to have the breadth of inhibitory effects necessary to control the full spectrum of growth factors that operate in the inflamed airway. Common pleiotropic intracellular effectors such as cAMP and activated glucocorticoid receptors appear to be insufficiently active to provide an optimal clinical response, possibly because inhibition by β_2-adrenoceptor agonists and glucocorticoids of the responses to growth factors using receptors with intrinsic tyrosine kinase activity is incomplete. In the case of the glucocorticoids, the

Table 2 Potential Drug
Targets for Antiremodeling
Agents

Growth factor release
Growth factor receptors
Intracellular signal transduction
Extracellular matrix remodeling
Cell migration
Phenotypic modulation

apparent failure to adequately control the remodeling process needs to be considered in the light of their additional ability to inhibit the release of many of the growth stimuli. The following areas are being explored for their potential to provide improved agents that target airway wall remodeling.

A. Signal Transduction Pathways

Much attention has been focused on the MAPK pathway as a site of inhibition of cell proliferation that may yield agents useful in the treatment of tumor growth. Inhibitors of ERK1/2 (PD98059) (55,61,95) and p38^{HOG} (SB203580; Ravenhall, Fernandes, and Stewart, unpublished observations) inhibit thrombin- and bFGF-induced proliferation of cultured airway smooth muscle. Similarly, inhibitors of the PI3K pathway (wortmannin, rapamycin) reduce proliferative responses to thrombin (95). The PI3K pathway is linked to p70 ribosomal S6 kinase activity and is inhibited by elevation of cAMP levels (96). Inhibitors of both PKC and PTK reduce fetal calf serum (FCS)-induced proliferation (59), and phospholipase C activity has also been implicated in the signal transduction pathways leading to airway smooth muscle proliferation (97). Treatment of human cultured coronary vascular smooth muscle with Raf-1 antisense oligodeoxynucleotides attenuates FCS-stimulated DNA synthesis (98). It remains to be established whether it is possible to specifically interfere with airway smooth muscle proliferation signal transduction pathways. The above-mentioned targets represent the more proximal components of the signal transduction cascades that are common to contractile and secretory responses. Thus, inhibition is likely to engender a wide range of adverse effects. Identification of essential, delayed intracellular signals leading to proliferative responses may provide targets of greater specificity.

B. Airway Smooth Muscle Phenotype

Early studies on the growth of vascular smooth muscle in culture identified that phenotypic modulation from a contractile to a synthetic phenotype was obligatory for proliferation (99). The most frequently documented aspect of this plasticity is the marked loss of contractile protein (actin, myosin, calponin) expression and increase in matrix synthetic activity of the noncontractile smooth muscle phenotype. Airway smooth muscle shows a similar phenotypic plasticity in culture (100) and heterogeneity in situ has now also been established (48). Thus, regulation of airway smooth muscle phenotype represents a potential mechanism for controlling proliferation (Fig. 3). The synthetic airway smooth muscle phenotype develops in cultured airway smooth muscle after approximately 5 days at which time proliferation commences (101). Extracellular matrix components such as collagen type I and fibronec-

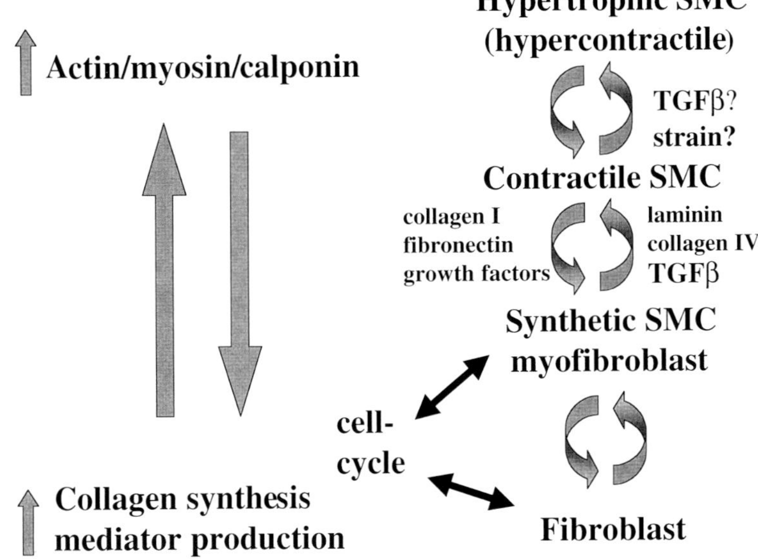

Figure 3 Airway smooth muscle can be considered to have phenotypic plasticity sufficient to range from a fibroblast-like cell to a hypercontractile smooth muscle cell. The extent of heterogeneity of smooth muscle phenotype in healthy individuals and asthmatics is not yet established.

tin promote this phenotype, whereas laminin and collagen type IV increase contractile protein expression and reduce proliferative responses (33). A further phenotype of hypercontractile airway smooth muscle with high levels of actin and myosin expression and increased size has been identified in freshly digested canine tracheal airway smooth muscle (48). Moreover, a recent study of allergen challenge of mild asthmatics suggested that rapid differentiation of airway subepithelial fibroblasts to a myofibroblast phenotype with migratory and proliferative capacity may contribute to the excess airway smooth muscle following chronic allergic inflammation (9) (Fig. 4). An alternative or additional possible explanation of the latter observations is that airway smooth muscle cells adjacent to the subepithelial region migrate from

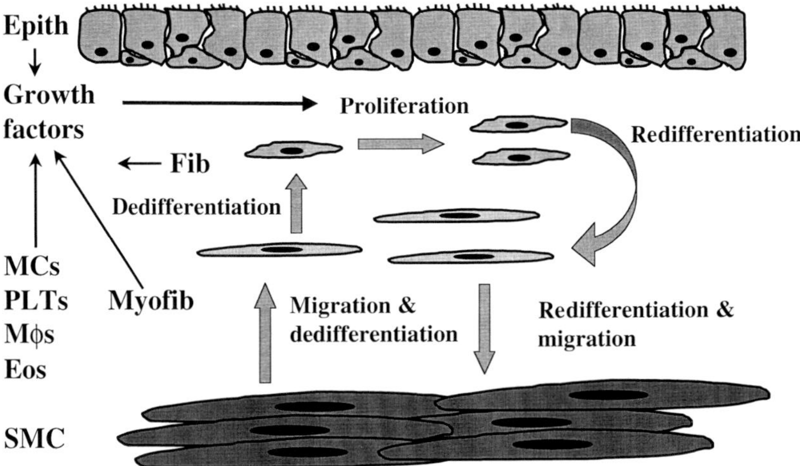

Figure 4 Possible mechanisms underlying increases in smooth muscle cell number. Inflammatory cells (MCs, mast cells; PLTs, platelets; Mφs, macrophages; Eos, eosinophils) and structural cells (Epith, epithelium; Fib, fibroblasts; Myofib, myofibroblasts; SMC, smooth muscle cells) express and release growth factors in inflamed airways. Under the influence of growth factors, two different mechanisms may lead to an increase in airway smooth muscle: subepithelial fibroblasts are stimulated to proliferate and differentiate into myofibroblasts and then migrate to the smooth muscle bundles in which further differentiation to the smooth muscle phenotype occurs. Alternatively or perhaps additionally, smooth muscle cells may escape the constraints of the extracellular matrix, migrate into the subepithelial space, and dedifferentiate initially into myofibroblasts and then fibroblasts before proliferation takes place.

the smooth muscle bundle and are liberated from the inhibitory signals to growth supplied by the normal ECM. It is envisaged that mast cells and infiltrating inflammatory cells may release the proteases necessary for this initial remodeling of the ECM, thus enabling these cells to migrate into the subepithelium and proliferate in a site that is known to contain an abundance of potential airway smooth muscle mitogens. Migration back to the smooth muscle layer and redifferentiation may contribute to the increase in muscle volume (Fig. 4).

The pharmacological regulation of these phenotypic changes has not been explored. In addition, it is not clear whether there would necessarily be a beneficial outcome from holding airway smooth muscle/fibroblasts in a particular phenotypic state. Increasing the proportion of airway smooth muscle in the contractile phenotype may prevent proliferation, but increase the rate or extent of force generated by airway smooth muscle. Conversely, promoting the synthetic phenotype of airway smooth muscle may diminish contractile capacity, but would be expected to increase the level of fibrosis (102), facilitate proliferation, and engender a higher level of proinflammatory mediator generation (23). A combination approach involving a ''phenotypic clamp'' and inhibition of the cellular activities would appear to offer a novel therapeutic strategy for asthma.

Solway and colleagues have identified a smooth-muscle-specific promoter, SM22α (103), which may be useful to regulate the expression genes transfected into airway smooth muscle (104). Microinjection of a decapeptide analog of the N-terminus of smooth muscle α-actin prevents polymerization of actin and represents a potential method for inhibition of the contractile process in both myofibroblasts and smooth muscle (105). In vascular smooth muscle, a ras- and eicosanoid -dependent, raf-independent pathway has been implicated in PDGF downregulation of smooth-muscle-specific α-actin expression (106). PGE$_2$ has been excluded as the effector, but the PLA$_2$ product responsible for this effect has not yet been identified. Characterization of this eicosanoid may provide a novel agent for regulation of airway smooth muscle contractility. Transfection of bovine tracheal smooth muscle or fibroblasts with smooth muscle calponin has a marked inhibitory effect on proliferation without increasing expression of contractile proteins such as actin or myosin (107). Migration of airway smooth muscle is an additional target for regulation of the phenotypic change (Fig. 4).

Further investigation of the pharmacology of phenotypic regulation may identify more selective drug targets as postdevelopment phenotypic change in airway smooth muscle and VSM appears to be restricted to disease processes.

Sex Steroid Metabolites

The estrogen metabolite 2-methoxyestradiol (2-MEO) is produced in a two-step pathway involving hydroxylation of estrogen, which is then methylated by catechol-*o*-methyl transferase (108). 2-MEO was considered to be biologically inactive until its antiangiogenic activities were described by Fotsis et al. in 1994 (109). Subsequently, 2-MEO has been shown to have antiproliferative effects in a variety of cell types including endothelial cells, fibroblasts, smooth muscle (109–111), and T lymphocytes (112). In addition, 2-MEO decreases tumor growth (113) and shows activity in a model of arthritis provoked by intra-articular type II collagen injection (112). 2-MEO has a greatly reduced affinity for the estrogen receptor in cytosolic preparation of rat uterus, but binds to tubulin at a site related to that for colchicine (114). The antiproliferative activities of 2-MEO and related molecules result from a functional deficit in tubulin causing a failure of the mitotic spindle and M-phase arrest of the cell cycle. However, in rabbit cultured vascular smooth muscle (115) and human airway smooth muscle (116), DNA synthesis is reduced by noncytotoxic concentrations of 2-MEO. The activities of 2-MEO have led to the suggestion that it may be an important endogenous metabolite protective against development of breast tumor (108). Our studies have indicated that 2-MEO, its precursor 2-hydroxyestradiol, and structural analogs of these natural estrogen metabolites inhibit airway smooth muscle proliferation via both G1 and M phase arrest of cell-cycle progression (116). Further work using in vivo models of airway wall remodeling is required to ascertain the therapeutic potential of this and related compounds.

The testosterone precursor dehydroepiandrosterone (DHEA) inhibits proliferation of airway smooth muscle at relatively high concentrations (>10 μM) (117) and inhibits tumor growth (118), as does 2-methoxyestradiol. DHEA reduces the transcriptional activity of AP-1, which has been implicated in cell cycle progression (119). However, the androgenic actions of DHEA preclude its direct therapeutic application.

VI. Conclusions

Smooth muscle hypertrophy and hyperplasia constitute rational targets for development of new antiasthma drugs that would reduce airway wall thickness, hyperresposiveness, and hence asthmatic symptoms. Glucocorticoids and β_2-adrenoceptor agonists attenuate proliferative responses of cultured airway smooth muscle, but appear not to have sufficient efficacy to prevent remodeling in chronically inflamed asthmatic airways. Thus, there is a need to examine agents that act in a complementary manner to existing antiasthma agents.

Acknowledgments

The author's work cited in this review has been supported by NHMRC (Australia), Glaxo Wellcome (UK), and AMRAD operations (Australia). The author thanks Dr. Malcolm Johnson (Glaxo Wellcome UK) for his interest and encouragement of this work.

References

1. Dunnill MS, Massarella GR. A comparison of the quantitative anatomy of the bronchi in normal subjects, in status asthmaticus, in chronic bronchitis, and in emphysema. Thorax 1969; 24:176–179.
2. Ebina M, Takahashi T, Chiba T, Motomiya M. Cellular hypertrophy and hyperplasia of airway smooth muscles underlying bronchial asthma: a 3- D morphometric study. Am Rev Respir Dis 1993; 148:720–726.
3. Hogg JC. Airway behavior and its regulation: how do structural changes affect airway behavior? Am J Respir Crit Care Med 1996; 153:S16–18.
4. Tilles SA, Bardana EJ. Seasonal variation in bronchial hyperreactivity (BHR) in allergic patients. Clin Rev Allergy Immunol 1997; 15:169–185.
5. Platts-Mills T. Dust mites: Immunology, allergic disease, and environmental control. J Allergy Clin Immunol 1987; 80:755.
6. Blyth DI, Pedrick MS, Savage TJ, Bright H, Beesley JE, Sanjar S. Induction, duration, and resolution of airway goblet cell hyperplasia in a murine model of atopic asthma: effect of concurrent infection with respirtory syncytial virus and response to dexamethasone. Am J Respir Cell Mol Biol 1998; 19:38–54.
7. Djukanovic R, Roche WR, Wilson JW, Beasley CR, Twentyman OP, et al. Mucosal inflammation in asthma. Am Rev Respir Dis 1990; 142:434–457.
8. Li X, Wilson JW. Increased vascularity of the bronchial mucosa in mild asthma. Am J Respir Crit Care Med 1997; 156:229–233.
9. Gizycki MJ, Adelroth E, Rogers AV, O'Byrne PM, Jeffery PK. Myofibroblast involvement in allergen-induced late response in mild atopic asthma. Am J Respir Cell Mol Biol 1997; 16:664–673.
10. James AL, Pare PD, Hogg JC. The mechanics of airway narrowing in asthma. Am Rev Respir Dis 1989; 139:242–246.
11. Stewart AG, Tomlinson PR, Wilson J. Airway wall remodelling in asthma: a novel target for the development of anti-asthma drugs. Trends Pharmacol Sci 1993; 14:275–279.

12. Hirst SJ, Twort CH. The proliferative response of airway smooth muscle. Clin Exp Allergy 1992; 22:907–915.

13. Eidelman DH, DiMaria GU, Bellofiore S, Wang NS, Guttmann RD, Martin JG. Strain-related differences in airway smooth muscle and airway responsiveness in the rat. Am Rev Respir Dis 1991; 144:792–796.

14. Zacour ME, Martin JG. Enhanced growth response of airway smooth muscle in inbred rats with airway hyperresponsiveness. Am J Respir Cell Mol Biol 1996; 15:590–599.

15. Hoshino M, Nakamura Y, Sim JJ. Expression of growth factors and remodelling of the airway wall in bronchial asthma. Thorax 1997; 53:21–27.

16. Zhang S, Howarth PH, Roche WR. Cytokine production by cell cultures from brochial subepithelial myofibroblasts. J Pathol 1998; 180:95–101.

17. Vignola AM, Chanez P, Chiappara G, Merendino A, Pace E, Rizzo A, LaRocca AM, Bellia V, Bonsignore G, Bousquet J. Transforming growth factor-b expression in mucosal biopsies in asthma and chronic bronchitis. Am J Respir Crit Care Med 1997; 156:591–599.

18. Person CA, Erjefalt JS, Erjefalt I, Korsgren MC, Nilsson MC, Sundler. Epithelial shedding—restitution as a causative process in airway inflammation. Clin Exp Allergy 1996; 26:746–755.

19. Ammit AJ, Bekir SS, Johnson PR, Hughes JM, Armour CL, Black JL. Mast cell numbers are increased in the smooth muscle of human sensitized isolated bronchi. Am J Respir Crit Care Med 1997; 155:1123–1129.

20. Stewart AG, Tomlinson PR, Fernandes DJ, Wilson JW, Harris T. Tumor necrosis factor alpha modulates mitogenic responses of human cultured airway smooth muscle. Am J Respir Cell Mol Biol 1995; 12:110–119.

21. Amrani Y, Panettieri RA, Jr., Frossard N, Bronner C. Activation of the TNF alpha-p55 receptor induces myocyte proliferation and modulates agonist-evoked calcium transients in cultured human tracheal smooth muscle cells. Am J Respir Cell Mol Biol 1996; 15:55–63.

22. Lazaar AL, Albelda SM, Pilewski JM, Brennan B, Pure E, Panettieri RA Jr. T lymphocytes adhere to airway smooth muscle cells via integrins and CD44 and induce smooth muscle cell DNA synthesis. J Exp Med 1994; 180:807–816.

23. Johnson SR, Knox AJ. Synthetic functions of airway smooth muscle in asthma. Trends Pharmacol Sci 1997; 18:289–292.

24. Cohen MD, Ciocca V, Panettieri RA Jr. TGF-beta 1 modulates human airway smooth-muscle cell proliferation induced by mitogens. Am J Respir Cell Mol Biol 1997; 16:85–90.

25. De S, Zelazny ET, Souhrada JF, Souhrada M. Interleukin-1 beta stimulates the proliferation of cultured airway smooth muscle cells via platelet-derived growth factor. Am J Respir Cell Mol Biol 1993; 9:645–651.

26. De S, Zelazny ET, Souhrada JF, Souhrada M. IL-1 beta and IL-6 induce hyperplasia and hypertrophy of cultured guinea pig airway smooth muscle cells. J Appl Physiol 1995; 78:1555–1563.

27. McKay S, de Jongste JC, Saxena P, Sharma HS. Angiotensin II induces hypertrophy of human airway smooth muscle cells: expression of transcription factorts and transforming growth factor-β1. Am J Respir Cell Mol Biol 1998; 18: 823–833.

28. Smith PG, Janiga KE, Bruce MC. Strain increases airway smooth muscle cell proliferation. Am J Respir Cell Mol Biol 1994; 10:85–90.

29. Smith PG, Moreno R, Ikebe M. Strain increases airway smooth muscle contractile and cytoskeletal proteins in vitro. Am J Physiol 1997; 272:L20–L27.

30. Wilson JW, Li X, Pain MC. The lack of distensibility of asthmatic airways. Am Rev Respir Dis 1993; 148:806–809.

31. Butt PR, Bishop JE. Mechanical load enhances the stimulatory effect of serum growth factors on cardiac fibroblast procollagen synthesis. J Mol Cell Cardiol 1998; 29:1141–1151.

32. Li Q, Muragaki Y, Hatamura I, Ueno H, Ooshima A. stretch-induced collagen synthesis in cultured smooth muscle cells from rabbit aortic media and a possible involvement of angiotensin II and transforming growth factor-b. J Vasc Surg 1998; 35:93–103.

33. Hirst SJ. Airway smooth muscle cell culture: application to studies of airway wall remodelling and phenotype plasticity in asthma. Eur Respir J 1996; 9: 808–820.

34. Solway J, Fredberg JJ. Perhaps airway smooth muscle dysfunction contributes to asthmatic bronchial hyperresponsiveness after all. Am J Respir Cell Mol Biol 1997; 17:144–146.

35. Macklem PT. A theoretical analysis of the effect of airway smooth muscle load on airway narrowing. Am J Respir Crit Care Med 1996; 153:83–89.

36. Skloot G, Permutt S, Togias A. Airway hyperresponsiveness in asthma: a problem of limited smooth muscle relaxation with inspiration. J Clin Invest 1995; 96:2393–2403.

37. Fredberg JJ, Inouye D, Miller B, Nathan M, Jafari S, Raboudi H, Butler JP, Shore SA. Airway smooth muscle, tidal stretches, and dynamically determined contractile states. Am J Respir Crit Care Med 1997; 156:1752–1759.

38. Tomlinson PR, Wilson JW, Stewart AG. Inhibition by salbutamol of the proliferation of human airway smooth muscle cells grown in culture. Br J Pharmacol 1994; 111:641–647.

39. Panettieri RA Jr, Goldie RG, Rigby PJ, Eszterhas AJ, Hay DW. Endothelin-1-induced potentiation of human airway smooth muscle proliferation: an ETA receptor-mediated phenomenon. Br J Pharmacol 1996; 118:191–197.

40. Panettieri RA Jr, Leonard T, Luttmann MA, Hay DWP. Pranlukast, but not zafirlukast, inhibits LTD_4-induced potentiation of human airway smooth muscle proliferation. Am J Respir Crit Care Med 1997; 155:A904.

41. Cohen P, Noveral JP, Bhala A, Nunn SE, Herrick DJ, Grunstein MM. Leukotriene D4 facilitates airway smooth muscle cell proliferation via modulation of the IGF axis. Am J Physiol 1995; 269:L151–157.

42. Rajah R, Nunn SE, Herrick DJ, Grunstein MM, Cohen P. Leukotriene D4 in-

duces MMP-1, which functions as an IGFBP protease in human airway smooth muscle cells. Am J Physiol 1996; 271:L1014–1022.

43. Panettieri RA, Yadvish PA, Kelly AM, Rubinstein NA, Kotlikoff MI. Histamine stimulates proliferation of airway smooth muscle and induces c-fos expression. Am J Physiol 1990; 259:L365–371.

44. Maruno K, Absood A, Said SI. VIP inhibits basal and histamine-stimulated proliferation of human airway smooth muscle cells. Am J Physiol 1995; 268:L1047–1051.

45. Noveral JP, Grunstein MM. Tachykinin regulation of airway smooth muscle cell proliferation. Am J Physiol 1995; 269:L339–343.

46. Noveral JP, Grunstein MM. Role and mechanism of thromboxane-induced proliferation of cultured airway smooth muscle cells. Am J Physiol 1992; 263:L555–561.

47. Noveral JP, Bhala A, Hintz RL, Grunstein MM, Cohen P. Insulin-like growth factor axis in airway smooth muscle cells. Am J Physiol 1994; 267:L761–765.

48. Halayko AJ, Rector E, MA X, Stephens DL, Stephens NL. Characterisation of airway smooth muscle cell phenotypes. Am J Respir Crit Care Med 1997; 155:A369.

49. Hirst SJ, Barnes PJ, Twort CH. PDGF isoform-induced proliferation and receptor expression in human cultured airway smooth muscle cells. Am J Physiol 1996; 270:L415–428.

50. Panettieri RA Jr, Hall IP, Maki CS, Murray RK. Alpha-thrombin increases cytosolic calcium and induces human airway smooth muscle cell proliferation. Am J Respir Cell Mol Biol 1995; 13:205–216.

51. Brown JK, Tyler CL, Jones CA, Ruoss SJ, Hartmann T, Caughey GH. Tryptase, the dominant secretory granular protein in human mast cells, is a potent mitogen for cultured dog tracheal smooth muscle cells. Am J Respir Cell Mol Biol 1995; 13:227–236.

52. Lew DB, Songu-Mize E, Pontow SE, Stahl PD, Rattazzi MC. A mannose receptor mediates mannosyl-rich glycoprotein-induced mitogenesis in bovine airway smooth muscle cells. J Clin Invest 1994; 94:1855–1863.

53. Pyne S, Chapman J, Steele L, Pyne NJ. Sphingomyelin-derived lipids differentially regulate the extracellular signal-regulated kinase 2 (ERK-2) and c-Jun N-terminal kinase (JNK) signal cascades in airway smooth muscle. Eur J Biochem 1996; 237:819–826.

54. Kelleher MD, Abe MK, Chao TO, Jain M, Green JM, Solway J, et al. Role of MAP kinase activation in bovine tracheal smooth muscle mitogenesis. Am J Physiol 1995; 268:L894–L901.

55. Karpova AY, Abe MK, Li J, Liu PT, Rhee JM, Kuo WL, et al. MEK1 is required for PDGF-induced ERK activation and DNA synthesis in tracheal myocytes. Am J Physiol 1997; 272:L558–565.

56. Xiong W, Pestell RG, Watanabe G, Li J, Rosner MR, Hershenson MB. Cyclin

D1 is required for S phase traversal in bovine tracheal myocytes. Am J Physiol 1997; 272:L1205–L1210.

57. Fernandes LB, Goldie RG. Co-axial bioassay of an epithelial relaxant factor from the guinea-pig trachea. Br J Pharmacol 1989; 97:117–124.

58. Stewart AG, Grigoriadis G, Harris T. Mitogenic actions of endothelin-1 and epidermal growth factor in cultured airway smooth muscle. Clin Exp Pharmacol Physiol 1994; 21:277–285.

59. Hirst SJ, Webb BL, Giembycz MA, Barnes PJ, Twort CH. Inhibition of fetal calf serum-stimulated proliferation of rabbit cultured tracheal smooth muscle cells by selective inhibitors of protein kinase C and protein tyrosine kinase. Am J Respir Cell Mol Biol 1995; 12:149–161.

60. Cano E, Mahadevan LC. Parallel signal processing among mammalian MAPKs. Trends Biochem Sci 1995; 20:117–122.

61. Fernandes DJ, Guida E, Koutsoubos V, Harris T, Vadiveloo P, Wilson JW. Glucocrticoids inhibit proliferation, cyclin D1 expression and retinoblastoma protein phosphorylation, but not activity of the extracellular regulated kinases (ERK) in human cultured airway smooth muscle. Am J Respir Cell Mol Biol 1999; 21:77–88.

62. Whelchel A, Evans J, Posada J. Inhibition of ERK activation attenuates endothelin-stimulated airway smooth muscle cell proliferation. Am J Respir Cell Mol Biol 1997; 16:589–596.

63. Sherr CJ. Cancer cell cycles. Science 1996; 274:1672–1677.

64. Brooks G, Poolman RA, Li JM. Arresting developments in the cardiac myocyte cell cycle—role of cyclin-dependent kinase inhibitors. Cardiovasc Res 1998; 39:301–311.

65. Sherr CJ. G1 phase progression: cycling on cue. Cell 1997; 79:551–555.

66. Vadas P, Stefanski E, Wloch M, Grouix B, Van Den Bosch H, Kennedy B. Secretory non-pancreatic phospholipase A2 and cyclooxygenase-2 expression by tracheobronchial smooth muscle cells. Eur J Biochem 1996; 235:557–563.

67. Vigano T, Habib A, Hernandez A, Bonazzi A, Boraschi D, Lebret M, et al. Cyclooxygenase-2 and synthesis of PGE2 in human bronchial smooth-muscle cells. Am J Respir Crit Care Med 1997; 155:864–868.

68. Belvisi MG, Saunders MA, Haddad el-B, Hirst SJ, Yacoub MH, Barnes PJ, et al. Induction of cyclo-oxygenase-2 by cytokines in human cultured airway smooth muscle cells: novel inflammatory role of this cell type. B J Pharmacol 1997; 120:910–916.

69. Pang L, Knox AJ. Effect of interleukin-1 beta, tumour necrosis factor-alpha and interferon-gamma on the induction of cyclo-oxygenase-2 in cultured human airway smooth muscle cells. B J Pharmacol 1997; 121:579–587.

70. Tomlinson PR, Wilson JW, Stewart AG. Salbutamol inhibits the proliferation of human airway smooth muscle cells grown in culture: relationship to elevated cAMP levels. Biochem Pharmacol 1995; 49:1809–1819.

71. Vlahos R, Stewart AG. Interleukin-1 alpha and tumour necrosis factor-alpha modulate airway smooth muscle DNA synthesis by induction of cyclo-oxygenase-2: inhibition by dexamethasone and fluticasone propionate. Br J Pharmacol 1999; 126:1315–1324.

72. Black PN, Young PG, Skinner SJ. Response of airway smooth muscle cells to TGF-beta 1: effects on growth and synthesis of glycosaminoglycans. Am J Physiol 1996; 271:L910–917.

73. John M, Hirst SJ, Jose PJ, Robichaud A, Berkman N, Witt C, et al. Human airway smooth muscle cells express and release RANTES in response to T helper 1 cytokines: regulation by T helper 2 cytokines and corticosteroids. J Immunol 1997; 158:1841–1847.

74. Saunders MA, Mitchell JA, Seldon PM, Yacoub MH, Barnes PJ, Giembycz MA, et al. Release of granulocyte-macrophage colony stimulating factor by human cultured airway smooth muscle cells: suppression by dexamethasone. B J Pharmacol 1997; 120:545–546.

75. Bellofiore S, Martin JG. Antigen challenge of sensitized rats increases airway responsiveness to methacholine. J Appl Physiol 1988; 65:1642–1646.

76. Padrid P, Snook S, Finucane T, Shiue P, Cozzi P, Solway J, et al. Persistent airway hyperresponsiveness and histologic alterations after chronic antigen challenge in cats. Am J Respir Crit Care Med 1995; 151:184–193.

77. Wang ZL, Walker BA, Weir TD, Yarema MC, Roberts CR, Okazawa M, et al. Effect of chronic antigen and beta 2 agonist exposure on airway remodeling in guinea pigs. Am J Respir Crit Care Med 1995; 152:2097–2104.

78. Wang CG, Du T, Xu LJ, Martin JG. Role of leukotriene D4 in allergen-induced increases in airway smooth muscle in the rat. Am Rev Respir Dis 1993; 148: 413–417.

79. Taki F, Suzuki R, Torii K, Matsumoto S, Taniguchi H, Takagi K. Reduction of the severity of bronchial hyperresponsiveness by the novel leukotriene antagonist 4-oxo-8-[4-(4-phenyl-butoxy)benzoylamino]-2-(tetrazol-5-yl)-4H-1-benzopyran hemihydrate. Arzneimittelforsch 1994; 44:330–333.

80. Fennessy MR, Stewart AG, Thompson DC. Aerosolized and intravenously administered leukotrienes: effects on the bronchoconstrictor potency of histamine in the guinea-pig. Br J Pharmacol 1986; 87:741–749.

81. O'Hickey SP, Hawksworth RJ, Fong CY, Arm JP, Spur BW, Lee TH. Leukotrienes C4, D4, and E4 enhance histamine responsiveness in asthmatic airways. Am Rev Respir Dis 1991; 144:1053–1057.

82. Schramm CM, Omlor GJ, Quinn LM, Noveral JP. Methylprednisolone and isoproterenol inhibit airway smooth muscle proliferation by separate and additive mechanisms. Life Sci 1996; 59:PL9–14.

83. Noveral JP, Grunstein MM. Adrenergic receptor-mediated regulation of cultured rabbit airway smooth muscle cell proliferation. Am J Physiol 1994; 267: L291–9.

84. Florio C, Martin JG, Styhler A, Heisler S. Antiproliferative effect of prostaglan-

din E2 in cultured guinea pig tracheal smooth muscle cells. Am J Physiol 1994; 266:L131–7.

85. Young PG, Skinner SJ, Black PN. Effects of glucocorticoids and beta-adrenoceptor agonists on the proliferation of airway smooth muscle. Eur J Pharmacol 1995; 273:137–143.

86. Stewart AG, Tomlinson PR, Wilson JW. β_2-Adrenoceptor agonist-mediated inhibition of human airway smooth muscle cell proliferation: importance of the duration of β_2-adrenoceptor stimulation. Br J Pharmacol 1997; 121:361–368.

87. Stewart AG, Tomlinson PR, Wilson JW. Regulation of airway wall remodelling: prospects for the development of novel anti-asthma Drugs. In: August JT, Anders MW, Murad F, Coyle JT, ed. Advances in Pharmacology. San Diego: Academic Press, 1995:209–254.

88. Stewart AG, Harris T, Fernandes DJ, Schachte LC, Koutsoubos V, Guida E, Ravenhall CE, Vadiveloo P, Wilson JW. Beta$_2$-adrenergic receptor agonists and cAMP arrest human cultured airway smooth muscle cells in the G(1) phase of the cell cycle: role of proteasome degradation of cyclin D1. Mol Pharmacol 1999; 56:1079–1086.

89. Choi YH, Lee SJ, Nguyen PM, Jang JS, Wu M-L, Takano E, Maki M, Henkart PA, Trepel JB. Regulation of cyclin D1 by calpain protease. J Biol Chem 1997; 272:28479–28484.

90. Stewart AG, Fernandes D, Tomlinson PR. The effect of glucocorticoids on proliferation of human cultured airway smooth muscle. Br J Pharmacol 1995; 116:3219–3226.

91. Kilfeather SA, Tagoe S, Perez AC, Okona-Mensa K, Matin R, Page CP. Inhibition of serum-induced proliferation of bovine tracheal smooth muscle cells in culture by heparin and related glycosaminoglycans. Br J Pharmacol 1995; 114: 1442–1446.

92. Johnson PR, Armour CL, Carey D, Black JL. Heparin and PGE2 inhibit DNA synthesis in human airway smooth muscle cells in culture. Am J Physiol 1995; 269:L514–519.

93. Halayko AJ, Rector E, Stephens NL. Airway smooth muscle cell proliferation: characterisation of subpopulations by sensitivity to heparin inhibition. Am J Physiol 1998; 274:L17–L25.

94. Stewart AG, Gillzan KM, Wilson JW, Schachte LC. Efficacy of beta2-adrenoceptor agonist-mediated anti-mitogenic effects on airway smooth muscle cells. Am J Respir Crit Care Med 1997; 155(4):A905.

95. Ravenhall CR, Guida E, Harris T, Koutsoubos V, Vadiveloo P, Stewart AG. The importance of ERK activity in the regulation of cyclin D1 levels in DNA synthesis in human cultured airway smooth muscle. Br J Pharmacol 2000. In press.

96. Walker TR, Moore SM, Lawson MF, Panettieri RA, Chilvers ER. Platelet-derived growth factor-BB and thrombin activate phosphoinositide-3-kinase

and protein kinase B: role in mediating airway smooth muscle proliferation. Mol Pharmacol 1998; 54:1007–1015.

97. De S, Zelazny ET, Souhrada JF, Souhrada M. Role of phospholipase C and tyrosine kinase systems in growth response of human airway smooth muscle cells. Am J Physiol 1996; 270:L795–802.

98. Schumacher C, Cioffi CL, Sharif H, Haston W, Monia BP, Wennogle L. Exposure of human vascular smooth muscle cells to Raf-1 antisense oligodeoxynucleotides: cellular responses and pharmacodynamic implications. Mol Pharmacol 1998; 53:97–104.

99. Campbell JH, Campbell GR. Culture techniques and their application to studies of vascular smooth muscle. Clin Sci 1993; 48:501–513.

100. Halayko AJ, Stephens NL. Potential role for phenotypic modulation of bronchial smooth muscle cells in chronic asthma. Can J Physiol Pharmacol 1994; 72:1448–1457.

101. Halayko AJ, Salari H, MA X, Stephens NL. Markers of airway smooth muscle cell phenotype. Am J Physiol 1996; 270:L1040–1051.

102. Brewster CEP, Howarth PH, Djukanovic R, Wilson J, Holgate ST, Roche WR. Myofibroblasts and subepithelial fibrosis in bronchial asthma. Am J Respir Cell Mol Biol 1990; 3:507–511.

103. Solway J, Seltzer J, Samaha FF, Kim S, Alger LE, Niu Q, et al. Structure and expression of a smooth muscle cell-specific gene, SM22 alpha. J Biol Chem 1995; 270:13460–13469.

104. Solway J, Forsythe SM, Halayko AJ, Vieira JE, Hershenson, MB, Trancriptional regulation of smooth muscle contractile apparatus expression. Am J Respir Crit Care Med 1998; 158:S100–S108.

105. Chaponnier C, Goethals M, Janmey PA, Gabbiani F, Gabbiani G, Vanderkerchove J. The specific NH2-terminal sequence Ac-EEED of alpha-smooth muscle actin plays a role in polymerisation in vitro and in vivo. J Cell Biol 1995; 130:887–895.

106. Li X, Putten VV, Zarinetchi F, Nicks ME, Thaler S, Heasley LE, Nemenoff RA. Suppression of vascular smooth muscle alpha-actin expression by platelet-derived growth factor in vascular smooth muscle cells involves Ras and cytosolic phospholipase A2. Biochem J 1997; 327:709–716.

107. Jiang Z, Grange RW, Walsh MP, Kamm KE. Adenovirus-mediated transfer of the smooth muscle cell calponin gene inhibits proliferation of smooth muscle cells and fibroblasts. FEBS Lett 1997; 413:441–445.

108. Zhu BT, Conney AH. Is 2-methoxyestradiol an endogenous estrogen metabolite that inhibits mammary carcinogenesis? Cancer Res 1998; 58:2269–2277.

109. Fotsis T, Zhang Y, Pepper S, Adlercreutz H, Montesaro R, Nawroth PP, Schweiger L. The endogenous oestrogen metabolite 2-methoxyoestradiol inhibits angiogenesis and suppresses tumour growth. Nature 1994; 368:237–239.

110. Seeger H, Mueck AO, Lippert TH. The anti-proliferative effect of 17b-estradiol

on human coronary artery smooth muscle muscle cells. Med Sci Res 1998; 26: 481–482.

111. Reiser F, Way D, Bernas M, Witte M, Witte C. Inhibitoiin of normal and experimental angiotumour endothelial cell proliferation and cell cycle progression by 2-methoxyestradiol. Proc Soc Exp Biol Med 1998; 219:211–216.

112. Josefsson E, Tarkowski A. Suppression of type II collagen-induced arthritis by the endogenous estrogen metabolite 2-methoxyestradiol. Arthritis Rheum 1997; 40:154–163.

113. Klauber N, Parangi S, Flynn E, Hamel E, D'Amato RJ. Inhibition of angiogenesis and breast cancer in mice by the microtubule inhbitors 2-methxyestradiol and taxol. Cancer Res 1997; 57:81–86.

114. Cushman M, He H-M, Katzenellenbogen JA, Lin CM, Hamel E. Synthesis, antitubulin and antimitotic activity, and cytotoxicity of analogs of 2-methoxyestradiol, an endogenous mammalian metabolite of estradiol that inhibits tubulin polymerisation by binding to colchicine binding site. J Med Chem 1995; 38: 2041–2049.

115. Anti-proliferative effect of 2-methoxyestradiol on cultured smooth muscle cells from rabbit aorta. Atherosclerosis 1995; 113:167–170.

116. Stewart AG, Harris T, Guida E, Vlahos R, Koutsoubos V, Hughes RA, Robertson A. The estradiol metabolite, 2-methoxyestradiol inhibits proliferation of human cultured airway smooth muscle. Am J Crit Care Med 1999; 159:A531.

117. Dashtaki R, Whorton AR, Murphy TM, Chitano P, Reed W, Kennedy TP. Dehydroepiandrosterone and analogs inhibit DNA binding of AP-1 and airway smooth muscle proliferation. J Pharmacol Exp Ther 1998; 285:876–883.

118. Schwartz AG, Pashko LL. Cancer prevention with dehydroepiandrosterone and non-androgenic structural analogs. J Cell Biochem 1995; 22(Suppl):210–217.

119. Krontiris TG. Oncogenes. N Engl J Med 1995; 333:303–306.

14

Growth Factor–Extracellular Matrix Interactions in Bronchial Tissue in Asthma

JANIS K. SHUTE

Southampton General Hospital
Southampton, England

I. Introduction

Within tissues, regulation of the biological effects of growth factor activity is dominated by mechanisms other than growth factor expression and receptor binding (1). While some growth factors, EGF and TGF-α for example, are synthesized as large precursors that remain bound to cell membranes where they are active as nondiffusible transmembrane species, others are secreted. However, growth factors that are secreted are no longer considered to be diffusible factors active in solution, but bound by components of extracellular and pericellular matrices. It is these interactions that determine the net activity and specific extracellular location of the secreted growth factors. Thus, the extracellular matrix plays a major role in the control of growth factor–mediated signaling, cell proliferation, and differentiation (2). A number of proteoglycans and proteins present within the extracellular matrix of bronchial tissue are known to bind growth factors that are considered to contribute to the pathogenesis of asthma, such as TGF-β, FGF-2, IGFs, PDGF, HB-EGF, and VEGF (3). Such binding influences not only the distribution of growth factors, but their potency, diffusion properties, and stability. Release of preformed growth factors from storage sites in the extracellular matrix or activation of latent complexes provides a means of rapid intercellular signaling, which is independent of de novo synthesis of the growth factors. Initiation of activation of these growth factors is therefore a posttranslational, extracellular process that depends on their release from inactive matrix-bound complexes.

The distribution of the extracellular growth factors and mechanisms potentially leading to the generation of active species, and the subsequent unscheduled tissue remodeling that accompanies inflammation, wounding, and repair leading to fibrosis in bronchial tissue, are discussed in this chapter.

II. Growth Factor Binding Molecules

A number of growth factor binding molecules (Table 1), both proteins and proteoglycans, have been described (reviewed in Refs. 1 and 2).

A. Proteoglycans

Proteoglycans are some of the most structurally complex and functionally diverse molecules in biology (4). They comprise a core protein and their hallmark, at least one glycosaminoglycan (GAG) side chain. GAG chains are heterogeneous, negatively charged polymers of repeating, highly sulfated disaccharide units (5). Based on core protein structure, the extracellular proteoglycans are classified in two broad categories: the small leucine-rich proteo-

Table 1 Growth Factor Binding Molecules

Growth factor propeptide precursor
TGF-β
Insulin-like growth factor binding proteins
IGFs
Proteoglycans
FGF-2, TGF-β, HB-EGF, PDGF, VEGF
Alpha$_2$-macroglobulin
EGF, NGF, PDGF, TGF-β1, TGF-β2, FGF-2
Soluble receptor
EGF, NGF, IGFII, FGF-2

glycans (SLRPs), which have a compact core protein, and the relatively large modular proteoglycans, which have multidomain core proteins. The former, decorin and biglycan for example, carry one to two GAG side chains, while the latter, perlecan, aggrecan, and versican for example, carry 10–100 GAGs. Among their many functions, proteoglycans bind, store, and deliver growth factors to target cells in normal and disease states. This can be a function of either the core protein or the GAG.

SLRP core proteins bind not only collagen and fibronectin, but also TGF-β and, for example, the core protein of decorin has been shown to inhibit both collagen fibril formation and TGF-β function (4). In addition to upregulation of its own expression (6), TGF-β downregulates expression of decorin, thereby amplifying the profibrotic potential of TGF-β in tissues. Unlike biglycan, which is typically associated with epithelial cell surfaces, decorin is found in connective tissue matrices where it influences both the distribution and function of TGF-β. Regulation of growth factor activity by the modular proteoglycans is, conversely, a property of heparan sulfate (HS) side chains (4). Perlecan, the most abundant extracellular HS-containing proteoglycan, is found in basement membranes where it binds and regulates the activity of a number of growth factors and cytokines (Table 2). Within the extracellular matrix distinct structural features in HS promote the binding of specific growth factors (2,7). Binding to proteoglycans provides a reservoir of inert matrix-associated growth factors and matrix degradation is required for the release of active,

Table 2 Heparin- or Heparan Sulfate–
Associated Growth Factors

Hematopoietic growth factors
GM-CSF, IL-3, IL-4
Neural factors
NT-6, HB-GAM, MK
Chemokines
IP-10, PF4, MCP-1, RANTES, IL-8
FGF family
FGFs 1–10
TGF-β and factors structurally related to TGF-β
TGF-β, VEGF, PDGF-A, PDGF-B
HB-EGF
HGF (scatter factor)

Source: Ref. 2.

free or HS-associated, growth factors (1,2). Importantly, the interaction of fibroblast growth factors with receptor tyrosine kinases (FGFRs) and signaling is facilitated by HS (4,8), which supports the concept that matrix-bound FGF is released as an active FGF-HS complex (Fig. 1).

B. Binding Proteins

Growth factor binding proteins may be products of the same or different genes as those of the growth factors to which they bind (1,2). In the former case, for example, the TGF-β latency associated peptide is synthesized as part of the growth factor precursor, while in the latter case IGF-binding proteins, the PDGF-binding glycoprotein SPARC, soluble receptors, and alpha$_2$-macroglobulin are separate gene products.

TGF-β Latency Associated Peptide

Active TGF-β is a 25-kDa homodimer. However, the transforming growth factors-β are synthesized and secreted as latent complexes (2,9). During secre-

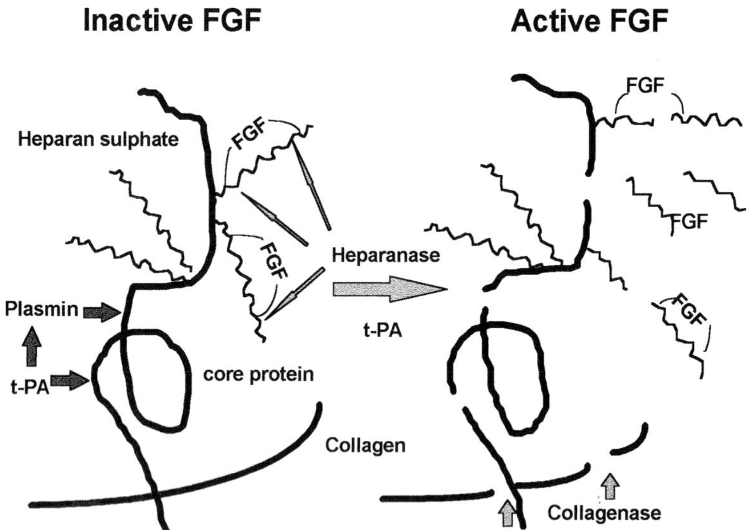

Figure 1 Scheme illustrating the binding of FGF-2 to heparan sulfate (HS)-containing proteoglycans in extracellular matrix and its release by heparanase and tissue plasminogen activator, which participate in the sequential degradation of HS-containing proteoglycans. (From Ref. 52.)

tion, active TGF-β is cleaved from its propeptide, the latency associated peptide (LAP), but the propeptide remains noncovalently associated with the growth factor (Fig. 2). This form, the small latent TGF-β complex, has a molecular weight of 110 kDa and is unable to bind to specific TGF-β receptors. The small latent TGF-β complex is targeted to the extracellular matrix by disulfide links with a second binding protein, the latent TGF-β binding proteins (LTBP 1–3), forming large latent TGF-β complexes with molecular weights of 280 kDa.

The concentration of free TGF-β in equilibrium with the small latent complex is thought to be physiologically negligible (9), thus activation of latent TGF-β is central to the regulation of TGF-β activity. In addition to rendering the growth factor inactive, LAP enhances the correct folding and secretion of TGF-β, while it is suggested that structural motifs in the LTBPs, such as EGF repeats, might direct the growth factor to specific cell or tissue targets (1).

IGF Binding Proteins

The insulin-like growth factors bind to a family of binding proteins, the IGFBPs, which were first identified in the circulation and subsequently in the

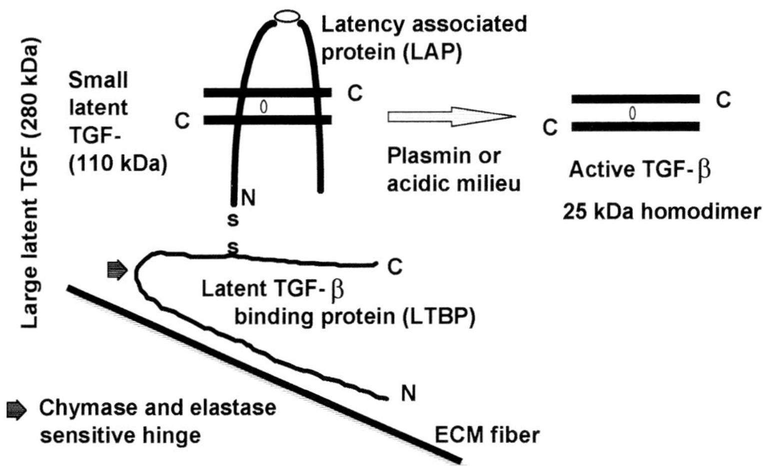

Figure 2 Structure of extracellular-matrix-associated latent TGF-β. Cleavage of the protease-sensitive hinge releases latent TGF-β from the matrix, whereas cleavage of LAP generates active TGF-β. (From Ref. 2.)

extracellular matrix of fibroblasts (1,2). The biological activity of IGFs may be enhanced or inhibited by binding to the IGFBPs (10). IGF-1 may be localized to the matrix by IGFBP-5, a binding protein that enhances the mitogenicity of IGF-1 to human fibroblasts. Alternatively, IGFBP-3 and -5 inhibit IGF activity. Within the circulation, the IGFBPs act as carrier proteins, increasing the half-life of free IGF from minutes to hours, and altering the potency of the growth factor. It is suggested that the amino acid sequence Arg-Gly-Asp (RGD), present in some IGFBPs, directs the growth factor to sites at cell surfaces where it may be released and activated.

SPARC

SPARC, secreted protein acidic and rich in cysteine, is a glycoprotein highly expressed in all tissues undergoing development and repair (11), and is a member of the matricellular class of antiadhesive proteins that includes tenascin and thrombospondin-1 (2,12). SPARC regulates cell proliferation by binding to the B chain of PDGF-BB or PDGF-AB and to VEGF, preventing the growth factors from interacting with their specific cell surface receptors on fibroblasts and endothelial cells, respectively. SPARC has also been shown to inhibit FGF-2-induced chemotaxis and proliferation of endothelial cells (13).

Soluble Receptors

Soluble receptors have been described for a number of growth factors (Table 1). The binding affinity and specificity of the soluble receptors are similar to those of cell surface receptors. Binding of growth factors to soluble receptors therefore inhibits binding to specific cellular receptors, and thus bioactivity, while prolonging the half-life of the growth factor. Soluble receptors arise either as the result of proteolytic activity, as in the case of TNF (14), or by genetic mechanisms, FGFs and EGF for example (15,16). Functional effects of soluble growth factor receptors have been shown in a number of studies; for example, FGF-stimulated angiogenesis is abrogated by high-affinity receptors in the basement membrane of endothelial cells (17). Similarly, murine fibroblast proliferative responses to IL-4 are regulated in an autocrine manner by the soluble form of the IL-4 receptor, which is encoded distinctly to the membrane-bound form (18).

Alpha$_2$-macroglobulin

Within the circulation a high-molecular-weight complex with the broad-spectrum protease inhibitor alpha$_2$-macroglobulin is the most abundant form of many growth factors. Via mechanisms that are distinct from proteinase trapping mechanisms, binding of TGF-β1, TGF-β2, PDGF, NGF-β, FGF-2, TNFα, and VEGF to native and proteinase-complexed (''fast'') alpha$_2$-macroglobulin has been described (19,20). Alpha$_2$-macroglobulin is present in plasma at 2–4 mg/mL and in lower concentrations in extravascular spaces including the inflamed asthmatic airway.

Proteinase-complexed, but not native, alpha$_2$-macroglobulin is rapidly cleared via the cellular alpha$_2$-macroglobulin receptor/low-density lipoprotein receptor-related protein; therefore, the native form of alpha$_2$-macroglobulin predominates in the circulation. The covalent binding of growth factors to native alpha$_2$-macroglobulin in vivo stabilizes the growth factors, decreases their susceptibility to proteinases, and retards their clearance from the circulation, thereby prolonging their half-life (21). The biological consequences of binding to alpha$_2$-macroglobulin are variable and inhibition of growth factor function may be limited to TGF-β2 (20) and FGF-2 (21). The glycosaminoglycan side chains of proteoglycans are important growth factor regulatory molecules (see above) and, in this respect, coregulation by heparin and alpha$_2$-macroglobulin of TGF-β function has been reported (22).

III. Mechanisms for Release and Activation of Matrix-Bound Growth Factors

It is evident that protein, proteoglycan, and glycoprotein molecules within the extracellular matrix of tissues bind and regulate the localization, stability, and potency of secreted, low-molecular-weight growth factors. These binding molecules allow the growth factors to accumulate in latent form at concentrations well in excess of the effective concentration of the free, low-molecular-weight growth factor. Growth factors encrypted in the extracellular matrix are released from latent complexes by processes, both enzymic and nonenzymic, that are critical determinants of cell proliferation and tissue remodeling responses.

A. Activation of Growth Factors by Nonenzymic Mechanisms

A number of such mechanisms have been described for the activation of latent forms of TGF-β (9) (Table 3). Extremes of pH are used to activate TGF-β in vitro, prior to assay of total TGF-β, and it has been suggested that acidic pH conditions at sites of inflammation may be a physiological stimulus for activation of TGF-β (9). Similarly, the association of PDGF with the inhibitory

Table 3 Mechanisms of Latent TGF-β Activation

	In vitro	In vivo
Nonproteolytic	Heat	
	Detergents	
	pH extremes	
	Radiation	?
	Thrombospondin-1	?
	Deglycosylation	
Proteolytic	Plasmin	?
	Cathepsin D	

protein SPARC is sensitive to pH, and mildly acidic conditions (pH ~ 6.0) in the extracellular space may induce dissociation and activation of these growth factors (2). Heat activation of TGF-β is also proposed to have a physiological parallel, at the edge of thermal burns (9). Ionizing radiation generates reactive oxygen species that activate TGF-β both in vitro and in tissues in vivo (9). However, it is not known whether physiological variations in redox potential in tissues are sufficient to activate this process.

Studies in mice have indicated that a physiologically important mechanism for TGF-β activation in vivo lies in the ability of the matricellular protein thrombospondin-1 to bind to the N-terminal region of the latency-associated peptide that normally binds and masks the activity of mature TGF-β. A conformational change takes place within the trimolecular complex that forms, such that the immunoreactivity of TGF-β is unmasked and the growth factor can bind to its specific receptor (23).

Growth factors bound and inactivated by association with glycosaminoglycans in the extracellular matrix may be displaced from binding sites by the more highly negatively charged heparin molecule, as has been shown for FGF-2 (1,2). This interaction of FGF-2 with heparin serves to protect the growth factor from proteolysis, significantly increasing its half-life in tissues and promoting diffusion of FGF. Similarly, extracellular matrix-bound VEGF can be released in a soluble and bioactive form by heparin (24).

B. Activation of Growth Factors by Enzymic Mechanisms

Enzymes that degrade the inhibitory growth factor binding proteins, glycoproteins or proteoglycans, promote the activation of growth factors. The regulation of TGF-β activity is outstanding in its complexity (Fig. 2). For example, deglycosylation of the latency-associated peptide activates TGF-β, and it is suggested that sialidases released from activated macrophages may play a role in this process (9). The large latent complexes of TGF-β are released (as latent TGF-β) from the extracellular matrix by a number of proteases, including plasmin, thrombin, neutrophil elastase, and mast cell chymase (25). Subsequently the action of plasmin and cathepsin D on the latency-associated peptide generates mature, active TGF-β (26). Finally, multiple mechanisms of TGF-β activation may operate simultaneously to generate free TGF-β, which is subsequently inactivated by binding to a number of soluble or matrix molecules, including alpha$_2$-macroglobulin, the core proteins of decorin, and betaglycan, heparin, and fucoidan (9). These latter interactions are believed to prevent TGF-β diffusing from the site of activation and causing inappropriate cell responses.

The degradation of heparan-sulfate-containing proteoglycans is a function of proteases that cleave the core protein, including matrix metalloproteinases (MMP-2, -3, -7, -9, MT1-MMP, MT2-MMP) (27,28), neutrophil elastase (29), and endoglycosidases (heparanases), which hydrolyze the glycosaminoglycan side chains (30). Release and activation of FGF-2 by a number of these mechanisms has been reported (Table 4). Plasmin-dependent proteolytic cleavage mobilizes proteoglycan fragments with the growth factor still bound (Fig. 1), these fragments forming active high-affinity trimolecular complexes with the FGF receptor (31,32). Release of bioactive VEGF from the extracellular matrix by plasmin has similarly been demonstrated (24). The effects of plasmin on proteoglycan degradation may be direct, or mediated via activation of MMPs in the proteolytic cascade shown in Figure 3 (33). Of the growth factor binding proteins, proteolysis of IGFBPs by smooth-muscle-derived MMP-1 was recently shown to be important in the autocrine upregulation of IGF-dependent smooth muscle proliferation (34). Thus, the integrity

Table 4 Factors That Release
FGF-2 from Basement Membranes

Stromelysin (MMP-3)
Collagenase
Plasmin
Thrombin
Heparanase
Heparin

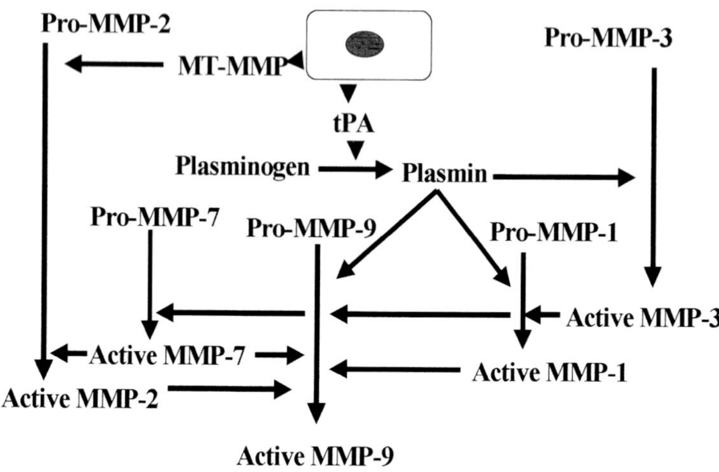

Figure 3 Proposed cascade for activation of the matrix metalloproteinases (MMPs) via plasmin-dependent activation of MMP-1, MMP-2, and MMP-3. MT-MMP, membrane-type matrix metalloproteinase: tPA, tissue plasminogen activator. (Adapted from Ref. 33.)

of the binding proteins is as much a determinant of net growth factor function as the expression of the growth factors per se. The potential for these proteolytic mechanisms to generate an increase in net growth factor bioactivity is balanced by the action of inhibitors, both specific inhibitors such as the plasminogen activator inhibitors, alpha$_2$-antiplasmin, and the tissue inhibitors of matrix metalloproteinases, and the broad-spectrum protease inhibitors such as alpha$_2$-macroglobulin and heparin. Net proteolytic activity and the generation of active growth factors may be self-regulatory. EGF, PDGF, and FGF-2, for example, upregulate expression of the matrix metalloproteinases, in synergy with inflammatory cytokines (27,35), while others such as TGF-β downregulate MMP expression while increasing synthesis of their inhibitors (36), contributing to the growth inhibitory function of TGF-β. Additionally, the importance of the inflammatory milieu in the generation of active growth factors is linked to MMP activation by proteolytic, oxidative, or other mechanisms dependent on leukocyte activation (27,37). High levels of nitric oxide in the inflammatory microenvironment may also contribute to these profibrotic processes by enhancing FGF-2 release from matrix via effects on MMP expression (38) and/or direct effects on heparan sulfate degradation (39).

IV. Growth Factors and Regulatory Mechanisms in the Asthmatic Airways

Both IGF immunoreactivity in bronchial tissue (40) and the number of epithelial and submucosal cells expressing TGF-β (41) have been demonstrated to correlate with the degree of subepithelial fibrosis. However, in the absence of unequivocal evidence for increased expression of profibrotic growth factors in association with atopy or asthma, conditions that are both associated with increased subepithelial fibrosis, it appears that posttranslational regulation of secreted growth factor activity may critically determine the degree of fibrosis that is seen in the airways (42).

Immunohistochemical analysis of the deposition of growth factors within the airways has provided clues as to the components of the extracellular matrix that may be involved in the regulation of growth factor function in vivo (42). Within bronchial tissue from both asthmatic and nonasthmatic subjects FGF-2 is localized to epithelial and endothelial basement membranes, where it colocalizes with heparan sulfate, presumably expressed as a component of perlecan, the most abundant of the heparan sulfate–containing proteoglycans. Release of FGF-2 from these binding sites is rapid following allergen bronchoprovocation and increased levels of FGF-2 were detected in bronchoalveolar lavage 10 min after exposure to allergen (42). The distribution of immunoreactive TGF-β in bronchial tissue colocalizes with immunostaining for decorin (43), suggesting that TGF-β is present largely in inactive form. In the light of these findings it was suggested that there is little relation between expression of immunoreactive TGF-β and biological availability of this growth factor (42,43). More recently, analysis of bronchial tissue homogenates has indicated that active 25-kDa TGF-β is present as only 1–2% of the total, although this is doubled following allergen challenge, most being present as high-molecular-weight complexes (unpublished observations). Following allergen bronchoprovocation, the concentration of total TGF-β in bronchoalveolar lavage fluids was increased, by unknown mechanisms, 24 hr after the exposure (42).

The growth-factor-regulating glycoproteins SPARC and thrombospondin-1, described earlier, are expressed in fibrotic airways disease, but their expression is not observed within healthy lung tissue (44). SPARC was observed within fibroblasts, whereas thrombospondin-1 was localized in the extracellular matrix immediately beneath reparative epithelium, suggesting that it may be synthesized by regenerating epithelium (44). Clearly, thrombospondin-dependent activation of TGF-β in this locale will profoundly influence epithelial cell proliferation and may stimulate collagen deposition by fibroblasts. However, immunoreactivity for SPARC and thrombospondin-1 within the asthmatic airways has not been described.

Alpha$_2$-macroglobulin leaking into the airway via plasma exudation will serve to affect growth factor function, both directly and indirectly, through the binding of growth factors and inhibition of protease activity. It is predicted that an increase in intravascular proteinase levels will shift the balance from native to proteinase-complexed forms of alpha$_2$-macroglobulin, with subsequent effects on the half-life of growth factors in the circulation. Clearly, the ratio of native to proteinase-complexed form of alpha$_2$-macroglobulin is likely to be different at extravascular sites compared to the circulation and the predominant form regulating growth factor function will depend on the tissue compartment being considered. Proteolytic and oxidative inactivation of alpha$_2$-macroglobulin in the airways are likely to influence growth factor function.

There are a number of reports of increased expression of MMP-9, at both the mRNA and protein level, in bronchial tissue from asthmatic subjects. MMP-9 immunoreactivity was found to be largely extracellular (45) and a correlation between the thickness of the collagen III layer and submucosal MMP-9 has been described (46). Activated macrophages and eosinophils were suggested to be sources of MMP-9. In our studies, eosinophils within bronchial tissue are depleted of MMP-9 compared to those remaining within blood vessels, suggesting the eosinophil is an important source of matrix-bound, submucosal MMP-9. The contribution of MMP-9 to bronchial tissue fibrosis may reflect a generic mechanism since MMP-9 levels in skin wounds predicted optimal collagen deposition (47). The latter study, and our own observations, indicate that active forms of the MMPs remain bound to the matrix and are not sampled in wound fluids or bronchoalveolar lavage fluids, respectively. While an in vitro study has demonstrated a direct relation between MMP-9 and MMP-3 activity and release of matrix-encrypted FGF-2 (38), effects on growth factors in vivo remain to be established.

In addition to inflammatory leukocytes, the resident tissue mast cells may also contribute to airway fibrosis. In a number of fibrotic lung disorders, mast cell numbers in lung biopsy specimens were significantly correlated with the degree of fibrosis ($r = 0.87, p < 0.001, n = 49$) (48). Thus it is conceivable that mast-cell-derived heparin or matrix-degrading enzymes may be involved in the rapid release of FGF-2 from proteoglycan-bound stores in the matrix following allergen challenge in asthma (42). It appears that mast cells are well equipped to mediate proteoglycan degradation since in addition to being a source of heparanase activity (49) we have also shown that mast cells contain

MMP-3, a potent proteoglycanase (45). Activated MMPs have been demonstrated in association with mast cell activation in athersclerotic plaques (50) and, applying in situ zymography to bronchial tissue sections from asthmatics, abundant gelatinolytic activity could be observed (unpublished observations). Mechanisms leading to MMP activation in vivo are largely unknown; however, it may be relevant that, uniquely, the mast cell constitutively expresses tissue plasminogen activator, in the absence of the plasminogen activator inhibitors (51). Baseline levels of FGF-2 and TGF-β are increased in asthmatic subjects (42), and this may be a reflection of increased mast cell activation previously reported in this disease.

In conclusion, via proteolytic activation cascades and/or the release of heparin and subsequent effects on growth factor activity, mast cells may play an important role contributing to the development of airway fibrosis.

References

1. Flaumenhaft R, Rifkin DB. The extracellular regulation of growth factor action. Mol Biol Cell 1992; 3:1057–1065.
2. Taipale J, Keski-Oja J. Growth factors in the extracellular matrix. FASEB J 1997; 11:51–59.
3. Vignola AM, Chiaparra G, Chanez P, Merendino AM, Pace E, Spatafora M, Bousquet J, Bonsignore G. Growth factors in asthma. Monaldi Arch Chest Dis 1997; 52:159–169.
4. Iozzo RV, Murdoch AD. Proteoglycans of the extracellular environment: clues from the gene and protein side offer novel perspectives in molecular diversity and function. FASEB J 1996; 10:598–614.
5. Hardingham TE, Fosang AJ. Proteoglycans: many forms and many functions. FASEB J 1992; 6:861–870.
6. Barnard JA, Lyons RM, Moses HL. The cell biology of transforming growth factor β. Biochim Biophys Acta 1990; 1032:79–87.
7. Salmivirta M, Lidholt K, Lindahl U. Heparan sulfate: a piece of information. FASEB J 1996; 10:1270–1279.
8. Filla MS, Dam P, Rapraeger AC. The cell surface proteoglycan syndecan-1 mediates fibroblast growth factor-2 binding and activity. J Cell Physiol 1998; 174: 310–321.
9. Munger JS, Harpel JG, Gleizes P-E, Mazzieri R, Nunes I, Rifkin DB. Latent transforming growth factor-β: structural features and mechanisms of activation. Kidney Int 1997; 51:1376–1382.
10. Murphy LJ. Insulin-like growth factor binding proteins: functional diversity or redundancy? J Mol Endocrinol 1998; 21:97–107.

11. Porter PI, Sage EH, Lane TF, Funk SE, Gown AM. Distribution of SPARC in normal and neoplastic tissue. J Histochem Cytochem 1995; 43:791–800.

12. Kupprion C, Motamed K, Sage EH. SPARC (BM-40, osteonectin) inhibits the mitogenic effect of vascular endothelial growth factor on microvascular endothelial cells. J Biol Chem 1998; 273:29635–29640.

13. Hasselar P, Sage EH. SPARC inhibits bFGF induced chemotaxis and proliferation in endothelial cells. J Cell Biochem 1992; 49:272–283.

14. Schall TJ, Lewis M, Koller KJ, Lee A, Rice GC, Wong GH, Gatanaga T, Granger GA, Lentz R, Raab H, Kohr WJ, Goeddel DV. Molecular cloning and expression of a receptor for human tumor necrosis factor. Cell 1990; 61:361–370.

15. Johnson DE, Lee PL, Lu J, Williams L. Diverse forms of a receptor for acidic and basic fibroblast growth factor. Mol Cell Biol 1990; 10:4728–4736.

16. Weber W, Gill GN, Speiss J. Production of an epidermal growth factor receptor-related protein. Science 1984; 224:294–297.

17. Hanneken A, Maher PA, Baird A. High affinity immunoreactive FGF receptors in the ECM of vascular endothelial cells-implications for the modulation of FGF-2. J Cell Biol 1995; 128:1221–1228.

18. Sempowski GD, Beckmann MP, Derdak S, Phipps RP. Subsets of murine lung fibroblasts express membrane-bound and soluble IL-4 receptors. Role of IL-4 in enhancing fibroblast proliferation and collagen synthesis. J Immunol 1994; 152: 3606–3614.

19. Crookston KP, Webb DJ, Lamarre J, Gonias SL. Binding of platelet-derived growth factor-BB and transforming growth factor-β1 to α2-macroglobulin in vitro and in vivo: comparison of receptor-recognized and non-recognized α2-macroglobulin conformations. Biochem J 1993; 293:443–450.

20. Crookston KP, Webb DJ, Wolf BB, Gonias SL. Classification of α2-macroglobulin-cytokine interactions based on affinity of noncovalent association in solution under apparent equilibrium conditions. J Biol Chem 1994; 269:1533–1540.

21. James K. Interactions between cytokines and α2-macroglobulin. Immunol Today 1990; 11:163–166.

22. McCaffrey TA, Falcone DJ, Du B. Transforming growth factor-β1 is a heparin-binding protein: identification of putative heparin-binding regions and isolation of heparins with varying affinity for TGF-β1. J Cell Physiol 1992; 152:430–440.

23. Crawford SE, Stellmach V, Murphy-Ullrich JE, Ribeiro SMF, Lawler J, Hynes RO, Boivin GP, Bouck N. Thrombospondin-1 is a major activator of TGF-β1 in vivo. Cell 1998; 93:1159–1170.

24. Park JE, Keller G-A, Ferrara N. The vascular endothelial growth factor (VEGF) isoforms: Differential deposition into the subepithelial extracellular matrix and bioactivity of extracellular matrix-bound VEGF. Mol Biol Cell 1993; 4:1317–1326.

25. Taipale J, Lohi J, Saarinen J, Kovanen PT, Keski-Oja J. Human mast cell chymase and leukocyte elastase release latent transforming growth factor β1 from

the extracellular matrix of cultured human epithelial and endothelial cells. J Biol Chem 1995; 270:4689–4696.

26. Lyons RM, Keski-Oja J, Moses HL. Proteolytic activation of latent transforming growth factor-β from fibroblast conditioned media. J Cell Biol 1988; 106:1659–1665.

27. Woessner JF. Matrix metalloproteinases and their inhibitors in connective tissue remodeling. FASEB J 1991; 5:2145–2154.

28. D'Ortho M-P, Will H, Atkinson S, Butler G, Messent A, Gavrilovic J, Smith B, Timpl R, Zardi L, Murphy G. Membrane-type matrix metalloproteinases 1 and 2 exhibit broad spectrum proteolytic capacities comparable to many matrix metalloproteinases. Eur J Biochem 1997; 250:751–757.

29. Klebanoff SJ, Kinsella MG, Wight TN. Degradation of endothelial cell matrix heparan sulphate proteoglycan by elastase and the myeloperoxidase-H_2O_2-chloride system. Am J Pathol 1993; 143:907–917.

30. Ishai-Michaeli R, Eldor A, Vlodavsky I. Heparanase activity expressed by platelets, neutrophils and lymphoma cells releases active fibroblast growth factor from extracellular matrix. Cell Regul 1990; 1:833–842.

31. Saksela O, Rifkin DB. Release of basic fibroblast growth factor-heparan sulfate complexes fron endothelial cells by plasminogen activator-mediated proteolytic activity. J Cell Biol 1990; 110:767–775.

32. Aviezer D, Hecht D, Safran M, Elsinger M, David G, Yayon A. Perlecan, basal lamina proteoglycan, promotes basic fibroblast growth factor-receptor binding, mitogenesis and angiogenesis. Cell 1994; 79:1005–1013.

33. Parsons SL, Watson SA, Brown PD, Collins HM, Steele RJC. Matrix metalloproteinases. Br J Surg 1997; 84:160–166.

34. Rajah R, Nachajon RV, Collins MH, Hakonarson H, Grunstein MM, Cohen P. Elevated levels of the IGF-binding protein protease MMP-1 in asthmatic airway smooth muscle. Am J Respir Cell Mol Biol 1999; 20:199–208.

35. Bond M, Fabunmi RP, Baker AH, Newby AC. Synergistic upregulation of metalloproteinase-9 by growth factors and inflammatory cytokines: an absolute requirement for transcription factor NF-κB. FEBS Lett 1998; 435:29–34.

36. Massague J. The transforming growth factor-β family. Annu Rev Cell Biol 1990; 6:597–641.

37. Schwartz JD, Monea S, Marcus SG, Patel S, Eng K, Galloway AC, Mignatti P, Shamamian P. Soluble factor(s) released from neutrophils activates endothelial cell matrix metalloproteinase-2. J Surg Res 1998; 76:79–85.

38. Sasaki K, Hattori T, Fujisawa T, Takahashi K, Inoue H, Takigawa M. Nitric oxide mediates interleukin-1-induced gene expression of matrix metalloproteinases and basic fibroblast growth factor in cultured rabbit articular chondrocytes. J Biochem 1998; 123:431–439.

39. Ghael D, Mileva M, Dweck HS, Rosenfeld L. The nitric oxide donor s-nitroso-*N*-acetyl-D,L-penicillamine degrades heparan sulfate and heparin. Biochem Mol Biol Int 1997; 43:183–188.

40. Hoshino M, Nakamura Y, Sim JJ, Yamashiro Y, Ichida K, Hosaka K, Isogai S. Inhaled corticosteroid reduced lamina reticularis of the basement membrane by modulation of insulin-like growth factor (IGF)-1 expression in bronchial asthma. Clin Exp Allergy 1998; 28:568–577.

41. Vignola AM, Chanez P, Chiappara G, Merendino A, Pace E, Rizzo A, la Rocca AM, Bellia V, Bonsignore G, Bousquet J. Transforming growth factor-β expression in mucosal biopsies in asthma and chronic bronchitis. Am J Respir Crit Care Med 1997; 156:591–599.

42. Redington AE, Sime PJ, Howarth PH, Holgate ST. Fibroblasts and the extracellular matrix in asthma. In: Holgate ST, Busse WW, eds. Inflammatory Mechanisms in Asthma. New York: Marcel Dekker, 1998:443–467.

43. Redington AE, Roche WR, Holgate ST, Howarth PH. Colocalisation of immunoreactive transforming growth factor-beta 1 and decorin in bronchial biopsies from asthmatic and normal subjects. J Pathol 1998; 186:410–415.

44. Kuhn C, Mason RJ. Immunolocalisation of SPARC, tenascin, and thrombospondin in pulmonary fibrosis. Am J Pathol 1995; 147:1759–1769.

45. Dahlen B, Shute JK, Howarth PH. Immunohistochemical localisation of the matrix metalloproteinases MMP-3 and MMP-9 within the airways in asthma. Thorax 1999; 54:590–596.

46. Hoshino M, Nakamura Y, Sim J, Shimojo J, Isogai S. Bronchial subepithelial fibrosis and expression of matrix metalloproteinase-9 in asthmatic airway inflammation. J Allergy Clin Immunol 1998; 102:783–788.

47. Agren MS, Jorgensen LN, Andersen M, Viljanto J, Gottrup F. Matrix metalloproteinase 9 level predicts optimal collagen deposition during early wound repair in humans. Br J Surgery 1998; 85:68–71.

48. Pesci A, Bertorelli G, Gabrielli M, Olivieri D. Mast cells in fibrotic lung disorders. Chest 1993; 103:989–996.

49. Bashkin P, Razin E, Eldor A, Vlodavsky I. Degranulating mast cells secrete an endoglycosidase that degrades heparan sulfate in subendothelial extracellular matrix. Blood 1990; 75:2204–2212.

50. Johnson JL, Jackson CL, Angelini GD, George SJ. Activation of matrix-degrading metalloproteinases by mast cell proteases in atherosclerotic plaques. Arterioscler Thromb Vasc Biol 1998; 18:1707–1715.

51. Valent P, Sillaber C, Baghestanian M, Bankl H-C, Kiener HP, Lechner K, Binder BR. What have mast cells to do with edema formation, the consecutive repair and fibrinolysis? Int Arch Allergy Immunol 1998; 115:2–8.

52. Vlodavsky I, Fuks Z, Ishai-Michaeli R, Bashkin P, Levi E, Korner G, Bar-Shavit R, Klagsbrun M. Extracellular matrix-resident basic fibroblast growth factor: implication for the control of angiogenesis. J Cell Biochem 1991; 45:167–176.

15

Is There an Animal Model of Airway Remodeling?

**JOHAN C. KIPS and
ROMAIN A. PAUWELS**

Ghent University and
Ghent University Hospital
Ghent, Belgium

**ELS PALMANS and
NELE VANACKER**

Ghent University Hospital
Ghent, Belgium

I. Introduction

Airway remodeling encompasses a number of changes to the airway structure, found in asthma. This includes goblet cell hyperplasia, pseudothickening of the basement membrane due to subepithelial fibrosis, neovascularization, changes in the composition of the extracellular matrix, and smooth muscle hyperplasia and/or hypertrophy (1–7). What exactly causes these structural changes to occur is unclear. The amount of mediators present in asthmatic airway that can activate and induce or enhance proliferation of fibroblasts and smooth muscle cells is seemingly endless (8–11), ranging from mediators such as leukotrienes, or proinflammatory cytokines including TNFα and IL-1β, to a variety of growth factors. These can be divided in nonfibrogenic mediators, such as GM-CSF, and fibrogenic ones, including epidermal growth factor (EGF), insulin-like growth factor (IGF), and transforming growth factor β (TGF-β). The exact functional importance of each of these mediators in the pathogenesis of remodeling is unknown. This is a first area to which data derived from in vivo models can contribute valuable information.

A second element with regard to remodeling that needs to be further evaluated is the impact of these structural changes on airway function. It has been hypothesized, largely based on mathematical models, that the remodeling process underlies bronchial hyperresponsiveness (12). The two main determinants of bronchial hyperresponsiveness are hypersensitivity and hyperreactivity of the airways (13). Hypersensitivity is reflected in a leftward shift of the dose-response curve toward a bronchoconstrictor agonist. This can be attributed, in adaptation of Poiseuille's law, to thickening of the airway wall, especially the area inner to the smooth muscle layer (14). Increased stiffness of the subepithelial layer could additionally contribute to this phenomenon, by influencing mucosal folding upon smooth muscle contraction (15). Hyperreactivity of the airways is reflected by an increased slope of the dose-response curve to methacholine and exaggerated maximal airway narrowing (16). This has been ascribed to an increased airway smooth muscle mass and/or changes in the adventitial matrix, leading to a loss of elastic recoil on contracting airway smooth muscle (14,16). These assumptions are based on superb mathematical models, but require further functional confirmation, an issue where in vivo animal models again can prove very useful. This in turn implies that the animal model displays not only morphological characteristics of remodeling, but also a degree of airway hyperresponsiveness, comparable to human asthma, and that from a methodological point of view, airway responsiveness is measured in such a way that both sensitivity and reactivity of the airways can be assessed. When combining both these morphological and physiological requirements, it is quite clear that the ideal animal model of airway remodeling does not yet exist. An obvious disadvantage is that animal models displaying naturally occurring asthma-like syndromes are nearly inexistent. Horses are known to develop airway obstruction after exposure to mold but the airway histology is different from asthma as it more closely resembles bronchiolitis (17).

The only species that seems to spontaneously develop an airway disorder that bears similarities to asthma, both functionally and histologically, are cats. Sensitization followed by repeated exposure to *Ascaris* has been shown to increase airway responsiveness in conjunction with histological changes that mimic those observed in naturally occurring feline asthma. This includes goblet cell hyperplasia, eosinophil infiltration in the airway mucosa, and an increase in the thickness of the airway smooth muscle layer. The overall airway wall thickness was not increased (18). However, the cat has not gained widespread acceptance as an animal model of asthma, and the vast majority of animal models of allergic airway inflammation have been experimentally induced in small rodents, mice in particular. This choice of animal species is in part dictated by economical and ecological considerations, but mainly attributable to the huge range of immunological tools available in mice. The development of monoclonal antibodies and, more recently, gene deletion technology makes it possible to effectively neutralize a given mediator or cell, thus fully establishing its functional importance in the disease process (19).

However, the degree of hyperresponsiveness obtained in most of the currently available models by no means compares to the generally far larger differences in airway responsiveness that exist between asthmatic and nonasthmatic individuals. This could relate at least in part to the pattern of airway inflammation induced in these models. In the murine models of allergic airway inflammation developed so far, only acute inflammatory changes have been induced, without any structural changes that might affect responsiveness to a larger degree. The distribution of the inflammation is also different from human asthma, concentrating not only in or around the airways, but frequently also including lung parenchymal, mainly perivascular, changes. Furthermore, in the vast majority of these currently available murine models, sensitivity as opposed to reactivity of the airways has not been specifically evaluated. This is predominantly due to methodological problems. No "gold standard" lung function test has been invariably accepted for small animal models, mice in particular. The indices used include lung resistance, based on the principles described by Amdur and Mead, overflow of insufflation pressure as described by Konzett and Rössler, sometimes expressed as the APTI (airway pressure over time index) or the penh value (20–23). These various indices reflect to a variable and ill-defined degree the changes in airway sensitivity and reactivity.

II. Rat Models of Airway Remodeling

Although as already explained, the ideal animal model of airway remodeling does not yet exist, the issue of structural airway changes has been addressed in a number of models. Most of these studies have been conducted in rats. In a series of studies conducted in Martin's laboratory, Brown Norway (BN) rats were sensitized to ovalbumin on day 0, injecting 1 mg of ovalbumin + 200 mg $Al(OH)_3$ subcutaneously, and 1 mL containing 6×10^9 *Bordetella pertussis* organisms intraperitoneally. The animals were then exposed to a number of inhalation challenges with ovalbumin, ranging from three to six, usually every 5 days, starting 2 weeks after sensitization (24–27). This protocol led to an increase in airway responsiveness in those animals that developed an early response to ovalbumin inhalation, as judged by the dose of inhaled methacholine required to double baseline resistance ($PD_{200}R_L$) in animals ventilated via a tracheal cannula (24). In one of these studies (25), the maximal increase in R_L that could be achieved was measured, revealing no difference between ovalbumin-exposed and control animals. Noteworthy is that the increase in airway responsiveness in some of these animals persisted for up to 17 days after the sixth challenge. The altered airway behavior in these rats was not accompanied by a clear eosinophil influx into the airways, nor increased airway wall thickness. The basement membrane thickness was not specifically measured. What was reported was an increase in the thickness of the smooth muscle layer when expressed as a percentage of the squared basement membrane length. Further analysis, using BrdU pretreatment to identify replicating cells, suggested this was due to smooth muscle hyperplasia (28). In these studies a weak correlation was found between the quantity of airway smooth muscle in the large airways and the $PD_{200}R_L$. No correlation was found with the maximal increase in R_L obtained in individual animals. Both the increase in airway smooth muscle mass and the increase in airway responsiveness could be blocked by pretreating animals with a $CysLT_1$-receptor antagonist (26).

In our hands, repeated allergen exposure of BN rats also induced components of airway remodeling, albeit somewhat different in nature. We sensitize animals by the intraperitoneal injection of 1 mg ovalbumin + 100 µg $Al(OH)_3$. A booster is given on day 7. The animals are then exposed to aerosolized ovalbumin 3 times a week for 2 weeks from day 14 onward (29). The protocol induces quite patchy inflammatory infiltrates, which are located predominantly around the airways and contain mononuclear cells in addition to eosinophils. Airway epithelium shows an increase in the relative proportion of goblet cells. In addition, the epithelium contains an increased number of $BrdU^+$ cells, indicating increased proliferative activity. The basement membrane does not appear thickened. Collagen deposition in the airway mucosa is slightly, but not significantly, increased. The smooth muscle layer is not thickened and, in contrast to the findings from Martin's group, does not show signs of hyperplasia, as judged by BrdU staining. However, morphometric analysis shows an overall increase in the thickness of the airway wall area, in both small and large airways. This coincides with an increase in airway responsiveness to aerosolized carbachol, as illustrated by a leftward shift of the dose-response curve. We could not reach a plateau. Of particular interest is that the increase in airway wall thickness and airway responsiveness persisted for at least 14 days after the last of seven ovalbumin exposures.

In addition, the airway changes induced in this model prove to be relatively insensitive to the effect of inhaled steroids. Pretreatment with inhaled fluticasone (FP) (10 mg), prior to each allergen inhalation, reduces the ovalbumin-induced peribronchial eosinophilic infiltration, the increase in BrdU$^+$ cells in airway epithelium, and the goblet cell hyperplasia. However, the increase in airway wall thickness and airway responsiveness are not fully prevented (30). Furthermore, once the increase in airway wall thickness and hyperresponsiveness have been induced, they remain unaffected to treatment with FP (10 mg) during the ensuing 14 days. These observations arguably add to the value of the model as this lack of responsiveness to steroids is quite similar to the limited and variable effect of steroids on airway hyperresponsiveness and subepithelial fibrosis observed in human asthma. This also seems to indicate that the thickening of the airway wall area and increase in airway responsiveness are not caused by acute inflammatory changes and cannot be readily reversed by steroids. What the exact pathophysiological mechanisms are causing both phenomena and whether they are causally linked remain to be further established.

However, that the increased airway wall area can indeed be the cause of this altered airway behavior is further suggested by experiments during which the sensitized BN rats were exposed to ovalbumin over more prolonged time periods. When animals are repeatedly exposed to ovalbumin over 12 weeks, as opposed to 2 weeks, the airway morphology further changes. Collagen deposition increases further in the mucosa, whereas in the adventitial area large amounts of fibronectin are present. The smooth muscle layer remains unaffected, showing no signs of hyperplasia or hypertrophy. Strikingly, the overall thickness of the airway wall is reduced in comparison to animals exposed to allergen over a 2-week period, and is not different from control animals. Correlating with these morphological observations, airway hyperresponsiveness also wanes, and even turns into a slight hyporesponsiveness of the airways, in comparison to control animals (31). These observations suggest not only that the elements in the remodeling process that cause an increase in airway wall thickness are indeed the cause of airway hyperresponsiveness, but also that when these elements are replaced by a scar-like tissue containing large amounts of collagen or fibronectin, this could possibly, through increased stiffness, appear to affect the airway smooth muscle, thus protecting against instead of enhancing increased airway responsiveness.

III. Other Animal Models of Airway Remodeling

A. Antigen-Induced Structural Airway Changes in Other Animal Species

The majority of the currently developed murine models have focused on acute inflammatory changes. However, in a few models, the effect of more prolonged allergen exposure has been evaluated. Blyth and co-workers reported that repeated intratracheal instillation of ovalbumin induced not only eosinophil infiltration in the airways, but also goblet cell hyperplasia in the airway epithelium. In contrast to the eosinophil infiltration, this was not influenced by treatment with dexamethasone. In this model, airway reactivity was not measured (32). Temelkovski and co-workers recently reported that repeated exposure of Balb/c mice to low-dose antigen over 6–8 weeks induced goblet cell hyperplasia as an early characteristic of airway remodeling, followed by epithelial thickening and subepithelial fibrosis. These changes are paralleled by increased sensitivity to methacholine. Of interest is that altered airway behavior was also observed in nonimmunized allergen-exposed control animals, despite the absence of clear inflammatory airway changes (33).

B. Non-Antigen-Induced Models of Remodeling in Genetically Manipulated Mice

Overexpression of cytokines in murine airway epithelium, using transgene technology, has been reported to induce structural airway changes. IL-11 overexpression causes subepithelial fibrosis, due to increased expression of collagen I and III (34). This is accompanied by an increase in airway responsiveness, as indicated by a decreased $PC_{100}R_L$ to inhaled methacholine. Others have reported some degree of subepithelial fibrosis in addition to eosinophil accumulation in IL-5 transgenic animals (35). In this model, penh as marker of airway caliber was used to demonstrate increased airway responsiveness. Others have reported that adenovector-mediated gene tranfer of TGF-β or GM-CSF induces widespread pulmonary fibrosis in rats (36,37).

These models obviously are of interest, illustrating the potential effect of high concentrations of a given cytokine in inducing structural airway changes. However, they do not address the role of physiological concentrations of endogenously released cytokines in the pathogenesis of the remodeling process.

C. Models of Remodeling, Using Nonantigenic Inhaled Substances

A number of models have exposed animals over prolonged periods to nonspecific irritants including SO_2 or endotoxin (38), thus inducing structural airway changes that resemble more similarities to the changes observed in chronic bronchitis than in asthma. In dogs, prolonged exposure to SO_2 increases the thickness of the epithelium and the smooth muscle layer as well as the size of the mucous glands. However, these changes are not accompanied by altered airway behavior (39). In contrast, in rats, increased airway responsiveness following chronic SO_2 exposure has been observed, together with histological changes that are quite similar to those reported in dogs (40). In addition to epithelial changes, the thickness of the airway smooth muscle layer is also increased provided C fibers are destroyed by neonatal capsaicin treatment (41).

To date the role of matrix-degrading enzymes, including collagenase and elastase, has been predominantly evaluated in animal models of emphysema, either by administering the enzymes exogenously or by evaluating the effect of cigarette smoke in genetically manipulated knockout mice (42–45). In most of these models, histological changes in the airways either were absent or were not specifically addressed. Likewise, altered airway reactivity was related to changes in the histology of the lung parenchyma (46). These models are therefore less suited for investigating the interrelationship between airway remodeling and bronchial responsiveness as observed in asthma.

References

1. Redington AE, Howarth PH. Airway wall remodelling in asthma. Thorax 1997; 52:310–312.
2. Laitinen A, Altraja A, Kämpe M, Linden M, Virtanen I, Laitinen LA. Tenascin is increased in airway basement membrane of asthmatics and decreased by an inhaled steroid. Am J Respir Crit Care Med 1997; 156:951–958.
3. Li X, Wilson JW. Increased vascularity of the bronchial mucosa in mild asthma. Am J Respir Crit Care Med 1997; 156:229–233.
4. Ebina M, Takahashi T, Chiba T, Motomiya M. Cellular hypertrophy and hyperplasia of airway smooth muscles underlying bronchial asthma. Am Rev Respir Dis 1993; 148:720–726.
5. Chetta A, Foresi A, Del Donno M, Bertorelli G, Pesci A, Olivieri D. Airways remodelling is a distinctive feature of asthma and is related to the severity of asthma. Chest 1997; 111:852–857.
6. Roche WR, Beasley R, Williams JH, Holgate ST. Subepithelial fibrosis in the bronchi of asthmatics. Lancet 1989; 2:520–524.
7. Jeffery PK, Wardlaw AJ, Nelson FC, Collins JV, Kay AB. Bronchial biopsies in asthma: an ultrastructural quantitative study and correlation with hyperreactivity. Am Rev Respir Dis 1989; 140:1745–1753.
8. Hirst SJ. Airway smooth muscle cell culture: application to studies of airway wall remodelling and phenotype plasticity in asthma. Eur Respir J 1996; 9:808–820.

9. Redington AE, Madden J, Frew AJ, Djukanovic R, Roche WR, Holgate ST, Howarth PH. Transforming growth factor-β1 in asthma. Am J Respir Crit Care Med 1997; 156:642–647.

10. Minshall EM, Leung DYM, Martin RJ, Song YL, Cameron L, Ernst P, Hamid Q. Eosinophil-associated TGF-β1 mRNA expression and airways fibrosis in bronchial asthma. Am J Respir Cell Mol Biol 1997; 17:326–333.

11. Vignola AM, Chanez P, Chiappara G, Merendino A, Pace E, Rizzo A, la Rocca AM, Bella V, Bonsignore G, Bousquet J. Transforming growth factor-β expression in mucosal biopsies in asthma and chronic bronchitis. Am J Respir Crit Care Med 1997; 156:591–599.

12. Paré PD, Bai TR. The consequences of chronic allergic inflammation. Thorax 1995; 50:328–332.

13. Woolcock AJ, Salome CM, Yan K. The shape of the dose-response curve to histamine in asthmatic and normal subjects. Am Rev Respir Dis 1984; 130:71–75.

14. Lambert RK, Wiggs BB, Kuwano K, Hogg JC, Paré PD. Functional significance of increased airway smooth muscle in asthma and COPD. J Appl Physiol 1993; 74:2771–2781.

15. Wiggs BR, Hrousis CE, Drazen JM, Kamm RD. On the mechanism of mucosal folding in normal and asthmatic airways. J Appl Physiol 1997; 83:1814–1821.

16. Macklem PT. A theoretical analysis of the effect of airway smooth muscle load on airway narrowing. Am J Respir Crit Care Med 1996; 153:83–89.

17. Derksen EJ, Robinson NE, Armstrong PJ, Stick JA, Slocombe RF. Airway reactivity in ponies with recurrent airway obstruction (heaves). J Appl Physiol 1985; 58:598–604.

18. Padrid P, Snook S, Finucane T, Shiue P, Cozzi P, Solway J, Leff AR. Persistent airway hyperresponsiveness and histologic alterations after chronic antigen challenge in cats. Am J Respir Crit Care Med 1995; 151:184–93.

19. Kips JC, Pauwels RA. Animal models of asthma. Clin Asthma Rev 1997; 1:45–53.

20. Amdur MO, Mead J. Mechanics of respiration in unanaesthetized guinea-pigs. Am J Physiol 1958; 192:364–368.

21. Konzett H, Rössler R. Versuchsanordung zur Untersuchungen an der Bronchialmuskulatur. Arch Exp Pathol Pharmakol 1940; 195:71–74.

22. Levitt RC, Mitzner W. Expression of airway hyperreactivity to acetylcholine as a simple autosomal recessive trait in mice. FASEB J 1988; 2:2605–2608.

23. Hamelmann E, Schwarze J, Takeda K, Oshiba A, Larsen GL, Irvin CG, Gelfand EW. Noninvasive measurement of airway responsiveness in allergic mice using barometric plethysmography. Am J Respir Crit Care Med 1997; 156:766–775.

24. Bellofiore S, Martin JG. Antigen challenge of sensitized rats increases airway responsiveness to methacholine. J Appl Physiol 1988; 65:1642–1646.

25. Sapienza S, Du T, Eidelman DH, Wang NS, Martin JG. Structural airway

changes in the airways of sensitized Brown Norway rats after antigen challenge. Am Res Respir Dis 1991; 144:423–427.

26. Wang CG, Du T, Xu LJ, Martin JG. Role of leukotriene D_4 in allergen induced increases in airway smooth muscle in the rat. Am Rev Respir Dis 1993; 148: 413–417.

27. Du T, Sapienza S, Wang CG, Renzi PM, Pantano R, Rossi P, Martin JG. Effect of nedocromil sodium on allergen-induced airway responses and changes in the quantity of airway smooth muscles in rats. J Allergy Clin Immunol 1996; 98: 400–407.

28. Panettieri RA, Murray RK, Eszterhas AJ, Bilgen G, Martin JG. Repeated allergen inhalations induce DNA synthesis in airway smooth muscle and epithelial cells in vivo. Am J Physiol 1998; 274:L417–L424.

29. Palmans E, Kips JC, Pauwels RA. Chronic allergen exposure causes structural airway changes in sensitized BN rats. Am J Respir Crit Care Med 2000; 161: 627–635.

30. Vanacker N, Palmans E, Kips JC, Pauwels RA. The effect of fluticasone on allergen induced structural airway changes in a rat model. Eur Respir J 1998; (suppl 28):62s.

31. Palmans E, Kips JC, Pauwels RA. The effect of chronic allergen exposure on airway structure and responsiveness in rats. Am J Respir Crit Care Med 1998; 157:A822.

32. Blyth DI, Pedrick MS, Savage TJ, Hessel EM, Fattah D. Lung inflammation and epithelial changes in amurine model of atopic asthma. Am J Respir Cell Mol Biol 1996; 14:425–438.

33. Temelkovski J, Hogan SP, Shepherd DP, Foster PS, Kumar RK. An improved murine model of asthma: selective airway inflammation, epithelial lesions and increased methacholine responsiveness following chronic exposure to aerosolised allergen. Thorax 1998; 53:849–856.

34. Tang W, Geba GP, Zheng T, Ray P, Homer RJ, Kuhn C, Flavell RA, Elias JA. Targeted expression of IL-11 in the murine airway causes lymphocytic inflammation, bronchial remodeling and airways obstruction. J Clin Invest 1996; 98: 2845–2853.

35. Lee JJ, McGarry MP, Farmer SC, Denzler KL, Larson KA, Carrigan PE, Brenneise IE, Horton MA, Haczku A, Gelfand EW, Leikauf GD, Lee NA. Interleukin-5 expression in the lung epithelium of transgenic mice leads to pulmonary changes pathognomonic of asthma. J Exp Med 1997; 185:2143–2156.

36. Sime PJ, Xing Z, Graham FL, Csaky KG, Gauldie J. Adenovector-mediated gene transfer of active transforming growth factor-β1 induces prolonged severe fibrosis in rat lung. J Clin Invest 1997; 100:768–776.

37. Xing Z, Tremblay GM, Sime PJ, Gauldie J. Overexpression of granulocyte-macrophage colony-stimulating factor induces pulmonary granulation tissue formation and fibrosis by induction of transforming growth factor-β1 and myofibroblast accumulation. Am J Pathol 1997; 150:59–66.

38. Stolk J, Rudolpus A, Davies P, Osinga D, Dijkman JH, Agarwall L, Keenan KP, Fletcher D, Kramps JA. Induction of emphysema and bronchial mucus hyperplasia by intratracheal instillation of lipopolysaccharide in the hamster. J Pathol 1992; 167:349–356.

39. Scanlon PD; Seltzer J, Ingram RH, Reid L, Drazem JM. Chronic exposure to sulfur dioxide. Physiologic and histologic evaluation of dogs exposed to 50 or 15 ppm. Am Rev Respir Dis 1987; 135:831–839.

40. Shore S, Kobzik L, Long NC, Skornik W, Van Staden CJ, Boulet L, Rodger IW, Pon DJ. Increased airway responsiveness to inhaled methacholine in a rat model of chronic bronchitis. Am J Respir Crit Care Med 1995; 151:1931–1938.

41. Long NC, Martin JG, Pantano R, Shore SA. Airway hyperresponsiveness in a rat model of chronic bronchitis: role of C fibers. Am J Respir Crit Care Med 1997; 155:1222–1229.

42. Otto-Verberne CJM, Ten Have-Opbroek AAW, Franken C, Hermans J, Dijkman JH. Protective effect of pulmonary surfactant on elastase-induced emphysema in mice. Eur Respir J 1992; 5:1223–1230.

43. Hautamaki RD, Kobayashi DK, Senior RM, Shapiro SD. Requirement for macrophage elastase for cigarette smoke-induced emphysema in mice. Science 1997; 277:2002–2004.

44. D'Armiento J, Dalai SS, Okada Y, Berg RA, Chada K. Collagenase expression in the lungs of transgenic mice causes pulmonary emphysema. Cell 1992; 71: 955–961.

45. Massaro GDC, Massaro D. Retinoic acid treatment abrogates elastase-induced pulmonary emphysema in rats. Nature Med 1997; 3:675–677.

46. Bellofiore S, Eidelman DH, Macklem PT, Martin JG. Effects of elastase-induced emphysema on airway responsiveness to methacholine in rats. J Appl Physiol 1989; 66:606–612.

16

Future Directions in Airway Remodeling

JOHN W. WILSON

The Alfred Campus
Monash University
Prahran, Australia

PETER H. HOWARTH

Southampton General Hospital
Southampton, England

I. Introduction

The phenomenon of airway wall remodeling has challenged investigators of airflow obstruction to define remodeling, identify its characteristics, describe the relevance of some of the many possible trophic factors to human disease, and then go forward to characterize the action of current and novel antiasthma drugs in the regulation of these changes. Many standard techniques of airway investigation, including airway biopsy, have limitations because of the dynamic nature of tissue remodeling. There has been renewed interest in noninvasive estimates of airway elasticity and the application of sophisticated animal models to the study of remodeling influences and asthma therapies. Future studies will need to encompass a broad range of invasive and noninvasive techniques in both human and animal systems.

II. Noninvasive Physiological Measurement of Airway Distensibility (Wilson, Johns, Li)

Airway distensibility, or airway elasticity, might be expected to be reduced in the presence of airway smooth muscle hypertrophy/hyperplasia, increased collagen deposition, vascularity, angiogenesis, edema, and cell infiltration.

The Fowler anatomical dead space (VD_F) increases with end-inspiratory lung volume (EILV) and the gradient of the relationship (ΔVD_F, mL/L) provides an index of airway distensibility (1). Wilson et al. were the first to show that ΔVD_F was significantly lower in asthmatics compared to normal subjects suggesting that asthmatic airways were stiffer, possibly owing to structural changes associated with inflammation-induced "remodeling" of the airway wall (2). Johns and colleagues have developed a rapid method for measuring ΔVD_F, compared ΔVD_F in mild asthmatics and control subjects, and determined the site within the conducting airways responsible for airway distension (3). A computerized CO_2 washout test was developed for use with tidal breathing at progressively decreasing lung volumes between TLC and RV. VD_F was measured from each expired breath and EILV measured from TLC. Sixteen control subjects (normal spirometry, $PD_{20} > 2$ mg methacholine) and 16 mild asthmatics (mean $FEV_1/FVC = 66\%$, $PC_{20} = 0.039$ mg) were recruited. Each subject inspired to TLC and then breathed tidally with progressively decreasing EILVs. VD_F and EILV were measured for each expired tidal breath and linear regression analysis was used to obtain the mean ΔVD_F. A breathing frequency of 25 breaths/min was used to exclude end-inspiratory pause. The site within the airways responsible for distension was determined by partitioning VD_F into an index of proximal airway volume (i.e., volume of phase 1, VD_{p1}) and peripheral airways (i.e., $VD_{p2} = VD_F - VD_{p1}$). The contribution of ΔVD_{p1} and ΔVD_{p2} to ΔVD_F was calculated (Table 1). The method proved rapid, with duplicate measurements of ΔVD_F taking less than 15 min.

Table 1 The Contribution of ΔVD_{p1} and ΔVD_{p2} to ΔVD_F in Asthmatic and Control Subjects (mean ± SEM)

	Control	Asthmatic	Significance
VD_F/TCL, mL/L	20.6 ± 1.18	20.9 ± 0.76	ns
ΔVD_F, mL/L	24.3 ± 1.69	18.8 ± 1.16	0.010
ΔVD_{p1}, mL/L	18.4 ± 1.24	13.1 ± 0.99	0.005
ΔVD_{p2}, mL/L	6.0 ± 1.49	5.7 ± 1.35	ns

The between-session reproducibility of ΔVD_F was 9.1% ΔVD_{p1} and contributed 76% of the observed change in ΔVD_F (Fig. 1). This suggests that most of the lung volume dependence of VD_F was due to distension of the proximal airways and not peripheral airways (VD_{p2}) as expected. A model was developed that shows that the unexpectedly large change in VD_{p1} with lung volume could be explained on the basis of the asynchronous pattern of lung emptying (a consequence of asymmetrical airway branching and the gravity-dependent topographical distribution of airway size). It is likely that the luminal volume of mild asthmatic airways is less dependent on lung volume compared with normal suggesting that their airways were stiffer. The changes in airway volume using this technique appear to reflect distension of the proximal airways although this may be due to the asynchronous pattern of lung emptying (3).

The gradient of the relationship between VD_F and EILV provides an index of airway stiffness or distensibility (ΔVD_F) and may prove to be a useful physiological test to quantify the functional significance of airway remodeling

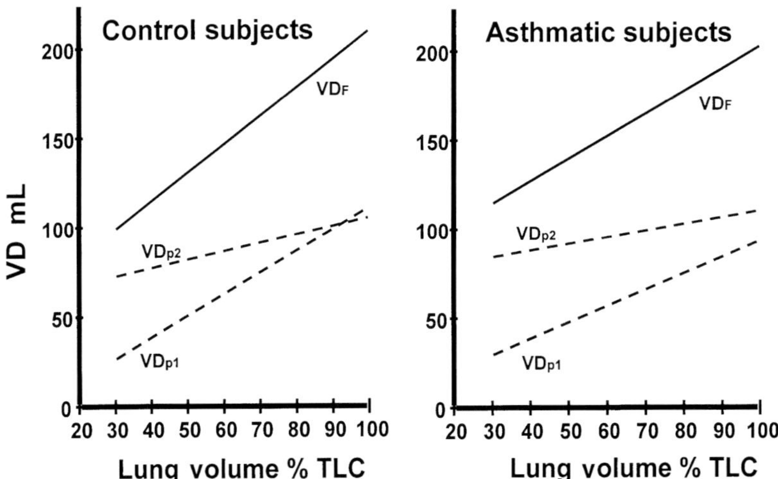

Figure 1 The slope of the VDF line represents airway distensibility. The higher slope in control subjects indicates that their airways are more distensible than those of asthmatics. VD_{p1} and VD_{p2} represent the components of VDF with VD_{p1} representing the dead space volume expired to the point where the CO_2 concentration increases to 0.2%. VD_{p2} is the remaining dead space. Thus, it was assumed that VD_{p1} represents the volume of the proximal airways and VD_{p2} the peripheral airway volume.

(2). However, the index may be affected by the breathing maneuver used to change EILV, and the dependence of VD_F and ΔVD_F on lung volume history has not been established. In a second study, Johns et al. measured anatomical dead space (1) using a tidal breathing CO_2 washout method. Dead space was measured at a number of known EILVs in two subject groups: 16 healthy control subjects (mean age 30 years, 10 males) with normal lung function and 16 asthmatics (mean age 41 years, 12 males, FER = 66%, PD_{20} = 0.039 mg methacholine). The VD_F at 50% TLC VD_F 50%) and ΔVD_F were measured and compared for three tidal breathing maneuvers (see Fig. 2): a) three discrete EILVs (TLC-FRC-RV); b) progressively decreasing EILVs from TLC to near RV (TLC to RV); c) progressively increasing EILVs from near RV to TLC (RV to TLC). Breathing frequency was regulated at 25 breaths/min using a metronome to eliminate end-inspiratory pause. Table 2 indicates that there were no significant differences in VD_F 50% and ΔVD_F between the three breathing maneuvers in either the control or asthmatic groups. Most subjects found the TLC to RV maneuver the easiest to perform and the RV to TLC the hardest. In healthy control subjects and asthmatics, airway distensibility and anatomical dead space at 50% TLC were independent of the breathing

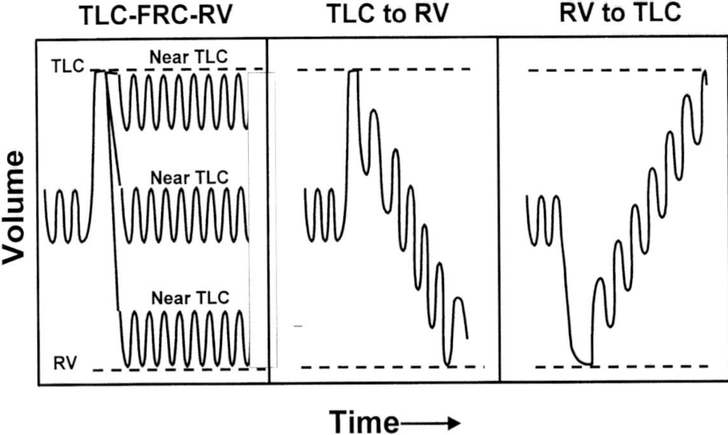

Figure 2   The three breathing regimes are shown as plots of respired volume versus time. TLC was taken as the volume reference point for the TLC-FRC-RV and TLC to RV regimens and RV was for used for the RV to TLC regimen. VDF was measured for each expiratory tidal breath.

Table 2 Relationship Between Breathing Maneuver, Airway Distensibility, and Dead Space Volume in Asthmatic and Control Subjects (mean $\pm$ SEM)

Breathing maneuver	ΔVD_F (mL/L)		$VD_F50\%$ (mL)	
	Control	Asthma	Control	Asthma
RV-FRC-TLC	25.3 ± 2.2	21.2 ± 1.7	128.4 ± 8.4	135.1 ± 6.8
TLC to RV	24.3 ± 1.7	18.8 ± 1.2	130.8 ± 8.3	141.3 ± 6.1
RV to TLC	23.3 ± 2.2	18.8 ± 1.7	130.5 ± 7.2	140.1 ± 5.9
Significance	ns	ns	Ns	ns

maneuver. Since the TLC to RV maneuver was the easiest of the three to perform, it is suggested that this be used for future studies.

III. Protease-Activated Receptor-2 (PAR-2) in the Activation of Airway Fibroblasts and Smooth Muscle Cells (Akers, Laurent, Sanjar, McAnulty)

The role of PAR-2 in mediating human mast cell tryptase-induced fibroblast proliferation has recently been studied by Akers and co-workers (4).

Subepithelial thickening in the airways of asthmatics and fibrotic lesions in patients with pulmonary fibrosis are characterized by fibroblast proliferation. Tryptase, a 134-kDa serine protease released from activated mast cells (5), is a potent mitogen for lung fibroblasts. However, the mechanism by which tryptase induces proliferation is unknown. Tryptase has recently been shown to activate PAR-2, but the functional significance of this is not known. Akers et al. have suggested that tryptase stimulates fibroblast proliferation via interaction with PAR-2. The mitogenic effects of tryptase and the PAR-2-activating peptides, SLIGKV and SLIGRL, were studied using human fetal and adult lung fibroblasts. The expression of PAR-2 on the cell surface was determined immunohistochemically using a polyclonal antibody to the N-terminal peptide sequence of PAR-2. Tryptase (0.7–17 mU/mL) caused concentration-dependent increases in cell proliferation in lung fibroblasts (fetal: 38 ± 3, adult 44 ± 2) and airway fibroblast (96 ± 4) as shown in Figure 3. The protease inhibitors Antipain (100 μM), BABIM (100 μM), and Benzamidine (100 μM) inhibited tryptase-induced cell proliferation in human fetal lung fibroblasts by $78 \pm 5\%$, $100 \pm 7\%$, and $70 \pm 6\%$, respectively. The PAR-2-activating peptides

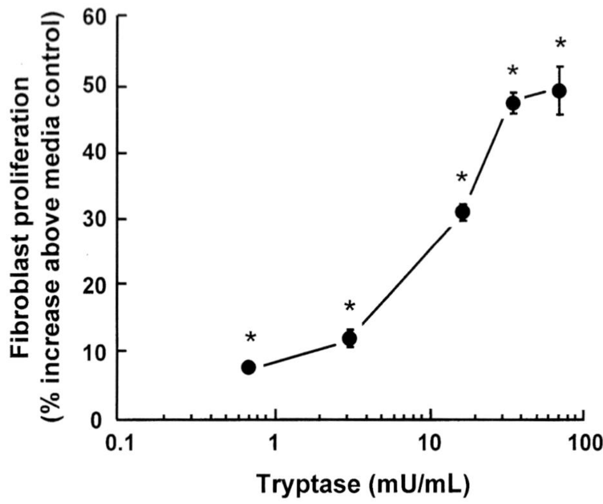

Figure 3   Effect of human mast cell tryptase on human fetal lung fibroblast proliferation. Cells were incubated with tryptase at concentrations of 0.7–17 mU/mL for 48 hr. Each point represents mean ± SEM of six observations from a representative experiment. Similar results were obtained in five separate experiments. Where errors are not shown, they are within the point. *$p < 0.01$ compared with media controls.

mimicked the effects of tryptase in fetal lung (SLIGKV, 39 ± 2%; SLIGRL, 31 ± 2%), adult lung (SLIGRL 39 ± 1), and airway (SLIGKV, 44 ± 4%; SLIGRL, 76 ± 2%) fibroblasts as shown in Figure 4. Immunohistochemical analysis demonstrated the presence of PAR-2 on the surface of fibroblasts. These results are consistent with the hypothesis that tryptase mediates its mitogenic effects via activation of PAR-2 and that the release of tryptase may play an important role in fibroblast proliferation and matrix deposition in the airways of asthmatics and the lungs of patients with pulmonary fibrosis (4). A comparison of protease-activated receptors and their activation in airway smooth muscle cells and fibroblasts may be useful to delineate the role of the PARs in airway remodeling (6).

Fibrosis and airway smooth muscle hyperplasia/hypertrophy are recognized to be important pathological features of chronic airway disease that are not well treated by current, standard therapies. Tryptase has been shown to play a role in the mitogenesis of airway smooth muscle cells, epithelial cells, and fibroblasts (5). We have investigated the effects of tryptase, other prote-

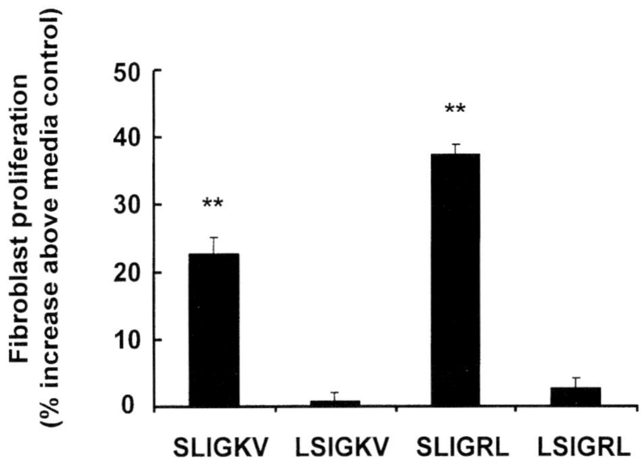

Figure 4 Effects of the PAR-2-activating peptides SLIGKV and SLIGRL on human fetal lung fibroblast proliferation. Fibroblasts were incubated with activating peptides corresponding to the human PAR-2 sequence, SLIGKV (0.01–1 mM), or the rat PAR-2 sequence, SLIGRL (0.01–1 mM). Increases in cell proliferation were assessed after 48 hr. Controls were performed using peptides (1 mM) in which the first two amino acids of the activating peptides had been reversed, LSIGKV and LSIGRL. Each value represents the mean ± SEM of six observations from a representative experiment. Similar results were obtained in four further experiments **$p < 0.01$ compared to media controls.

ases, and protease-activated receptor (PAR)-activating peptides on the proliferation of human airway smooth muscle cells (ASMC) and fibroblasts, and have initiated studies to identify potential receptor or signaling pathway targets for controlling airway smooth muscle cell and fibroblast proliferation that contribute to airway thickening and remodeling in asthma (7,8).

ASMC and fibroblast proliferation was stimulated by the proteases tryptase, thrombin, and trypsin, but not by human sputum elastase, PAR-2 peptide, or tartrate-resistant acid phosphatase (TRAP) peptide at the concentrations tested. Figure 5 shows that in each case the ASMCs responded more strongly than the fibroblasts (e.g., tryptase at 1 µg/mL stimulated the growth of ASMCs by 386% compared to 76% and 30% for the lung fibroblast cell line 34LU and NHLF, respectively). This cannot be explained by the expression of the PARs, since all three cell lines expressed PAR-1, PAR-2, and PAR-3, at the mRNA level, determined by RT-PCR. MagiCAL analysis of ASMCs showed

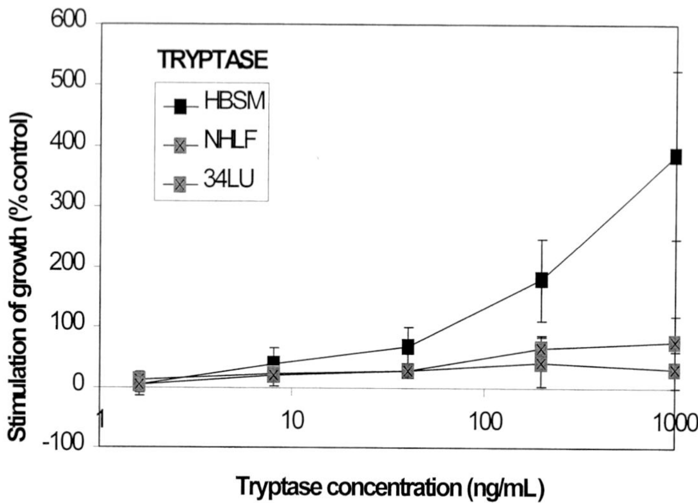

Figure 5   Effect of tryptase on growth of airway smooth muscle and fibroblasts in vitro.

that thrombin was a potent initiator of calcium flux, but no signal was seen with tryptase indicating that there are differences in the PAR signaling initiated by these proteases. Further investigation of PARs and their signaling pathways needs to be undertaken, but initial studies suggest that tryptase may play an important role in airway remodeling, and may provide novel approaches to currently untreatable aspects of lung disease.

The proliferation of human airway smooth muscle cells stimulated by mast cell tryptase may be significant. Any response to the suppressive effects of fluticasone propionate and dexamethasone would indicate a reversible component of airway remodeling.

Increased airway smooth muscle (ASM) cell hypertrophy and/or hyperplasia is also an important component of the airway remodeling observed in asthma that may contribute to airways hyperresponsiveness (9). The response of early-passage ASM cells to a variety of cytokines, growth factors, and other inflammatory mediators has been studied in vitro. Methylene blue staining was used to measure proliferation of cells stimulated in the presence of 1% FCS, and the degree of proliferation was calculated as a percentage of the growth in 1% FCS. Growth was stimulated at 100 ng/mL (% control) by the growth factors PDGF (240%), IGF-I (73%), TGF-α (245%), EGF (268%),

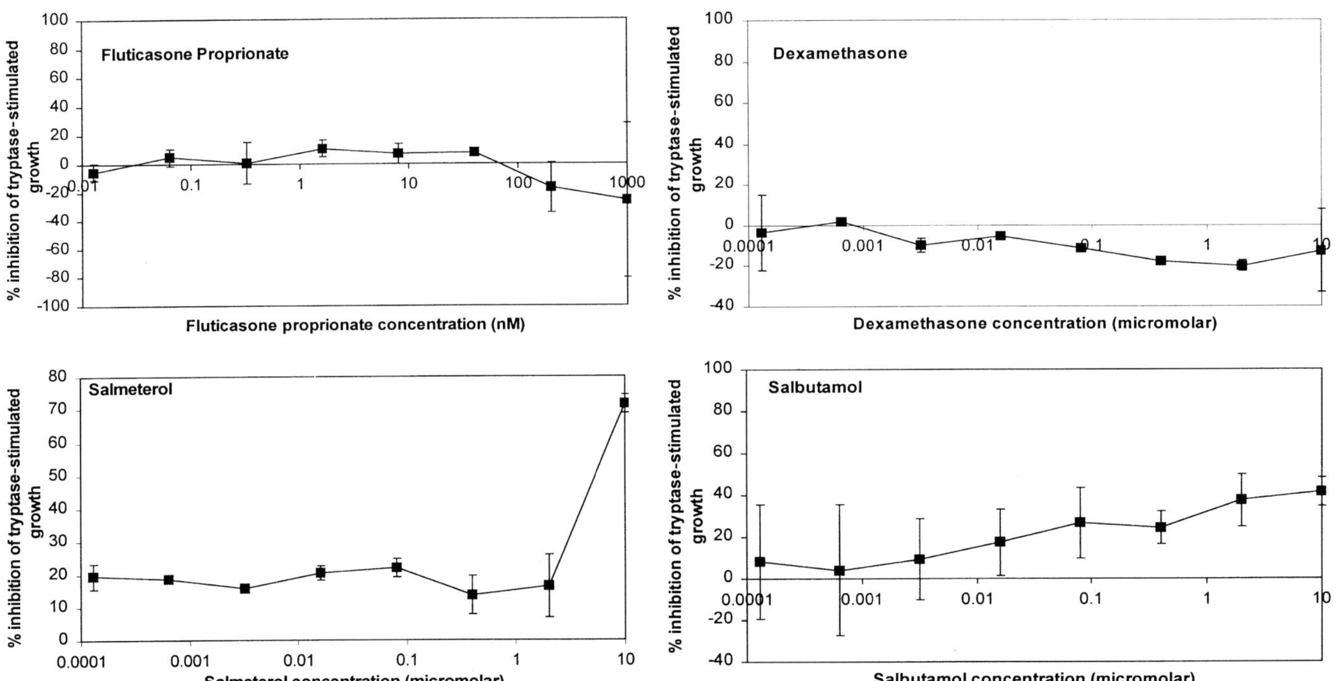

Figure 6 Effect of salbutamol, salmeterol, dexamethasone, and fluticasone propionate on airway smooth muscle cell growth in response to stimulation with tryptase.

and b-FGF (419%). Proliferation was also induced significantly by the proteases mast cell tryptase (386% at 1 µg/mL), thrombin (181% at 1000 mU/mL), and trypsin (100% at 10 µg/mL). The potent proliferative effect of tryptase was confirmed by cell counts. The sensitivity of cells stimulated by tryptase to growth modulation by corticosteroids and β_2-adrenoceptor agonists was tested (Fig. 6). Fluticasone propionate (FP) and dexamethasone had no effect at concentrations up to 1 µM. Salmeterol inhibited growth by only 20% at 2 µM. Salbutamol inhibited growth in a dose-dependent manner, with maximal inhibition of 41% at 10 µM. These findings support the observations of Tomlinson et al. and suggest that tryptase could play an important role in ASM thickening observed in asthma (10). Being steroid insensitive, it suggests an avenue for the development of novel therapies.

IV. Fibrogenic Factors and Metalloproteinases in Airway Remodeling (Warner, McConnell, Shute, Howarth)

Matrix metalloproteinases (MMPs) are present in bronchoalveolar lavage following allergen challenge, and may be suppressed by fluticasone propionate (11).

MMPs are involved in airway remodeling and leukocyte migration through tissues. MMPs were measured in BAL from 20 allergic asthmatic subjects before, and 24 hr after, allergen challenge. Levels of MMPs were low before allergen (median = 0 ng/mL), but rose significantly 24 hr later (median = 139 ng/mL, $p < 0.05$) as shown in Figure 7. The majority of the activity was MMP-9, confirmed by Western blot and immunoprecipitation. There was an increase in the MMP-9 inhibitor TIMP-1, from a median value of 35.5 ng/mL to 181.3 ng/mL ($p < 0.05$) after allergen and a strong positive correlation between MMP-9 and TIMP-1 (rho = 0.679, $p < 0.001$). MMP-9 levels correlated with both eosinophils (rho = 0.522, $p < 0.001$) and neutrophils (rho = 0.611, $p < 0.001$) in the BAL while TIMP-1 correlated with eosinophils (rho = 0.521, $p < 0.001$) but not neutrophils (rho = 0.328, $p =$ NS). Patients then received either 500 µg fluticasone propionate (FP) twice daily by inhalation or placebo for 6 weeks and allergen challenge was repeated. There was a significant increase in MMP-9 in both groups after allergen (median = 51 ng/mL for FP-treated patients vs. 125 ng/mL in the controls) possibly because the neutrophil remains a key source of MMP-9 and there was no change in neutrophil numbers in BAL after FP though eosinophils were reduced ($p < 0.05$). Intriguingly, there was no significant increase in TIMP-1

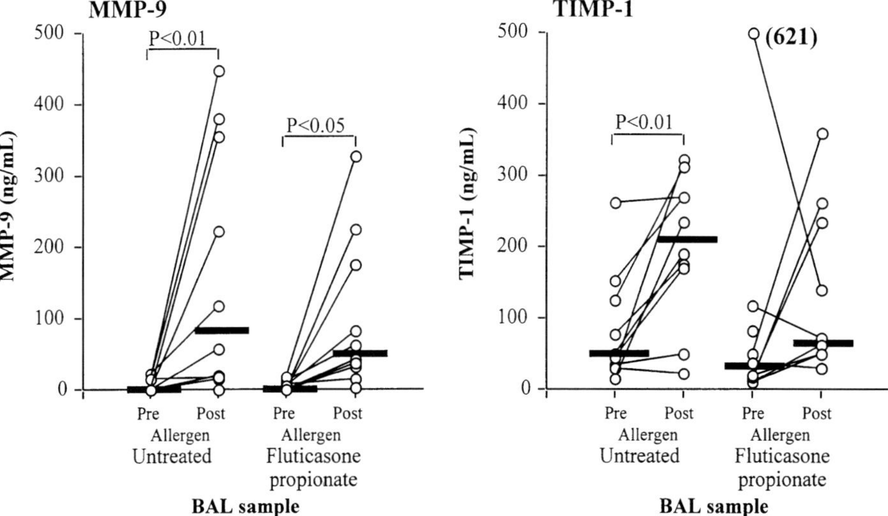

Figure 7 Effect of fluticasone propionate on MMP-9 and TIMP-1 levels following allergen challenge. Ten patients with mild asthma underewent BAL followed by segmental allergen challenge and a second BAL 24 h later. They then received 500 μg fluticasone propionate bid for 6 weeks and then underwent a second BAL and allergen challenge. MMP-9 and TIMP-1 were measured in the cell-free supernatant of the BAL by gelatin zymography and ELISA, respectively. Individual responses are shown as open circles with the median as a solid bar. The effect of allergen challenge was assessed using a Wilcoxon signed rank test and a value of $p < 0.05$ accepted as significant.

following allergen in patients treated with FP (median = 71 ng/mL for FP vs. 150 ng/mL in control), which may reflect the role of eosinophils as a source of TIMP-1 in the lung following allergen challenge. FP thus appears to modify MMP-9/TIMP-1 balance in the BAL mainly by modulating eosinophil recruitment.

Many fibroproliferative factors may be found in bronchoalveolar lavage and in vitro systems have become an important tool in the assessment of bioactivity.

Airway remodeling in asthma is characterized by thickening of the subepithelial collagen layer associated with increased numbers of myofibroblasts in asthma (7). These cells may be responsive to TGF-β_1 (12), thrombin (13), and bFGF (14). McConnell and co-workers have studied the effects of BAL from 10 asthmatic patients on the proliferation in serum-free medium of a human fetal lung fibroblast cell line (MRC-5) in vitro, using ^{3}H-thymidine incorporation as an indicator of cellular proliferation (15). Thymidine uptake in the presence of asthmatic BALF was 363% (range 118–979 %, $p = 0.0004$) of that with phosphate-buffered saline control. In the three most fibroproliferative samples of BAL, BAL-induced fibroblast proliferation was significantly inhibited by blocking antibody to basic fibroblast growth factor (bFGF) (inhibition 27 $\pm$ 2.3%, $p = 0.0002$). There was no significant effect with anti-PDGF, anti-TGFβ, anti-IGF-1, anti-IGF-2, or a combined endothelin A and B receptor antagonist. Marked inhibition of BAL-induced fibroblast proliferation was observed with TGF-β_1 (50 ng/mL) and with a broad-spectrum protease inhibitor cocktail. Use of specific protease inhibitors demonstrated significant inhibition of BAL-induced proliferation with α_2-antiplasmin (inhibition 37 $\pm$ 3.89%, $p < 0.0001$) but no significant effect from hirudin or plasminogen activator inhibitor-1 (Fig. 8). Blocking antibodies to MMP-3 and MMP-9 caused significant stimulation of proliferation in the presence of BAL. These results suggest a role for plasmin in airway remodeling, possibly through release of stored bFGF. MMPs may cause inhibition of proliferation by activa-

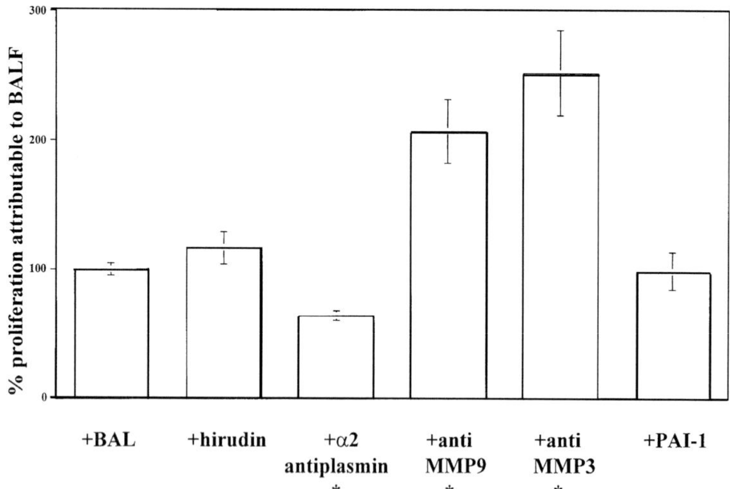

Figure 8 Effects of blocking antibodies and antagonists to various proteases on the fibroblast proliferation induced by asthmatic bronchoalveolar lavage fluid ($n = 9$, *p < 0.05).

tion of stored TGF-β_2 in asthma (12), which displays antiproliferative properties toward fibroblasts.

V. The Regulatory Effect of Eosinophils on Fibroblasts and Collagen Synthesis (Levi-Schaffer)

Eosinophils and mast cells have been associated with fibrosis (16,17). To investigate their direct role in fibrosis and matrix deposition (18), human peripheral blood eosinophil sonicates were added to human lung, foreskin, or intestine fibroblasts and fibroblast proliferation ([^{3}H]-thymidine), collagen synthesis ([^{3}H]-proline), metalloproteinase activity, and collagen lattice contraction were evaluated.

Proliferation was enhanced significantly in all the monolayers in a dose-dependent manner. The activity of the eosinophil fibrogenic factor(s) remained unaltered when heated (56°C, 30 min). Supernatants of cultured eosinophils (20 min or 18 hr) also enhanced lung fibroblast proliferation, indicating that

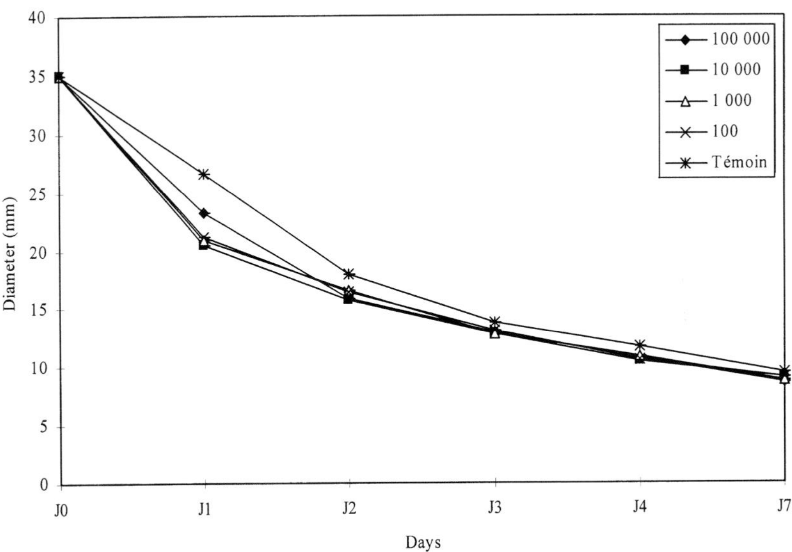

Figure 9 Effect of eosinophil sonicates on fibroblast-mediated collagen lattice contraction.

the preformed mitogenic factor(s) can be released both promptly and with a longer kinetic profile.

Eosinophil sonicate significantly decreased collagen production in lung and intestine fibroblasts while increasing it in foreskin fibroblasts. However, eosinophil sonicate, which was found to possess metalloproteinase-9 (zymography) in latent form, did not significantly influence either lung or foreskin fibroblast metalloproteinases. Eosinophil sonicate added to skin fibroblasts in tridimensional collagen lattices was found to significantly enhance their contraction (Fig. 9). Since TGF-β enhanced both proliferation and collagen synthesis, the eosinophil sonicate was preincubated with anti-TGF-β neutralizing antibodies. This treatment partially inhibited proliferation of lung and collagen synthesis of foreskin fibroblasts, indicating the fibrogenic role of eosinophil-associated TGF-β. In summary, eosinophils have been shown to directly modulate fibroblast properties. This observation corroborates the important role of eosinophils in fibrotic conditions.

VI. Animal Models of Airway Remodeling (Palmans, Kips, Pauwels)

The exact mechanisms underlying airway remodeling remain to be fully characterized. In vivo animal models could provide relevant information in this respect (19). Kips et al. have previously reported that repeated exposure of sensitized BN rats to aerosolized allergen over a period of up to 2 weeks induced an increase in airway responsiveness, in addition to acute inflammatory response, as well as structural airway changes that include epithelial hyperplasia and thickening of the smooth muscle layer (19–21). Collagen deposition was not increased. Morphometric analysis revealed an increase in the total airway wall area of large, medium, and small airways (Fig. 10c). These histological changes were accompanied by an increase in airway responsiveness to aerosolized carbachol (Fig. 10c). In the present study, allergen exposure was prolonged over a 3-month period. BN rats were actively sensitized to ovalbumin (OA) on day 0 and exposed to aerosolized PBS or OA from day 14 to day 96. Outcome measures were assessed 24 hr after the last exposure. The epithelium of OA-exposed animals contained increased numbers of goblet cells ($9.65 \pm 1.11\%$ goblet cells vs. $1.49 \pm 0.32\%$ goblet cells; $p < 0.001$). In the OA-exposed group the number of infiltrating eosinophils around bronchi and bronchioles was increased (740 ± 161 cells/mm^2 airway wall vs. 124 ± 57 cells/mm^2 airway wall; $p < 0.001$). The total amount of

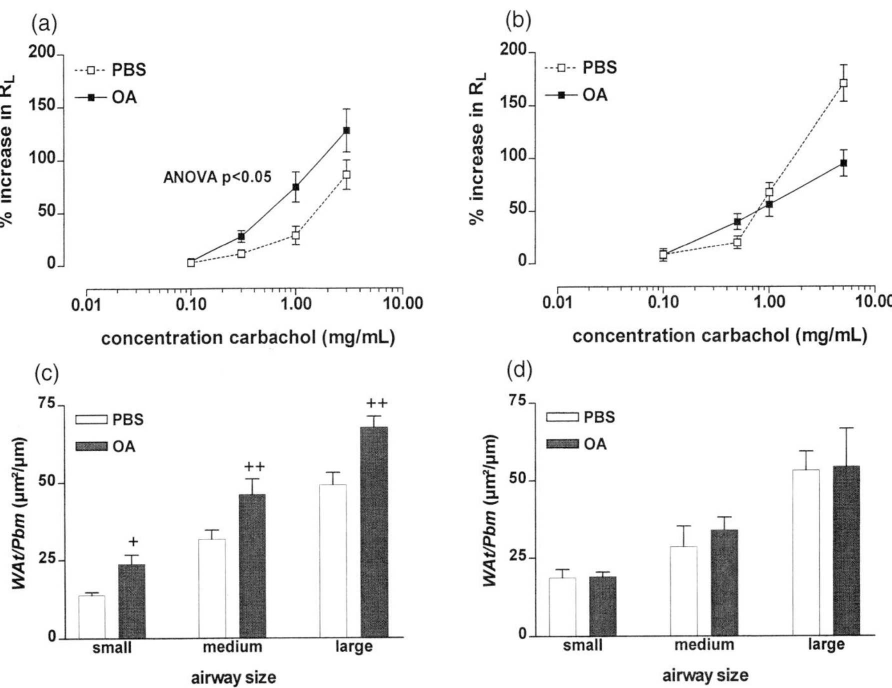

Figure 10 Bronchial responsiveness to aerosolized carbachol (a and b) and total airway wall area normalized to the length of basement membrane (WAt/Pbm) (c and d) in sensitized BN rats exposed to PBS or OA during 2 weeks (a and c) or 12 weeks (b and d). $^{+}p < 0.01$ vs. PBS; $^{++}p < 0.05$ vs. PBS.

collagen was increased in large airways of OA-exposed animals ($p < 0.05$) and prolonged exposure to OA also induced an increased deposition of fibronectin ($p < 0.001$) around the smooth muscle layer. The total area of the airway wall was not different between OA- and PBS-exposed animals (Fig. 10d) nor was the airway responsiveness to carbachol (Fig. 10b).

These observations suggest that during prolonged allergen exposure changes occur within the airways that protect against the increase in airway responsiveness despite the persistence of airway inflammation. The loss of these protective mechanisms could contribute to the altered airway behavior observed in chronic asthma.

VII. Intracellular Pathways Through Which Smooth Muscle Remodeling May Occur (Stewart, Wilson)

Hyperplasia and hypertrophy of airway smooth muscle (ASM) contributes to airway wall thickening and hyperresponsiveness in asthma. Numerous tyrosine kinase receptor-linked growth factors and other inflammatory mediators have been shown to be mitogenic for human ASM. A complex signal transduction pathway regulates the subsequent growth and division of ASM cells. The known components of this pathway include mitogen-activated protein kinase (MAPK/ERK), and cyclin D1, which partners cyclin-dependent kinase 4 to phosphorylate the restriction protein, retinoblastoma (pRb), enabling progression of cells into the S phase of the cell cycle (22). Work by Stewart and colleagues examines the importance of changes in cyclin D1 protein levels and the requirement for persistent MAPK/ERK activation for mitogenesis in human ASM cells using the MAPK kinase (MEK1) inhibitor PD98059. MAPK/ERK activity in cell lysates was assessed by incorporation of ^{32}P-ATP into an ERK-specific substrate (22). MAPK/ERK activity was also measured by immunoprecipitation kinase assays. Cyclin D1 protein levels and the phosphorylation states of MAPK/ERK and pRb were assessed using Western blotting. DNA synthesis was assessed by the incorporation of [^{3}H]-thymidine. Changes in cell number and cell cycle progression were measured by cell counts and flow cytometry. Both bFGF (0.3–3.0 nM), and thrombin (0.3–3.0 U/mL) increased DNA synthesis and cell number in cultured airway smooth muscle cells. There was a consistent relationship between the mitogenic potential of each agent, its ability to phosphorylate pRb, to increase both cyclin D1

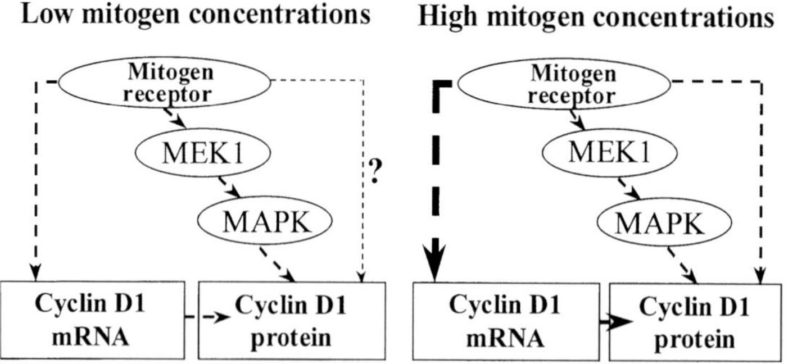

Figure 11 Effect of high-dose mitogen stimulation of human airway smooth muscle cells indicates a decreasing dependence on MAPK/ERK pathways.

protein and mRNA levels, and to induce persistent activation (2+ hr) of MAPK/ERK. DNA synthesis, increases in cyclin D1 protein levels, and MAPK/ERK activity in response to low mitogen concentrations were completely inhibited by PD98059 (30 μM). PD98059 completely inhibited DNA synthesis and increases in MAPK/ERK activity (2 hr) stimulated by a higher concentration of thrombin (3.0 U/mL), but cyclin D1 levels were unaffected. bFGF- (3.0 nM) induced MAPK/ERK activation was blocked by PD98059, DNA synthesis was attenuated, but cyclin D1 levels were unaffected. It appears that the MAPK/ERK-dependence of mitogenesis signaling decreases with increasing mitogen concentration indicating the existence of additional, uncharacterized pathways (Fig. 11).

VIII. Microvascular Remodeling and Plasma Leakage (Baluk, McDonald)

The traditional view of the microvasculature as ''fixed plumbing'' has recently evolved into the concept of a dynamic system of blood vessels controlled by a balance of angiogenic and angiostatic factors. This view is reflected in the realization that changes in airway mucosal vasculature can be a manifestation of disease. It has been possible to characterize the patterns of vascular remodeling and plasma leakage in health and in disease, using infection of mouse airways with *Mycoplasma pulmonis* as an experimental model of chronic inflammation (23). When blood vessels are stained histologically by perfusion of biotinylated lectins and observed in whole-mount preparations of the trachea, the pattern of the entire vasculature is revealed in detail. In pathogen-free mice, the mucosal blood vessels form a characteristic two-dimensional plexus of arterioles, capillaries, and venules with segmental repeats over the cartilage rings. Pathogen-free mice have a low baseline plasma leakage as assessed spectrophometrically by the Evans blue technique, and morphologically by lectin staining. Unlike rats and guinea pigs, the vessels of pathogen-free mice are particularly resistant to leakage induced by capsaicin or substance P, unless the enzymes that normally degrade tachykinins (NEP and ACE) are first inhibited. Mice with *M. pulmonis* infection develop lifelong inflammation of the respiratory tract, manifested by a chronic remodeling of the vasculature and epithelium, airway fibrosis, and influx of lymphocytes and neutrophils into the tissues and airway lumen. In some strains of mice (e.g. C57BL/6), the dominant process in response to *M. pulmonis* infection is angiogenesis, or the formation of new capillaries (Fig. 12). In other strains, (e.g.,

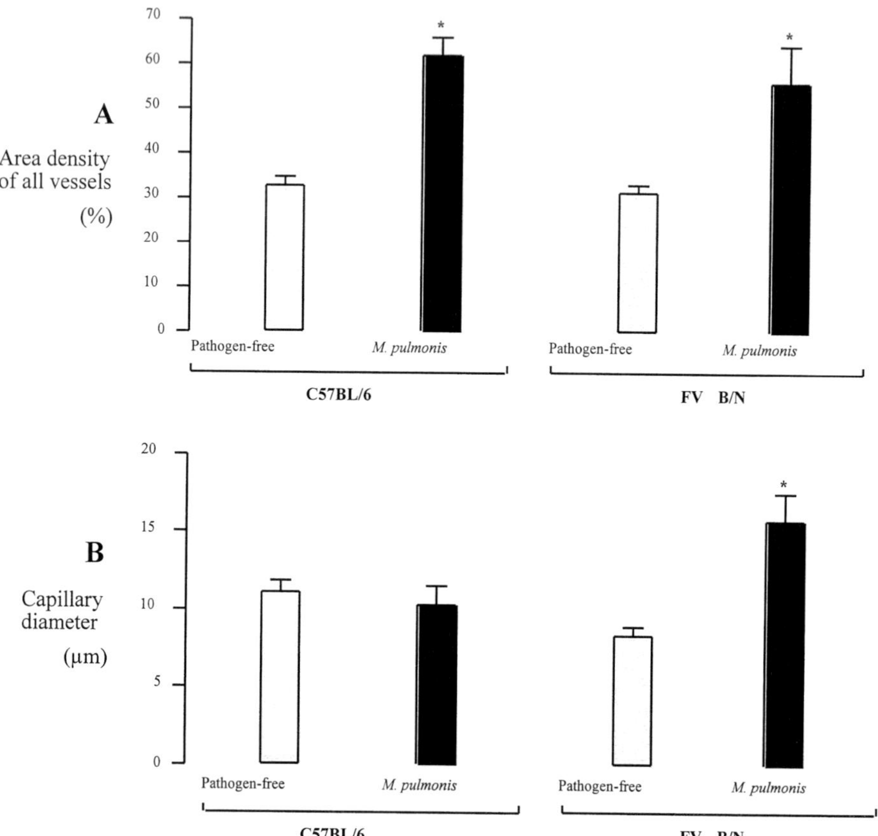

Figure 12 Effect of infection on airway vessel density and size in mice and rat models. *, p < 0.5.

FVB/N), the main change is microvascular dilatation, in which existing blood vessels enlarge their diameter. Although tracheas of infected mice do not have an increased baseline leakage of Evans blue, lectin staining can reveal focal sites of plasma leakage in newly formed capillaries. Similar to the situation in rats, tracheal blood vessels of mice become more sensitive to substance P after *M. pulmonis* infection, and significant leakage can be induced in the absence of inhibitors of NEP and ACE. We conclude that different patterns of angiogenesis are induced in different strains of mice by *M. pulmonis* infection, and may be genetically determined. Plasma leakage is minimal in pathogen-free mice, but is increased after infection.

Acknowledgments

The authors most gratefully acknowledge contributions from the following participants who enabled the compilation of this chapter: IA Akers, GJ Laurent, and RJ McAnulty from The Centre for Cardiopulmonary Biochemistry and Respiratory Medicine, The Rayne Institute, London, England; S Sanjar, Respiratory Diseases Unit, Glaxo Wellcome R&D Ltd., Medicines Research Centre, Herts, England (supported by Glaxo Wellcome R&D Ltd.); DP Johns, JW Wilson, X Li, C Ingram, EH Walters, Department of Respiratory Medicine, Alfred Hospital, Melbourne, Victoria, Australia; R Harding, Monash University Medical School, Melbourne, Victoria, Australia (supported by the NHMRC and Glaxo Wellcome Australia); F Levi-Schaffer, E Garbuzenko, R Reich, Department of Pharmacology, Hebrew University of Jerusalem, Jerusalem, Israel; A Rubin, P Gillery, F-X Maquart, CNRS UPRESA 6021, Faculty of Medicine, Reims, France; SJ Pearce, JA Warner, School of Biological Sciences, University of Southampton, Southampton, England; WC Moore, ER Bleecker, University of Maryland School of Medicine, Baltimore, MD; K Affleck, V Norman, R Shaw, S Sanjar, Respiratory Diseases Unit, Glaxo Wellcome Ltd., Medicines Research Centre, Herts, England; E Palmans, NJ Vanacker, JC Kips, RA Pauwels, Department of Respiratory Diseases, University Hospital Ghent, Ghent, Belgium; P Baluk, G Thurston, and DM McDonald, Cardiovascular Research Institute, and Department of Anatomy, University of California, San Francisco, CA (funded in part by NIH Program Project Grant HL-24136); WD McConnell, JK Shute, PH Howarth, University Medicine, Southampton General Hospital, Southampton, England.

References

1. Fowler WS. Lung function studies. II. The respiratory dead space. Am J Physiol 1948; 154:405–416.
2. Wilson JW, Li X, Pain MCF. Lack of airway distensibility in asthma. Am Rev Respir Dis 1993; 148:806–809.
3. Johns DP, Wilson JW, Augustin S, Li X, Harding R, Ingram C, Walters EH. Lung volume history does not affect airway distensibility or anatomical deadspace measurements in healthy subjects. Am J Respir Crit Care Med 1997; 155:A543.
4. Akers IA, Laurent GJ, Sanjar S, McAnulty RJ. Human mast cell tryptase and protease-activated receptor-2 (PAR-2) activating peptides induce lung and airway fibroblast proliferation. Eur Respir J 1998; A1129.
5. Brown et al. Tryptase, the dominant secretory granular protein in human mast cells, is a potent mitogen for cultured dog tracheal smooth muscle cells. Am J Respir Cell Mol Biol 1995; 13:227–236.
6. Affleck K, Norman V, Sanjar S. Proliferation of human airway smooth muscle cells stimulated by mast cell tryptase is insensitive to fluticasone propionate and dexamethasone. Am J Respir Crit Care Med 1999; 159:A529.
7. Wiggs et al. A model of airway narrowing in asthma and chronic obstructive pulmonary disease. Am Rev Respir Dis 1992; 145:1251–1258.
8. Brewster et al. Myofibroblasts and subepithelial fibrosis in bronchial asthma. Am J Respir Cell Mol Biol 1990; 3:507–511.
9. Lambert et al. Functional significance of increased airway smooth muscle in asthma and COPD. J Appl Physiol 1993; 74:2771–2781.

10. Tomlinson et al. Inhibition by salbutamol of the proliferation of human airway smooth muscle cells grown in culture. Br J Pharmacol 1994; 111:641–647.

11. Moore WC, Pearce SJ, Himielski RR, Rogenes PR, Reed KD, Bleecker ER, Warner JA. Matrix metalloproteases (MMPs) in bronchoalveolar lavage (BAL) following allergen challenge: effect of fluticasone propionate (FP). Am J Respir Crit Care Med 1998; 157:A872.

12. Redington AE, Madden J, Frew AJ, Djukanovic R, Roche WR, Holgate ST, Howarth PH. Transforming growth factor-β1 in asthma. Measurement in bronchoalveolar lavage fluid. Am J Respir Crit Care Med 1997; 156:642–647.

13. Hernandez-Rodriguez NA, Cambrey AD, Harrison NK, Chamber RC, Gray AJ, Southcott AM, duBois RM, Black CM, Scully MF, McAnulty RJ, Laurent GJ. Role of thrombin in pulmonary fibrosis. Lancet 1995; 346:1071–1073.

14. Saksela O, Rifkin DB. Release of bFGF-heparan sulfate complexes from endothelial cells by plasminogen activator-mediated proteolytic activity. J Cell Biol 1990; 110:767–775.

15. McConnell WD, Shute JK, Howarth PH. The fibroproliferative properties of asthmatic bronchoalveolar lavage fluid: the contribution of proteases and growth factors. Am J Respir Crit Care Med 1999; 159:A196.

16. Levi-Schaffer F, Rubinchik E. Activated mast cells are fibrogenic for 3T3 fibroblasts. J Invest Dermatol 1995; 104:999–1003.

17. Levi-Schaffer F, Weg VB. Mast cells, eosinophils and fibrosis. Clin Exp Allergy 1997; 27:64–70.

18. Loimeir S, Gillery P, Hornebeck W, Chastang F, Laurant-Maquin D, Bouthors S, Droulle C, Potron G, Maquart FX. Tissue origin and extracellular matrix control neutral proteinase activity in human fibroblast three dimensional cultures. J Cell Physiol 1996; 168:188–198.

19. Kips JC, Palmans E, Pauwels RA. Repeated antigen exposure leads to structural airway changes in rats. Am J Respir Crit Care Med 1997; 155:A546.

20. Sapienza S, Du T, Eidelman DH, Wang NS, Martin JG. Structural changes in the airways of sensitized Brown Norway rats after antigen challenge. Am Rev Respir Dis 1991; 144:423–427.

21. Panettieri RA, Murray RK, Eszterhas AJ, Bilgen G, Martin JG. Repeated allergen inhalations induce DNA synthesis in airway smooth muscle and epithelial cells in vivo. Am J Physiol 1998; 274:L417–424.

22. Stewart AG, Harris T, Fernandes DJ, Schachte LC, Kalafatis V, Gillzan KM, Ravenhall CE, Tomlinson PR, Wilson JW. β_2-adrenergic agonists and cAMP arrest human cultured airway smooth muscle cells in G1 phase of the cell cycle: role of mitogen-activated protein kinase, Cyclin D1 and p27[Kip1]. Mol Pharmacol 1999; 56:1079–1086.

23. Thurston G, Murphy TJ, Erwin J, Lindsey JR, McDonald DM. Changes in endothelial cell phenotype in chronic inflammation of mouse airways. Am J Respir Crit Care Med 1997; 155:A124.

INDEX

T

V